Becoming an Advanced Healthcare Pr

CW00926365

We dedicate this book to our students. Many from the past are already advanced practitioners, and those with whom we work currently, carry the seeds of future advanced practice.

For Butterworth Heinemann:

Commissioning Editor: Heidi Allen
Project Development Editor: Robert Edwards
Project Manager: Joannah Duncan
Design Direction: George Ajayi
Illustration Manager: Bruce Hogarth

Becoming an Advanced Healthcare Practitioner

Edited by

Gillian Brown MSc, DipCOT, SROT
Head Occupational Therapist, Barking Havering and Redbridge NHS Trust
Senior Lecturer, University of East London, London, England, UK

Susan A. Esdaile PhD, MAPS, AccOT, OTR, SROT
Professor, Department of Occupational Therapy, Eugene Applebaum College of Pharmacy and Health
Sciences, Wayne State University, Detroit, Michigan, USA

Susan E. Ryan MS, B App Sc, OTR, SROT, AccOT
Professor, School of Occupational Therapy, University College, Cork, Ireland

Foreword by

Orvill Adams MA (International Affairs), MA (Economics), BA Hons (Economics)
Director, Department of Health Service Provision, WHO, Geneva

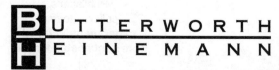

EDINBURGH LONDON NEW YORK OXFORD PHILADELPHIA ST LOUIS SYDNEY TORONTO 2003

BUTTERWORTH-HEINEMANN
An imprint of Elsevier Science Limited

© 2003, Elsevier Science Limited. All rights reserved.

No part of this publication may be reproduced, stored in a retrieval
system, or transmitted in any form or by any means, electronic,
mechanical, photocopying, recording or otherwise, without either the
prior permission of the publishers or a licence permitting restricted
copying in the United Kingdom issued by the Copyright Licensing
Agency, 90 Tottenham Court Road, London W1T 4LP. Permissions
may be sought directly from Elsevier's Health Sciences Rights
Department in Philadelphia, USA: phone: (+1) 215 238 7869, fax: (+1)
215 238 2239, e-mail: healthpermissions@elsevier.com. You may also
complete your request on-line via the Elsevier Science homepage
(http://www.elsevier.com), by selecting 'Customer Support' and then
'Obtaining Permissions'.

First published 2003

ISBN 0 7506 5441 4

British Library Cataloguing in Publication Data
A catalogue record for this book is available from the British Library

Library of Congress Cataloging in Publication Data
A catalog record for this book is available from the Library of
Congress

Notice
Medical knowledge is constantly changing. Standard safety
precautions must be followed, but as new research and clinical
experience broaden our knowledge, changes in treatment and drug
therapy may become necessary or appropriate. Readers are advised to
check the most current product information provided by the
manufacturer of each drug to be administered to verify the
recommended dose, the method and duration of administration, and
contraindications. It is the responsibility of the practitioner, relying on
experience and knowledge of the patient, to determine dosages and
the best treatment for each individual patient. Neither the Publisher
nor the authors/editors/contributors assumes any liability for any
injury and/or damage to persons or property arising from this
publication.

The Publisher

 your source for books,
journals and multimedia
in the health sciences
www.elsevierhealth.com

The
Publisher's
policy is to use
**paper manufactured
from sustainable forests**

Printed in the UK

Contents

Foreword   vii

Preface   ix

Contributors   xi

Acknowledgements   xiii

1. **Appreciating the big picture: you are part of it!**   1
   Susan E. Ryan, Susan A. Esdaile and Gillian Brown

2. **Developing competencies for advanced practice: how do I get there from here?**   30
   Helen M. Madill and Vivien Hollis

3. **Integrating theory and practice: using theory creatively to enhance professional practice**   64
   Maralynne D. Mitcham

4. **Evidence-based practice: informing practice and critically evaluating related research**   90
   M. Clare Taylor

5. **Enhancing reflective abilities: interweaving reflection into practice**   118
   Gillian Brown and Susan E. Ryan

6. **Do you reason like a (health) professional?**   145
   Joy Higgs

7. **Creating scholarly practice: integrating and applying scholarship to practice**   161
   Susan A. Esdaile and Linda M. Roth

8. **Creating occupational practice: a multidisciplinary health focus**   189
   Clare Hocking

9. **Using adult education theories: facilitating others' learning in professional practice settings**   216
   Lindy McAllister

10. **Role models and mentors: informal and formal ways to learn from exemplary practice**   239
    Linda M. Roth and Susan A. Esdaile

11. **The leading edge of competence: developing your potential for advanced practice**   260
    Auldeen Alsop

12. **Consultancy and advanced teaming: promoting practice beyond the healthcare environment**   282
    Gwilym Wyn Roberts

Epilogue   **300**

Index   **301**

Foreword

'The great thing in this world is not so much where we are but in what direction we are moving' (Oliver Wendell Holmes)

It has been enlightening to write the foreword for this visionary book which takes the reader on a journey along the path to advanced practice in, explaining, *en route,* what advanced practice is and why, in today's challenging health care world, it is important.

The authors are drawn from different rehabilitation therapy areas, bringing a fresh perspective to the issues of advanced practice and start by reflecting on the drivers for change in the current health care arena. The economic imperative in most countries is to keep costs down while continuing to meet growing demand, often resulting in changes to the structure of the health system. Because of this, there is a need for professionals who are able to work within ever-changing health care systems as well as a growing interest in the links between education, provider performance and quality of care. These challenges provide an apt backdrop against which to consider the potential contributions of advanced health care practitioners.

Human resources in health care are central to delivering health services, and yet the *World Health Report 2000* noted that determining and achieving the 'right' mix of health personnel is a major challenge for most health systems. The knowledge and skills that staff have, and the ways in which they are managed so that they can use them effectively and efficiently, affects not only the satisfaction of health care practitioners, but even more crucially, determines the quality of care they provide.

One of the challenges of skills utilization has been finding ways to use, define and regulate 'advanced' practice. There are several reasons why this is so: it is difficult to functionally define the exact level of practice which stops being 'ordinary' and becomes advanced: education may not have kept up with the needs of practice, so that practitioners learn from experience and in-service professional development, and none of this is regulated: or there may be turf wars, over who 'owns' particular pieces of practice. These are difficult issues, but this book tackles them all in a practical way, using worked examples to show different routes to advanced practice, likely obstacles and ways of overcoming them. The book acknowledges that in many ways the title of advanced practitioner cannot be given, it has to be taken, and this readiness for practice is acquired not only through formal learning. The reflective practitioner is one who can look at their own quality of practice, and consider to what extent it is evidence based, how theory can be applied to it, and whether they can teach others.

Having a level of self-awareness which results in increased motivation to improve knowledge and skills, and put these into practice to improve quality of care, is the cornerstone of empowerment as a practitioner. With self-efficacy comes inner power to make decisions comfortably, to take calculated risks and to tackle the unexpected in everyday practice. This is the sustainable professional development for which all those involved in human resources development are seeking. It is not easily taught, but it is encouraging to find it discussed in this book in all its dimensions.

Over the past few years, there has been a growing debate about the role of health in the development of societies. Work done by WHO has shown that a healthy population is a prerequisite for growth, rather than an expensive option for developing countries. Healthy people, supported by a functioning health sector, can ensure that their societies develop, and sustain their development. For this reason, loss of health is a loss not only to the person but also to families and societies.

Improving the health of an individual, or the population as a whole, does not mean only reducing premature death due to disease and injury, but also about maximizing the capacity of individuals to live a full life in society. Health is the ability to live life to its full potential, and to realise this potential, rehabilitation therapists have a key role.

In Chapter 8 of this book, Clare Hocking discusses the advanced occupational practice skills needed by health care practitioners in order to help people follow their occupations, and thus lead a fulfilling and productive life. She uses the WHO's *International Classification of Functioning Disability and Health*, which is a common international framework for describing and measuring health, to define activity and participation. Hocking notes that in using this framework practitioners will have to have the skills and knowledge to measure health outcomes in an individualised way, over the long term – skills she identifies with advanced practice. To achieve this goal, she suggests that professionals must increasingly work together, each with a unique contribution.

This is the new world of health care. Such an approach – teamwork using the skills of a range of professionals, and measuring health and not only illness in a population – is vital both to developing countries struggling to improve health conditions despite severe financial and human resources limitations, and to industrial countries working to provide fair and responsive health services in a time of changing expectations among their populations, and with limited financial resources.

The journey is only beginning, but this book provides an essential map to all serious travellers. I commend it to all those looking to advance their practice.

Orvill Adams
WHO, Geneva, 2003

Preface

The impetus for writing this text came firstly from numerous recent government publications, particularly in the UK and the USA. These papers emphasize the need for health professionals to be collaborative, innovative, evidence-based and creative in developing new, integrated areas of practice. The concept of a highly qualified, advanced practitioner and specialist, who can act as, and is, officially recognized as a *consultant* is an important feature of the government directives, especially in the UK. We became challenged and inspired by the notion of developing a *map* that could guide an early-career healthcare practitioner to become an advanced practitioner, who could effectively fill a consultant position at some later time.

Our second source of inspiration came from our own experience as clinicians, managers and educators of undergraduate and postgraduate students. Between us, we have worked as clinicians and/or educators in seven countries, where we had to adapt to different concepts of health and culture, in the delivery of services (public and private) and the education of healthcare professionals. Also, we have worked with students who have come to our programs from many countries and cultures. Each one had a different slant on healthcare. These perspectives stemmed from each country having other priorities and needs. Furthermore, each profession had developed slightly differently, so there were many diverse ways of working and interpreting practice. There are few universal truths and yet there are some common principles and processes. The chapters in this text give you several ways in which you could examine the needs of your own place of work while at the same time putting your service into a wider context. These are skills that an advanced practitioner needs to acquire and to be sensitive about.

Our own professional development has gone through many stages, becoming honed often through trial and error but also through deliberate planning and further study. Now, in different ways, we have reached a stage where we can operate on expert knowledge, supported through lifelong learning, until we hit the next big learning curve. Given the fast rate at which all aspects of health-care are changing, we believed that it would be helpful to provide you with a guide as an early-career practitioner so that you can accelerate the process of becoming an advanced practitioner. This notion follows the same line of thinking that is advocated in teaching clinical reasoning in order to enhance the process of moving from novice to expert. Processes like these take a considerable amount of time—often many years—so the sooner you are aware of your career path the better you can plan and follow your own map.

We also bring our own perspective on, and belief about, healthcare professionals. Deliberately, we have not referred to them as *allied* despite the fact that many documents do. We believe that the term *allied* suggests dependency, and this is not compatible with the notion of autonomy that we are advocating. However, we accept that in some contexts, the term *allied* refers to the operational relationship of the allied health professional groups to each other and to that of medicine.

All the chapters in this text were written by experienced and advanced healthcare professionals. These authors come from Australia, Canada, New Zealand, the UK and the USA. They represent a rich diversity of experiences from cultural and professional perspectives that include health promotion, medical education, occupational therapy and physiotherapy and speech-language therapy/pathology. As this text is published in the UK, we have used UK spelling, with some modifications. However, we have used both UK and North American terms to describe professionals, depending on their country of origin and/or the literature being cited. Thus, North American physical therapists and their publications have not been turned into physiotherapists, or vice versa. We have also kept references to speech and language therapists or pathologists, depending on their countries of origin. The majority of the references we have cited, and examples we have used are about occupational therapists, physio/physical therapists, and speech-language pathologists, therapists. But we have also included examples and references that relate to many other health professionals, such as dieticians, dental hygienists, nurses, medical technologists, psychologists, physicians, and pharmacists.

Figure 1.1 is our map. It represents the context of healthcare practice from the perspective of the practitioner. It is repeated as a key for each chapter. We invite you to use the figure and the text reflectively, as a guide for developing your own career plan, and adding your own questions and ideas. We see this text as a working map to which you can constantly return at different stages in your career as well as using it for different purposes such as working with and supervising students or for developing your role as a mentor. It can also be used as a plan for a department to progress to becoming more scholarly and research-focused. We hope that you will find the text valuable, and that collectively we have inspired you to learn more and to add your own insights and scholarship as you move along in your career.

Gillian Brown, Susan A. Esdaile, Susan E. Ryan
2003

Contributors

Auldeen Alsop, MPhil, BA, DipCOT, SROT,
Discipline Leader for Occupational Therapy
Sheffield Hallam University, School of Health
and Social Care, Sheffield, England, UK

Gillian Brown, MSc, DipCOT, SROT,
Head Occupational Therapist, Barking Havering
and Redbridge NHS Trust, and Senior Lecturer,
University of East London, London, England, UK

Susan A. Esdaile, PhD, MAPS, AccOT, OTR, SROT,
Professor, Department of Occupational Therapy,
Eugene Applebaum College of Pharmacy and
Health Sciences, Wayne State University, Detroit,
Michigan, USA

Joy Higgs, PhD, MPHEd, GradDipPhty, BSc, Professor,
School of Physiotherapy, Director, Centre for
Professional Education Advancement, Faculty of
Health Sciences, University of Sydney, NSW,
Australia

Clare Hocking, MHSc(OT),
Principal Lecturer, School of Occupational
Therapy Auckland University of Technology,
Auckland, New Zealand

Vivien Hollis, PhD, MSc, T Dip, COT, OT(C),
Professor and Chair, Department of Occupational
Therapy, Faculty of Rehabilitation Medicine,
University of Alberta, Edmonton, Alberta, Canada

Lindy McAllister, PhD, MA BSpThy,
Course Coordinator Speech Pathology, School of
Community Health, Charles Sturt University,
Albury, NSW, Australia

Helen M. Madill, PhD,
Professor and Graduate Programs Coordinator
Centre for Health Promotion Studies, University
of Alberta, Edmonton, Canada

Maralynne D. Mitcham, PhD, DipCOT, OTR/L
FAOTA,
Professor and Director, Occupational Therapy
Educational Program, Department of
Rehabilitation Sciences, College of Health
Professions, Medical University of South
Carolina, Charleston, SC, USA

Gwilym Wyn Roberts, MA DipCOT SROT AMICPD,
Head of Department, Department of Occupa-
tional Therapy Education, School of Health Care
Studies, University of Wales College of Medicine,
Cardiff, Wales, UK

Linda M. Roth, PhD,
Associate Professor and Education Coordinator,
Department of Family Medicine, Faculty of
Medicine, Wayne State University, Detroit,
Michigan, USA

Susan E. Ryan, MS, BAppSc, OTR, SROT, AccOT,
Professor, School of Occupational Therapy,
University College, Cork, Ireland

M. Clare Taylor, PhD, DipCOT, SROT, BA (Hons), MA
(Dist),
Principal Lecturer, Occupational Therapy Subject
Group, School of Health and Social Sciences
Coventry University, England, UK

Acknowledgements

We would like to express our gratitude to the colleagues listed below for reviewing earlier chapter drafts and providing us with valuable feedback.

Barbara Hooper MS, OTR/L
Diane Hamilton OTR
Ida Canini OTR
Jennie C. Ariail Ph D
Karen Fron MPT

We are pleased that we were able to include suggestions from people representing several health professions and from early-career practitioners.

Mary E. Wilcox BSc (Pharm), BA, Dip J
Niall Fitzpatrick Dip COT, SROT
Petra J. Klompenhouwer-Meijer MS, OTR, SROT
Stephanie Fade BSc(Hons), SRD
Todd Wolney MT(ASCP)

1

Appreciating the big picture: you are part of it!

The socio-political influences on health practice in the public and private sphere

Susan E. Ryan, Susan A. Esdaile and Gillian Brown

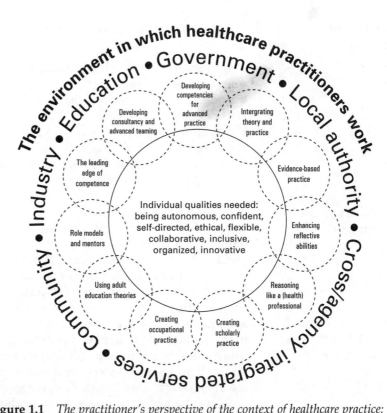

The environment in which healthcare practitioners work

Education • Government • Local authority • Cross/agency integrated services • Community • Industry

Developing competencies for advanced practice

Developing consultancy and advanced teaming

Intergrating theory and practice

The leading edge of competence

Evidence-based practice

Individual qualities needed: being autonomous, confident, self-directed, ethical, flexible, collaborative, inclusive, organized, innovative

Role models and mentors

Enhancing reflective abilities

Using adult education theories

Reasoning like a (health) professional

Creating occupational practice

Creating scholarly practice

Figure 1.1 *The practitioner's perspective of the context of healthcare practice: individual qualities needed and key aspects of professional development to become an advanced practitioner*

Chapter outline

We have separated this chapter into two parts that examine the major influences on healthcare in the public and the private sphere. The first part looks at the present challenges to healthcare professionals, including, in particular, the definitions and role requirements of the newly created position of the advanced practitioner. The reasons for the creation of this role are outlined in subsequent sections that look at the factors driving healthcare changes, the changing healthcare scenarios and the consequent need for different ways of working. These factors are coupled with the recognition that other forms of knowledge and different capabilities are required. Ways of maintaining professional standards that will support these changes with various regulations are contrasted between professions and between countries. International and global issues that impact on practice in the various countries represented in this book are discussed and implications are suggested. The factors shaping the private sphere of the individual and how each practitioner works in this changing climate are featured in three ways: *how to shape ideas, how to manage power*, and *how to organize time* to avoid stress. The chapter concludes with a summary.

Key words   Advanced practice, vision, leadership, power structures

Anticipated outcomes   As a result of reading this chapter we anticipate that you will be able to:

- appreciate the complex breadth of factors that impact on national and local healthcare services
- understand the need for vision and leadership from advanced practitioners
- realize the implications for altered service structures that the proposed changes will generate
- formulate strategies to progress your career-path towards becoming an advanced practitioner.

Perspectives on the big picture   Healthcare practitioners are being challenged on several different fronts. Many governments in developed countries are demanding fundamental re-organizations of all aspects of their healthcare. This includes all levels of education, the diversification and distribution of health programs, other ways of working with patients/clients and the promotion of particular forms of research. Various commissions have been set up in different countries to examine national requirements and many of these reports are referenced in this book. At the same time, evolutionary changes are being generated from within health professions as a natural result of the developing maturity of some relatively young professions. Research capabilities and study findings are also contributing to practice changes.

Some challenges often seem contradictory. Certain changes appear to suggest that healthcare practitioners should work at lower technical levels to formulated patterns of practice. At the opposite end of this continuum is the advanced practitioner, a new career role that is being carved out that has a different combination of skills and knowledge. This role is the focus of this book.

Called variously by other titles such as consultant therapist and nurse specialist, the definition of an advanced practitioner remains cloudy and is developing. You can become part of this development and this book will give you ways to follow and ideas to use. Figure 1.1 illustrates multiple and overlapping layers that we believe constitute the crucial parts that will develop this role. Centred by personal qualities and ringed by different working environments, the key aspects for becoming an advanced practitioner form the inner circle—the chapters of this book. The qualities that you will need in order to become an advanced practitioner and the many types of knowledge (Higgs and Titchen 2001) that you will need to develop are inter-locked and inter-related. Each person will have a different configuration and we hope that as you read this book or dip into particular chapters you will be more aware of the factors needed to appraise, evaluate and create your career-path. When we were putting this book together we included the full range of mainstream healthcare practitioners in our thinking and searches. We were also aware that others from complementary and alternative healthcare practices will become interested in the future in certain aspects of professional development as their contribution to healthcare is being increasingly recognized (see the section on Complementary Healthcare at the end of this chapter). The writers of this book also come from a range of countries and disciplines and the chapters they have written show different styles and perspectives which meld into the big picture. You may find that particular styles resonate with you more than others. It would be beneficial to notice these reactions. You will get to know yourself better in this way.

Briefly, the roles and responsibilities of an advanced practitioner go beyond what is understood as normal practice and it is these extra advanced skills that will be recognized with higher profiles, responsibilities and salary structures. For example, in the UK the requirements extend to and encompass a broader notion of professional competence, with greater priority being placed on non-clinical aspects of care in six key areas in the education, training and continuing professional development of healthcare professionals. These areas are:

- skills in communicating with patients and colleagues
- education about the principles and organization of the National Health Service (NHS), about how care is managed, and the skills required for this management
- the development of teamwork
- shared learning across professional boundaries
- clinical audit and reflective practice
- leadership.

It is always easier to list aims like those above than to interpret the capabilities required in these key areas and it is these abilities that we would like to tease out in this book. In fact, the varied chapter titles provide you with the complex range of skills (taken in the broadest sense of the meaning) that we believe could constitute advanced practice. Realistically, you will have a combination of talents and these will constantly shift as you use and develop them. These changes may happen naturally through the demands of your job or you may actively seek to alter them yourself. This is a challenge but it is also very exciting and opportunities abound for those, like yourself, who are willing to try.

Previously, health practitioners were collectively described in terms of their work setting and their grades in that setting. Some would be referred to as, for example, a *physical therapy expert clinician in orthopedic and neurological practice,* others as a *senior two in hand therapy.* Their real expertise in and beyond contact practice was never really elaborated. As we have noted above, the title of advanced practitioner assumes skills beyond direct practice. Although expertise in practice and leadership qualities in the health professions have been promoted for some time in a bottom-up approach (Martin et al 1992, Roberts and Machon 2000), the main thrust of inspiration and change has come from top-down government initiatives in most countries. In the next section we will look at these socio-political drivers that form the overarching umbrella environment shown in Figure 1.1.

Driving healthcare changes

One of the major drivers that has persuaded governmental change has been the demand-driven system. This is based on the enormous financial power of healthcare markets in most developed English-speaking countries (H M Treasury (UK) 2001, National Forum on Health (Canada) 1995, Pew Health Professions Commission (USA) 1995, US Department of Health and Human Services 1999). These countries have different healthcare organizations. Some have national health services, others have a high percentage of private healthcare while others have or are developing a mixture of both public and private care. All of them are driven to make changes because of the increasing costs of healthcare. Because of these differences, each country's immediate priorities are not the same; their level and speed of implementation of new styles of services are not synchronized but the general trends in their vision for change are similar. These include: principles of universality in healthcare (for most countries, not all), accessibility, comprehensiveness, portability and public administration for medical services. There will be a greater awareness of health promotion and wellness, more emphasis on primary healthcare, more community and home-care, better pharmaceutical management, wider health information and communication and greater equity in the portioning of health equipment in the overall infrastructure.

Funding levels to organizations have been affected and cuts have been made. This has put pressure on these organizations in health and social services. When this rationing is coupled with the cost of new diagnostic procedures and treatment techniques, expensive new drugs, and a subsequent increase in client expectations, managers have been forced to review their efficiency and effectiveness in response to these economic pressures. In turn this has led to job cuts, job restructuring based on the need to provide less specialized or professionally focused care, and a reduction in profession specific managers of services. The increase in part-time employment is also economically driven. The consequence is that employee benefits are reduced and employers can exercise greater flexibility in scheduling for peak times. These trends can be expected to continue, as healthcare cost containment becomes an issue around the world. We should expect continual change as health and social care organizations respond to demographic shifts and to political, economic, social and technological demands.

Other change is happening in the workplace. These factors driving healthcare, outlined above, are forcing certain professions to change their roles and their places of work (Adamson et al 2000). Many rehabilitation professionals, such as those in Canada, have left the system and have become self-employed. In turn, they contract their services back to the government health services they left (von Zweck 1999).

Other factors driving healthcare change come from the general public. Attitudes towards social conditions such as homelessness and begging for money on the streets, sexual morality and orientation, gender roles and responsibilities, tolerance or otherwise of different faiths, and health rationing continue to alter between decades, between generations and between sexes (Jowell et al 2000). As an advanced practitioner you would need to be conversant with the latest reports and trends in the country where you are working currently. You will need to incorporate this knowledge into any planned changes you propose to make and be able to articulate your reasons. Your remit is therefore much wider than it was previously. In fact, in the UK, 60% of the public want doctors and healthcare workers to make health-related decisions 'as they see best' rather than have administrators and politicians make these decisions (Bryson and New 2000). Furthermore, public involvement in decision-making is happening increasingly. In New South Wales, Australia, there is already greater consumer and community involvement in planning services (Reid 2001) and this trend is being echoed in other countries, causing sometimes radical changes (see NHS Plan website, p. 456). Some of the public wish to be more involved in decision-making as they become better informed about health-related matters through the various media. Many voice their opinions and concerns—sometimes quite vociferously. Litigation surrounding poor practice continues to increase. At the local work-face level, health practitioners are being exhorted to alter their ways of working to make their interventions more client-centred so that clients become involved and take responsibility and ownership for their care and for what happens to them. The new visions that are being proposed have different orientations to healthcare from those of the past, so these changes are not merely maximizing present practice but they are changing practice structurally across established boundaries. The advanced practitioner is seen as being a leader who is instrumental in implementing and shaping these ideas.

Changing healthcare—changing practice

Change has always been present but it has been endemic to most healthcare structures in the last decade and, rather than settling down, the pace is gathering momentum, with new ideas generating new plans. In fact, the pace of change in healthcare is so great that the ideas outstrip the abilities of many of those trying to implement them. This produces great strains on both persons and organizations (website: The National Committee of Inquiry into Higher Education, 1997). Sometimes new procedures that have taken 2 years to put in place and to recruit and train staff for have been superseded before they have even got off the ground. Hence the need for a cadre of health professionals who are comfortable with and can work with change. Do you feel comfortable with these turbulences? We are persuaded that you would not be reading this book if you were not intrigued to find out if you could be one of these players. How much do you incorporate change already? Try this exercise.

Activity box 1.1

- Is your service integrated—does it include primary, secondary and tertiary care across all groups that access your service?
- Is your service financially sound?
- Do you include various and innovative ways of educating the public, your staff, and students? Do these methods include the principles of lifelong learning?
- Do you encourage interdisciplinary and interagency collaborations?

(Department of Health 2000)

Those with abilities to put these changes in motion have never been so sorely needed.

Changing roles

As Figure 1.1 illustrates, the arenas where healthcare practices will be delivered are changing rapidly and so the way you work will need to change accordingly and roles will inevitably alter. In some countries, the numbers of hospital beds are being cut because of the high cost of care and as a consequence, hospitals are closing. The Pew Health Professions Commission (1995) report in the USA anticipated that in the future 60% of hospital beds would be closed. This trend is being mirrored in other countries. With the massive expansion into other areas of practice such as ambulatory care and community settings, the roles of healthcare workers will change. Because of these changes some countries like the USA will have surpluses of staff such as physicians, nurses and pharmacists, although not necessarily in some states, or in many rural areas, where shortage of these professionals will continue (Pew Health Professions Commission 1995). To be more competitive, these healthcare professionals will have to change their present way of working and take on different roles such as those of the advanced practitioner. Alternatively, they may consider moving to countries experiencing shortages of healthcare professionals, such as the UK, although the pay-scale level is often not comparable. Moving to another country, the practitioner will need to become more conversant with other systems and societies, as discussed in the preceding sections. Changing within disciplines and between professions will be a new feature of career planning that has not been contemplated or made possible before. Health practitioners will be able to step on, step off and step over at different points in their education and in their career (Department of Health 2000). To enable this to happen certain benchmarks or points of reference were developed between disciplines and in the UK these have happened in stages.

Benchmarking

Benchmarking is a term that evaluates or assesses performances (Pearsall 1998). As described in the preceding sections, new ways of thinking about health and education have emerged from the numerous consultations that have taken place in the past years. Benchmarks are needed in order to understand the issues and to provide a way forward with ideas. For instance, initial work in the UK has been developed in collaboration with the health professions that include dietetics, health visiting, midwifery, nursing, occupational therapy, orthoptists, physiotherapy, podiatry/chiropody, prosthetics and orthotics, radiography, and speech and language therapy. Working first in subject-specific groups, an early analysis identified a number of features that all the groups shared. It became clear that there was considerable overlap as well as a set of common beliefs. In this first phase a common healthcare framework started to emerge (The Quality Assurance Agency for Higher Education 2001). This emerging framework has the potential to include in the next phase other health-related disciplines such as social work, dentistry, medicine and other therapies not listed above. This further work could lead to an overarching health professions' framework. Common features would include:

- the need to put the client/patient at the centre of a student's learning experience,
- the need to promote that experience within a team's way of thinking
- the need for cross-professional collaboration and communication.

From this work there is now acknowledgement and agreement that there are common skills and knowledge shared by the range of healthcare professionals and another set of profession-specific knowledge and skills. Figure 1.2 illustrates how these facets of knowledge overlap and inter-relate with the worlds of the people that use health services.

This configuration illustrates that 'practice' does not exist without the interaction between the healthcare professional and the person who is the service user. This is all the more pertinent when the patient's or client's pathway is seen as fundamental and central to patterns of service delivery. These services have to be moulded to fit these expectations.

As an advanced practitioner you would need to know about and be able to facilitate these changes in small and larger ways. Now you can begin to appreciate how the 'big picture' is changing radically and how you could be a part of these changes. But, even though there are changes, standards must be maintained while these are happening. The next part of the picture looks at the current information and the issues surrounding the standards and regulations that are being implemented and the tensions these cause. Issues around power structures in the workplace together with some stress-related solutions will help to guide you through this maze and these aspects will be addressed in the final part of this chapter.

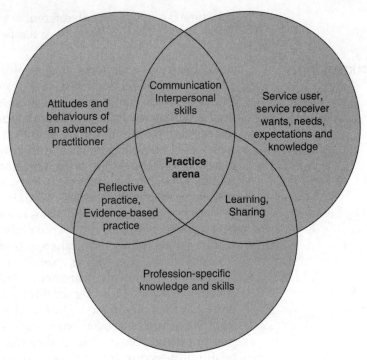

Figure 1.2   *The inter-relationship between clients and practitioners in practice.*

Professional standards and regulations

Professional standards initiatives are so complex and have such far-reaching implications that they have to be inter-twined with regulatory procedures. Are you familiar with the disciplinary procedures where you work? At this point it may be appropriate for you to stop and consider these. Try the following questions.

Activity box 1.2

- Is there a national reporting system in place that analyses unexplained occurrences in practice?
- Do you know if members of the public are invited to your professional regulatory body when disciplinary activities take place?
- Is there a local committee that hears disciplinary procedures and which takes into account the wider contributing factors beyond the individual?
- Do you know the maximum hours allowed before reporting unusual occurrences in practice?
- Is there opportunity to report an offence in confidence?
- What is written in your contract of employment about regulatory proceedings?

Standards and regulations are important—and even essential—to continuous quality control that is demanded of us as professionals. However, we need to be vigilant in ensuring that standards and regulations reflect needs that enhance future scholarly, ethical professional practice, and enable, not constrict, the education of future practitioners. Practice has to be dynamic and continually modified in order to meet the changing needs of society and the changing, diverse needs of individual communities. Regulations that focus on educational preparation for practice that is current when the regulations are determined, and do not make provisions for future practice, yet to be determined, can become disadvantageous. Guidelines, standards and examinations that reflect best practice, as recognized and approved by those who pay the practitioners, exert a major influence on educators (Esdaile and Roth 2000). External pressures on health professionals have led to a focus on defining professional competence in terms of skills, which may or may not be associated with scholarship. This situation is evident in the USA (Gourley 2001, Smith 2001, US Department of Health and Human Services 1999) and the UK (Department of Health 2000; Greatbach and Morris 2001) where educational and professional standards are monitored and controlled by the national association and/or certifying bodies, as can be seen from Table 1.1 on pages 11–13.

Grossman's (1998) study of the forces driving continuing competence in the health professions included literature and document reviews and telephone interviews with key informants representing 13 professions: chiropractic, dentistry, dietetics, nursing, occupational therapy, optometry, pharmacy, physical therapy, podiatry, psychology, speech-language pathology and audiology, social work, and veterinary medicine. Most of us believe, or hope that professionals are internally motivated to ensure best practice, and that they develop a mechanism to assess this process. However, as we have seen in earlier parts of this chapter, external pressures, often driven by economic imperatives, demand other levels of regulation and control. There is a delicate balance between public accountability and professional self-regulation and autonomy. Grossman (1998) suggests that creating and maintaining this balance requires partnership between regulatory boards, professional associations, and certification programs as well as member support for new initiatives. Professional leadership is essential 'to meet the changing needs of society and the concerns of multiple stakeholders' (p. 714). Being active in your professional association is a good starting point. Think about the following questions.

Activity box 1.3	Consider whether your profession makes its own decisions about its practice and the education of practitioners, or whether some outside authority makes some, or all of these decisions for your profession.
	Take time to answer the following questions and reflect on your responses. If you don't know the answer, we suggest that you find out where you can get this information.
	1. What is your profession?
	2. Did you take a certification examination? Who sets this examination?

Continued

Activity box 1.3 *cont'd*	3. Did you take a registration and/or licensure examination? Who sets this examination?
	4. How are these professional certification and registration examinations financed?
	5. Are you required to provide proof of continuing professional development to be able to practice your profession?
	6. Do you know how the professional course that you took at your college or university is accredited? Who is responsible for maintaining this accreditation?

Regulations in different countries

Perhaps your responses to the exercise above have alerted you to consider the position of your own profession and to realize your part in this picture. As with other thinking about the health changes previously described, many countries are at different points along the regulatory road, as seen from Table 1.1. And, as with all the other aspects of healthcare, there is no consistent agreement with terminology or processes. These will take time to develop. But behind all the ideas the paramount importance is that of being accountable to the public for health programs and services and the quality of the practitioners who deliver these.

Regulatory practices differ considerably between countries, often reflecting how the status of each profession is viewed. There are usually three parties involved: the university, the professional association and the registering body (Alsop and Ryan 1996). Often, but not always, academic qualifications are separated from professional qualifications and as in most other areas, there is much current debate about these procedures and structures (Waters 2001). If you are unsure about this area we suggest you become conversant with the different international regulatory procedures in your own profession as mobility between countries is increasing. Here are some examples. In the USA a national registration examination, Occupational Therapist Registered (OTR) happens in occupational therapy after the completion of the degree course. In the UK the student passes the validated university qualifying course, and then applies for registration, becoming a State Registered Occupational Therapist (SROT). This process is being reviewed and new structures and procedures will be shortly in place. Some countries, e.g. Canada, the UK and the USA, require that foreign entrants take their national registration examination before being allowed to practice. This regulatory area is constantly changing within and between countries. Table 1.1 illustrates a sample of countries and professions that have different regulations. Further regulatory procedures beyond qualification will be described later.

Standards can be viewed in other ways. Most countries are developing statewide frameworks to ensure a more equitable delivery of care. In New South Wales, Australia, for example, a statewide quality framework has been put in place with advances in performance monitoring. There has been an increase in the number of women and

Table 1.1   International sample of regulatory procedures for different health professions

	Entry qualifications	Registration after qualifying	Licensure	Accreditation	Continuing professional development (CPD) requirements
Australia					
Occupational therapy	BAppSc, BSc, BOT, MSc A number of universities offer double degrees	Registration in: Queensland, Western Australia, Northern Territory, South Australia No registration in: NSW, Victoria, Tasmania		Personal accreditation—introduced for individual therapists in May 2001—not compulsory	To maintain accreditation, 60 CPD points must be gained in 2 years—sample audit
Physiotherapy	BappSc, BSc, MSc	By application on completion of course accredited by ACOPRA			
Speech and language therapy	Bachelors degree level	Met the requirements for competencies (entry level) Speech Pathology Association of Australia (SPAA), Melbourne	Overseas therapists must demonstrate their competence by the standards of SPAA	Accreditation of programs by SPAA by teleconference—site visits are rare	
Canada					
Occupational therapy (OT)	BSc OT—will change to a Master's degree entry in 2010	On completion of college program and national certification exam Healthcare Professionals in Canada will be regulated under Health Professions Act enforced July 2002. Registration for each individual profession will be established.	Each province has a regulatory body	Each university program is accredited—no personal accreditation	Colleges establish, maintain and enforce standards for CPD under HPA 2002
Physiotherapy (PT)	BSc PT—will change to a Master's degree entry in 2010		Most, but not all, provinces have a regulatory body, College of PT requires evidence of PCE	Each university program is accredited—no personal accreditation	
Speech-language pathologist/ audiologist pathology	MA		Each province has a regulatory body		

Continued

Table 1.1 *International sample of regulatory procedures for different health professions—cont'd*

	Entry qualifications	Registration after qualifying	Licensure	Accreditation	Continuing professional development (CPD) requirements
Netherlands					
Occupational therapy	Diploma Occupational Therapy (equal to BSc)	Do not need official registration *but* the professional body has set up registration procedures—a basic register has come into effect in 2000	Licensure is considered to be the degree plus the registration	No set requirements yet—being developed for 2005	No set requirements yet
Physiotherapy	Diploma Physiotherapy (equal to BSc)	Central Physiotherapy Register	The diploma and the registration are considered to be licensure	Reregistration will be required by 2005—this will require some training—in the process of being developed	CPD will be linked to reregistration
Speech and language therapy	Diploma Speech Therapy (equal to BSc)	Do not need official registration *but* the professional body has set up registration procedures—a basic register has come into effect in 2000	Licensure is considered to be the degree plus the registration	No set requirements yet—being developed for 2005	No set requirements yet
South Africa					
Occupational therapy/ physiotherapy/ speech and language therapy	BOT, BSc, (4 years)	Register with Health Professions Council of South Africa and the Professional Boards for Health Professions—annual registration	No	No	No
United Kingdom					
Occupational therapy	BSc (3 years) BSc Hons (4 years)	Formal registration with Health Professions Council on completion of an accredited course	No	No	Recommendations exist to develop professional portfolio of competencies
Physiotherapy Speech and language therapy	BSc Hons (3 years) BSc (3 years)				Mechanisms for formal monitoring under development

USA					
Occupational therapy	BS, MOT, MA(OT) or MS(OT); from 2007 entry-level Master's degree	National certification examination, administered by NBCOT	Each state has regulatory body; some also have licensure	Each program is accredited by its own institution and ACOTE (AOTA)	Requirement of licensure in some states; may become a requirement of recertification by NBCOT in the future
Physical therapy	Post-baccalaureate, masters or clinical doctorate	National certification exam, administered by FSBPT	All states have licensure	Each program is accredited by its own institution and the Commission on Education in Physical Therapy	According to state determination; not national
Speech—language-hearing pathology	Entry-level Master's degree, MS, MA, MEd, MCD, in speech- and language-related field	National certification exam, administered by PRAXIS	Each state has regulatory body; some also have licensure	Each program is accredited by its own institution and ASHA	Will be required for audiology in 2003, and speech pathology in 2005

BOT, Bachelor in Occupational Therapy; ACOPRA, Australian Council for Physiotherapy Regulation; MOT, Master of Occupational Therapy (USA); NBCOT, National Board of Certification for Occupational Therapy (USA); ACOTE, Accreditation Council for Occupational Therapy Education (USA); AOTA, American Occupational Therapy Association; FSBPT, Federation of State Boards for Physical Therapy (USA); ASHA, American Speech-and-Hearing Association; PRAXIS, the organization that administers the certification exam for ASHA.

clinicians at senior management level and greater recognition for consumer involvement has occurred (Reid 2001). Similar work is happening in Canada, the UK and the USA in different ways.

Another way of regulating quality is by making sure that there are sufficient numbers, types and grades of staff to do the work. In the UK significant expansions in the numbers of practitioners is planned by 2004. Universities will expand their student numbers considerably and efforts will be made to retain staff in practice settings or re-train staff through work-based learning programs, often in association with a university. Therapists who have left the profession for various reasons are being re-called and people from other walks of life are being enticed to join health as a career. In the section of the NHS (2000) document *Meeting the Challenge*, specific mention is made of recruiting black and ethnic-minority members 'both to delivering the increased workforce that is needed and providing effective, accessible and culturally sensitive services to diverse communities' (p. 19). Universities are widening their access policies in order to recruit students who are representative of the diverse and complex societies where many practitioners work (Edmonds 1998). Other ways of improving the practice of those already in post are through various clinical governance regulations, with continuing professional development and lifelong learning being situated at the heart of regulatory planning, as we shall see in the following section.

Continuing professional development

A main criterion for professions is that of 'being up to date' and 'using evidence wisely' (Fish and Coles 1998, p. 5). Regrettably, this has not always happened and increasingly, politicians are sensing that the public wants more or different things from professional people (Fish and Coles 1998). Regulations to 'prove' continuing competence have come into being at various stages in different countries, as shown in Table 1.1 above. In the USA licensure (L) is required in some states. This could be from examinations but other times it is from evidence of continuing professional updating. In 2000/2001 Australia launched accreditation in occupational therapy (AccOT) in order to give individual therapists recognition for their continuing learning and professional development. Divided into seven areas and through a portfolio collection they must show:

- practice development
- private study
- mentoring/supervision
- professional activities
- non-assessed studies
- assessed studies and, courses
- research and publications.

These areas promoting reflection and life-long learning are being addressed in varying degrees in most of the countries represented in this book. However, there are other international considerations of which you will need to be aware in the future. The next section will look at some of these.

International perspectives

As you read on you will begin to realize that, although you can borrow ideas and procedures from other countries, the larger cultural context where you are working needs to be understood. This is far from easy. In fact, this is another outer layer of understanding that is not illustrated in Figure 1.1. It is all-embracing and we believe it will become more so in different ways in future work. This book is rich with examples of health professionals managing and working together from different countries. The writers come from several continents. Even the fact that we have put this book together without all of us meeting is an example of mutual working across vast divides. But there are other considerations of which you will need to be aware.

One of us worked in India for several years and she realized that she could import certain principles of practice, although some had to be used differently, particularly in the psycho-social and activities of daily-living spheres. These adjustments were in contrast to the intrinsic medical aspects of her work. Many of the assessments and protocols did not fit into another culture, yet others did. It was only because she had lived in India for several years that she had become aware of the areas of practice that needed great sensitivity and prolonged discussions were needed in an effort to understand. Differences in language, translations and consequent understandings about terminology also happen. In formal meetings in the USA an item that is *tabled* is taken off the agenda. Thus confusion can be created for or by someone from another country (e.g. Australia or UK) where *tabled* at a meeting means that the item is put on the agenda. There is a growing body of literature in the health professions that is addressing these issues related to improving intercultural interaction (Brislin and Yoshida 1994).

An understanding of the different belief systems related to illness is a particularly important aspect of healthcare delivery. Therefore, health professionals need to understand different models and frameworks related to illness. Mullavey-O'Byrne's chapters in the Brislin and Yoshida (1994) text provide useful training exercises to assist healthcare professionals. She also provides a comprehensive discussion to explain the theoretical rationale that supports and facilitates intercultural interactions in welfare work. Given the psychosocial affects of any illness experience, it is important for healthcare professionals to have an understanding of transcultural issues in mental health (Fitzgerald et al 1997).

Being aware of other cultures' values about health and social issues can affect advanced practice in a myriad of ways. Understanding these issues is important, and not only for those working with patients or clients from other cultures. With the continental barriers opened in Europe and greater mobility of health professionals globally, these differences will become more apparent. Also, with the shortages of trained personnel, health workers are literally being imported from one country to another and patients are being sent abroad for treatment. Britain has approached Spain for more medical practitioners to work in the NHS. Developed countries are being more considerate with respect to taking health practitioners from less developed countries where their expertise and skills are urgently needed back home. While the professional bodies in each country take overall care of the entry qualifications and regulations, it will be one feature of an advanced practitioner that inter-disciplinary work is promoted. This will be from a different perspective to that of merely practice skills, thinking and application as cultural awareness should also be incorporated into these dynamics.

We could imagine different ways of working and different ways of reasoning between members of teams being facilitated to come to some common understanding by a sensitive advanced educator. As noted above, future practice must not be compromised by current regulations and an advanced practitioner could advocate changes at community and national levels and with policy makers, business leaders and other non-medical organizations. Entrepreneurial qualities will be part of this new picture that is evolving (Higgs and Edwards 1999).

The healthcare systems of different countries operate from distinct knowledge bases and belief systems about health practice and its underlying foundations of art and/or science. Their levels of education, particularly among the therapists, are very disparate as well. While some European countries have diploma (associate degree)-level courses, others, at the opposite end of the spectrum, are pushing for Master's degrees as entry-level qualifying programs (Allen et al 2001), and other countries already have these in place. Because of continuing shortages of health personnel in general, other ways of managing the problem are being tried. Professional courses are being shortened with fast-track syllabi and the doors are already opened for mature people, some of whom have first degrees while others have no family history of university education (Baty 2001). It is for this last group that special attention needs to be paid by providing enabling educational climates of support and acceptance.

In the UK this factor is of great concern and it is recognized presently that these systems are not in place (Ryan 2001). For advanced practice this has tremendous implications and there is much work to do. Those qualifying from particular schools will certainly have advantages over those from other programs. Potential students will become more discerning in their selection of programs if that is a possibility they could consider. Advanced educators will need to be acutely aware of these differences and programs of continuing professional development must take the learners' stances and levels of knowledge into account when courses are designed. Continuing professional development courses are also viable options for making up shortfalls in knowledge for those from less academic programs.

In education, more health professionals use adult learning theories and principles where the past experiences of the students are considered and included into the program to make learning more personally relevant and enjoyable. These are elaborated in Chapter 9. These theories need to be integrated with those from the Higher Education sector that have more critical and cognitive demands. Many post-professional Master's-level students have entered university with a diploma or associate degree. They have succeeded just as well as those from Bachelor's degree programs (courses), although their learning curve at the beginning of such courses is much steeper as they lack research knowledge and academic writing skills. These differences and divergences make the central work of the World Health Organization (WHO) even more critical. Their classification of Functioning and Disability, ICIDH-2, provides frameworks that can help individuals, services, economies, scientists and society in general make sense of the differences (website: World Health Organization 2001). Chapter 8 elaborates on this work.

You can see from the many factors above that you must hold in your mind different images of health, practice and programs at different levels and use both universal and particular aspects together. Henriksson's (1994) comments regarding occupational therapy in Sweden are also applicable to other health professionals:

> Development can be described on different levels. The global level considers the development of occupational therapy as a worldwide profession with a common knowledge base. Professional, theoretical knowledge in occupational therapy is rapidly increasing and globally available. [But] another local level deals with the development of the profession as a result of interaction between praxis, education and knowledge development. This is dependent on the structure and advancement of the healthcare system of the surrounding society, the organization and development of the educational system, healthcare needs and policies, priorities and the allocation of economic resources (p. 165).

Being aware of all these dimensions will enrich your way of working at whatever level you are at this present time. This might be an area to which you will return much later in your career. Let us now look at other global perspectives.

Global perspectives

There are many advantages from international developments that you will be able to use, if you are not already doing so. Some countries are far more advanced than others with electronic technology and the balance is changing between countries because of this phenomenon. For instance, Finland is a small country yet a high proportion of its population (40%) is using the Internet, and it is becoming a global developer in cell phones and other electronic apparatus. The Finnish government is committed to making it an information society (Salminen 2000) which will change the daily living habits of its inhabitants as their lives become re-organized. Similarly, countries like India and China with their vast populations will be increasingly accessible to e-learning programs. This access will level some universal knowledge while at the same time it might create local difficulties when cultures, values and customs are not considered in the course design. The types of educational programs designed by advanced educators or health professionals must then be examined from these global perspectives. What might be easy in the USA might be impossible elsewhere due to the medical facilities available or other such constructs.

The Internet, and its extensive use for communication and information exchange, especially in the more affluent countries of the world by a large number of professionals, indeed made Marshall McLuhan's (1967) concept of a 'Global Village' a reality. People separated by half a world, two seasons, and speaking together on different dates and different calendars can hold a teleconference or videoconference. Living in such complex, multiple realities can be challenging to a point of saturation and dislocation (Gergen 1991). Professional leaders in health sciences are aware of the juggling act we need to perform, and are working to provide guidelines for current practice. Later in this chapter we will look at ways of combating the stress and burnout that these realities sometimes cause.

In discussing the need to move beyond parochialism in the higher education of physical therapists, Schmoll (2000) identified four major shifts that drive quality in higher education. They are:

- competition between for-profit and not-for-profit sectors in education
- increasing costs
- the need to demonstrate accountability
- a move to adopt a service orientation.

Educational institutions are increasingly required to be like companies and continually re-design their systems to improve their process of delivering educational excellence. This in turn ensures that professionals who graduate from these proactive programs can effectively meet the needs of the communities that they serve.

From the perspective of enthusiastic, recent graduates in the health professions, the possibilities offered by an international community of colleagues may be less daunting and more inviting than the demands on educators. In their article about using electronic mail to facilitate nursing scholarship, Ribbons and Vance (2001) wrote:

> The traditional attributes of nursing scholarship, such as critical thinking, reflection, creativity, critical analysis and an openness to new thinking may also be considered in the light of the linguistic concept of a *discourse community* (p. 105).

For busy professionals who are already active electronic mail users, using the Internet to share ideas with colleagues is an attractive option. Miller (1989) calls these networks *invisible colleges*. One disadvantage that the three of us have discovered when we communicated about this book is that our other lives seem disembodied from the reality of the person sending the message. The sender has no way of knowing what we are doing, what pressures we are experiencing and how we are feeling. For those of you contacting each other frequently, it is really necessary to make some ground rules about messages. Think of things like how often you will look at your e-mail, letting the other person know when you will be away for several days, being mindful of the other person's tasks and being reasonable in your requests.

There are other ways that you can help your career with electronic contact. DHNet is an example of using web-based Internet resources, in this case to encourage research collaboration and sharing of clinical observations among dental hygiene professionals and others interested in collaboration (Forrest and Koopman 1998). These ways of working over long distances eliminate personal supervisory visits to placements and are thus time- and cost-effective. They can take place over long distances, they can assist the clinical reasoning of the health workers and students by collaborating with the academe at the learning base and they can provide expert advice relatively easily.

Use of international faculty/student exchange programs is another way to enhance learning beyond a more traditional arena. Concern to increase opportunities for biomedical research for graduate and post-graduate students in a Mid-West USA college of health professions, led to a successful collaboration with a British university that resulted in several joint student publications (Gallicchio et al 1998). Many examples of Internet-based resources are listed at the end of this chapter, as well as others in this book. You can add them to your reservoir of information. But, how to manage all the ideas that these and other facts might generate is the focus of the next section. As the title of this chapter suggests this last part changes direction from looking at the public sphere to enhancing the private one. It adds extra dimensions to the inner circle of Figure 1.1, shown at the beginning of this chapter. It addresses aspects like shaping ideas, managing power issues and coping with stress. We believe that awareness of these factors will be advantageous for you in your journey towards becoming an advanced practitioner.

Shaping your ideas

We said in the earlier parts of this chapter that the ideas in this book can be used in several ways. We hope that as you read through various parts you will focus on a particular area that you want to develop. And, because of the plethora of ideas and the complexity of differing knowledge at this advanced level, we would like to share some investigative ways of sorting through and sorting out ideas into workable solutions. Table 1.2 on page 20, indicates some practical procedures that have worked for us.

Managing power issues

As an advanced practitioner you will have to implement change and influence others in various ways by being inclusive and collaborative. 'Power is the ability to take one's place in whatever discourse is essential to action and the right to have one's part matter' (Heilbrun 1988, p. 18). Reframing your perceptions about what another has to offer so that your interaction and relationship are seen as an opportunity and a challenge is a very effective way of taking control and using power. You will find that you cannot force change and that you have to help others grow to value and respect the ideas you have to offer. The following narrative talks about power from several perspectives.

When one of us was growing up her godmother used to say 'Don't forget that poise is power'. She had not forgotten her advice, even though it was not easy to follow it at all times. At the same time, her grandmother used to remind her of a Latin proverb, which, loosely translated, says that what Jupiter can do the ox can't. She came to realize that, between them, these two ladies summed up all the major issues that relate to personal power. We think that most of the important things we need to learn in life are flagged for us in

Table 1.2   *Practical procedures to investigate ideas*

Brainstorming with a partner(s)
- Be creative and think laterally to make a list that will cover most eventualities
- You could let the list be written in a free-form way, just jotting down all ideas randomly
- You could write the ideas into groups immediately—this works well for more limited ideas

Conceptualizing your ideas
- Create concept maps or decision trees (Gelb 1995) to group your ideas and to show the relationship between sections

Concentrate your data
- Develop your first lead tasks or particular questions
- Phrase them in such a way that it will be easy to look for answers

Talk to people
- Examine and use your own past experience
- Make sure your ideas are clear
- Ask for advice or supervision
- Revisit your question(s)

Search the professional literature
- Conduct a computer search using key words
- Hand-search relevant journals if you can be specific about years and dates
- Examine library text books

Search the internet
- Use a search engine like www.google.com or www.yahoo.com
- Key in target words to start the search
- Try list servers
- Discover e-mail groups of special interest

Contact people involved in this area—formally
- Organize a focus group
- Send out a questionnaire
- Interview people on a one-to-one basis
- Present your ideas to a formal meeting and ask for feedback
- Ask people on networks for their feedback

Appraise all your findings
- Are your findings relevant?
- Do they really apply to what you are looking for?
- Can you sort them into meaningful categories?

Apply your findings
- Try the findings out—play with them until you are satisfied they are what you want to do or ask and they are in the correct order
- Carry out the next move in your plan

childhood, but we rarely heed them enough, and need to keep learning them, sometimes for a very long time till they hit that 'aha' spot.

We can now expand on what the godmother said by saying that, in our opinion, the first rule to learn if you want to have any personal power is not to empower anyone else by complaining about them. Complaining about someone is an acknowledgment that they have influence over you. Mary MacKillop, the 19th-century Australian nun, had a terrible time with the local bishops who wanted to control all her activities; at one point she was even excommunicated. In all her extensive correspondence she never complained about the bishops. She always wrote about them with great respect, stressed how hard the poor bishops worked, and urged her sisters to pray for the bishops and do whatever they could to assist them. She did not own the problems the bishops created for her, and eventually, she got what she wanted. There is no guarantee that retaining your poise will get you what you want, but it does increase the probability. Try not to complain about people with whom you work, especially the people in charge. You have much to gain and nothing to lose by following this dictum.

The second rule relates more to what the grandmother said, in that it acknowledges the fact that some individuals in an organization have more power than other individuals, and this must be faced, not denied. Remember, never go to anyone in a position of power in an organization with just a complaint; always go with a plan. If things are not working well, you may have genuine reasons to complain. However, if you just complain, the situation may not change, because your problem may not be at the top of the supervisor's or manager's list of issues. Or, if changes are made they may not be the changes you want. Take time to work out a plan. Then you can make an appointment and outline how you believe things in your workplace could be improved. You may find it easier to do this with a small group of your colleagues. However, we would suggest that the group is made up of not more than two or three of you, unless you have a very well-worked-out, detailed plan and you are sure, because you have evidence, that what you are suggesting is a really 'good thing'. By having a big group, it becomes a big issue. Think about it carefully, collect all the information you may need and then act.

In a recent literature review Griffin (2001) described a range of viewpoints concerning power discussed in health literature, and reviewed research and discussions related to the concept of power. She found that this concept is most often discussed in health-related publications in terms of a trait approach to professionalization, in terms of medical dominance, and in terms of the organization of healthcare work-places. The bases of power may be viewed positively or negatively. Willey (1987) has described these bases of power in different configurations or terms that include the following:

- reward power through the ability to bestow gifts or create opportunities
- coercive power through the ability to punish or withhold
- power through legitimate authority
- referrent power from identification with sources of power
- expert power derived from knowledge
- informational power from having access to important sources of knowledge
- charismatic power derived through personal attractiveness.

We agree with Griffin's (2001) statements that it is important for healthcare professionals, and particularly those aspiring to become advanced practitioners, to be comfortable with the concept of power, and learn to develop strategies for exerting influence in their workplace. This involves understanding the political climate in which you work, knowing how to be assertive without being aggressive, having good negotiating and conflict resolution skills and having the capabilities and relevant knowledge to influence decision-making in the healthcare team. Money and knowledge are two major sources of power, as this example from medicine illustrates.

The medical dominance of the healthcare professions is to a large extent related to the fact that in many situations doctors perceive themselves, and are perceived, as having the largest knowledge base. This enables the medical profession to obtain favorable funding. Then, as more medical knowledge is generated through research, the positive cycle is repeated. But, don't forget that healthcare is delivered through multi- or inter-disciplinary teams, and the sources of funding are also administered by teams of people with diverse qualifications appropriate to current societal needs. The knowledge, funding potential and therefore, power base of the healthcare professions are not static. You can be part of the team that helps to build power bases to support your work.

If thinking about power issues is new for you, it would be a good idea to read more. A number of additional references are listed at the end of this chapter, including significant publications related to management and working in teams. Some people have said that individuals who have played contact sports have a better appreciation of the politics of power. They know that when someone knocks you over and thumps you in the back, it isn't because they dislike you, it's just that they want the ball. Power issues are rarely personal. As you read all the other chapters in this text, you will develop a better understanding of yourself, and have a clearer idea of what kind of advanced healthcare practitioner you want to become. This knowledge will help you to decide where and how you want to exert your power, and whether it is through having specialist knowledge and skills as a clinician, as a researcher, or as an administrator. You will need to decide how much power you want and why. Some people really want to change the world in which they live and are prepared for the work it takes. Others may just want to live in the world, doing their best within a more limited sphere. Only you can decide where you want to be on this continuum. Try to avoid getting stuck on the fence, being unhappy about things, but not prepared to develop the skills and spend the time it will take to make the changes. Try this exercise.

Activity box 1.4

Reflect on power in your workplace
1. Who convenes the meetings?
2. Who sets the agenda?
3. When you attend meetings, who talks and who listens?
4. Have you noticed whether there is anyone who has difficulty making a point, and even when he/she does, others don't listen?
5. Who are the seemingly more powerful people? Why do you think they are more powerful?
6. Do people listen to you and act on suggestions you make?
7. Is there anything you would wish to change?

Organizing time and coping with work-related stress

Finally, the last part of the private sphere relates to two inter-related factors: the way you organize your time, and how you look after yourself. Paying attention to these two facets, we believe, will help you as you try to institute change in your working environment. Creative processes have their price to pay and work-related stress and burnout are enemies in this constantly frantic and busy world.

Learning how to organize their time can help most people to cope better and reduce their level of stress. We have found that using Covey's work has been helpful (Covey 1990, Covey et al 1994). The concept of using his four quadrants is a powerful tool. These quadrants are:

- important non-urgent
- important urgent
- non-important urgent
- non-important non-urgent

Covey et al (1994) suggest that in order to be effective people need to spend 65–80% of their time doing the important non-urgent things that build the future; 20–25% doing the important urgent things that need attention immediately so that work gets done; about 15% of their time doing the non-important urgent things that crop up in every workplace; and only less than 1% of time doing non-important non-urgent things, or the trivia that can often swamp us. Learning how to prioritize your work into these categories may take time and practice. Covey (1990) describes using a compass, not a clock, to guide you when developing your personal mission and vision statements that you may or may not share with others. We would add that sometimes you have to use the concept of a concave and convex lens to focus on detail, or on the big picture. Again, this is an examination of both small and big issues. For example, if planning to submit an abstract for review at a professional conference that is due in 3 weeks, you have to plan in detail what has to be done by when, so you will need a concave lens to focus small. When you are planning your career development for the next 5 years, you will need the convex lens to see the big picture.

Organizing your time, and setting realistic priorities are important, but you will need to consider other factors as well in coping with work-related stress. As a healthcare professional you must provide quality care in a rapidly changing environment, often with resources that are being cut, rather than increased, so you need to be aware of the risks of burnout in certain situations (DiGiacomo and Adamson 2001). New professionals, making the adjustment from using text book knowledge and supervised practice, often find their more autonomous, fast-paced work situation very stressful. Staff development programs that include orientation, burnout appraisal, individual counseling and provisions for on-going staff support are recommended by experts (DiGiacomo and Adamson 2001). Learning relaxation techniques, having relaxation breaks and having a mentor to assist the transition to the demands and expectations of a job can help prevent and reduce work-stress. We all have different ways to re-balance our energies. Much depends also on what is happening in your life at the time. Make sure that you have considered some of these ways of organizing your work so that you do not become over-whelmed as you begin your journey towards advanced practice. Remember that life is not linear and that cycles of enthusiasm should be interspersed with times of fun, rest and leisure at work and outside. In fact, the more creative you become with yourself and your work, the more essential it is to have a different set of creative outlets (McMeekin 2000).

Summary

The major, overarching theme of this text is the discussion and explo-ration *of expert* and/or *advanced practice*, what this means in different contexts, and the steps involved in achieving these levels. This topic is investigated from different perspectives by us, and all the contributing authors. The theme is like a ribbon: it is continuous, with similar ideas, but the focus shifts as different aspects are highlighted. This ribbon of ideas and concepts is woven in, emerging and submerging throughout the text. In Chapter 1, we introduce you to, and place you within the *big picture* that embraces this topic. In subsequent chapters you are provided with a variety of information, guidelines, tools and activities that can assist your planning and learning related to a range of issues about this topic.

Increasing your self-knowledge and *knowledge about others*, are major sub-themes. Using a range of strategies to achieve these attributes is discussed in Chapters 1, 2, 3, 5 and 7–11. In Chapter 1, we have dis-cussed ways to shape your ideas, how to manage power and how to organize time in order to avoid stress. Chapter 2 includes specific information about using checklists and standardized tests to learn about your personality type, work values and preferences, as well as those of others. You are also given information about emotional intel-ligence, and locus of control, to assist you to plan and acquire skills for the career-path that best suits your needs and talents. Chapter 5 focuses on increasing self-knowledge through reflection, while Chapter 7 highlights ways to relate your scholarly development to your needs and preferences. Chapter 8 will increase your understand-ing of occupations and the meaning assigned to them by different peo-ple in different contexts. In Chapter 9, you are given the opportunity to increase your self-knowledge through understanding and applying theories and principles of adult learning. You should make informed decisions about the mentors you need to advance your personal and professional development. How to work effectively within the men-tor–protégé framework is described in Chapter 10. Planning, organiz-ing, and recording your Continuing Professional Development and Higher Education relate to the application of your self-knowledge, so that others, especially your employers or supervisors, can know and appreciate your skills. This is discussed in Chapter 11.

The sub-theme of *planning your career* is explored in different ways throughout the text. In Chapter 1, we have written about this in terms of the opportunities and constraints offered within the socioeconomic and political context of your situation, and how you may work effec-tively to manage change and demands on your time and personal resources. In Chapter 2, you are provided with examples of career tra-jectories and information you can use to decide on the pros and cons of further education and specialization relevant to your preferences and needs. Chapter 7 outlines the importance of incorporating schol-arship at all levels of your practice, and describes the process of including these elements in your career plans. Understanding and using theories to advantage, to inform and enhance your practice, is described and demystified in Chapter 3. An understanding of adult learning theories, and related reflections, described in Chapter 9, will assist you in the process of implementing your formal and informal learning, understanding your preferences, documenting your reflec-tions, and acknowledging and valuing your insights. You can also use Chapter 5 to learn more about reflection as a valuable part of career-planning. Chapter 11 provides more detailed information about continuing professional development; in particular, how to ensure that you plan for this activity and develop the skills and process for meeting your profession's continuing professional development requirements.

The provision of healthcare is evolving, and increasing in complex-ity. Chapter 4 explores the strategies available for the evidence-based practitioner. Chapter 6 discusses the dimensions of professional rea-soning. In delivering healthcare services we all need to consider the fact that humans are occupational beings, and attach different mean-ing and value to their occupations. This is discussed in Chapter 8. More is demanded from healthcare professionals working at all levels and within different structures. An outcome is a greater demand for more expert consultants within the healthcare field. This topic, and what you need to do to become a successful advanced practitioner, then a consultant, is discussed in Chapter 12.

Throughout the text we have used cues, like flags that you can fol-low, as concepts are woven in and out to explicate a topic. Examples include the six characters, in search of advanced practitioners, whose careers are described in Chapter 2. The shopping flag in Chapter 3 guides you through the selection of theories for your advanced prac-tice wardrobe. The story of Daniel is used to explain the process, the-oretical rationale and application of reflection in Chapter 5. In Chapters 7 and 10, the scholarship of practice, and finding the right mentor, then working in the mentor–protégé relationship, are dis-cussed with four early-career health practitioners: a medical technolo-gist, an occupational therapist, a physical therapist and a radiation therapist; their perspectives and experience guide you through these topics.

We are giving you a map: it is your journey! We hope that you will enjoy it and find that being a life-long learner is a meaningful occupa-tion, and that reading this text will make it easier for you to set goals and achieve them.

References

Adamson B, Lincoln M, Cant R 2000 An analysis of managerial skills for the current and future healthcare environment. Journal of Allied Health 29:203–213

Allen S, Strong J, Polatajko H 2001 Graduate-entry master's degrees: launch-pad for occupational therapy in this millennium. British Journal of Occupational Therapy 64:572–576

Alsop A, Ryan S 1996 Making the most of fieldwork education: a practical approach. Stanley Thornes, Cheltenham

Baty P 2001 No A levels? No problem . . . . The Times Higher Educational Supplement 7 September: 1

Brislin R, Yoshida T (eds) 1994 Improving intercultural interactions. Modules for cross-cultural training programs. SAGE Publications, Thousand Oaks, CA

Bryson C, New B 2000 Health care rationing: a cut too far? In: Jowell R, Curtice J, Park A, Thomson K, Jarvis L, Bronley C, Stratford N (eds) British social attitudes: focusing on diversity. The 17th report: 2000–2001 edn. National Centre for Social Research, Sage Publications, London

Covey S R 1990 The seven habits of highly effective people. Powerful lessons in personal change. Simon & Schuster, New York

Covey S R, Merrill A R, Merrill R R 1994 First things first. Simon and Schuster, New York

Department of Health 2000 A health service of all the talents: developing the NHS workforce. Consultation document on the review of workforce planning. Department of Health, London

DiGiacomo M, Adamson B 2001 Coping with stress in the workplace: implications for health professionals. Journal of Allied Health 30:106–111

Edmonds M 1998 The call for nurturing leaders for the rapidly changing diverse, global society of the 21st century. Journal of Physical Therapy 12:39–43

Esdaile S, Roth L 2000 Viewpoint. Education not training: the challenge of developing professional autonomy. Occupational Therapy International 7:147–152

Fish D, Coles C 1998 Developing professional judgement in health care. Butterworth-Heinemann, Oxford

Fitzgerald M H, Beltran R, Pennock J, Williamson P and Mullavey-O'Byrne C 1997 Occupational therapy, culture and mental health. Transcultural Mental Health Centre, Parramatta, NSW, Australia

Forrest J L, Koopman A 1998 DHNet: a model of international collaboration. Journal of Allied Health 27:39–44

Gallicchio V S, Kirk P, Birch N J 1998 Use of an international faculty/student exchange program as a process to establish and improve graduate education and research within an allied health discipline. Journal of Allied Health 27:31–34

Gelb M 1995 Thinking for a change: discovering the power to create, communicate, and lead. Aurum Press, London

Gergen K J 1991 The saturated self. Dilemmas of identity in contemporary life. Basic Books, New York

Gourley M 2001 Maintaining career competence. OT Practice 6:14–16

Greatbach D, Morris S 2001 Simple yet complex: a different approach to competence. Occupational Therapy News 6:15

Griffin S 2001 Occupational therapists and the concept of power: a review of the literature. Australian Journal of Occupational Therapy 48:24–34

Grossman J 1998 Continuing competence in the health professions. American Journal of Occupational Therapy 52:709–715

Heilbrun C G 1988 Writing a woman's life. Ballentine Books, New York

Henriksson C 1994 The development and future of occupational therapy in Sweden. British Journal of Occupational Therapy 57:165–169

Higgs J, Edwards H (eds) 1999 Educating beginning practitioners: challenges for health professional education. Butterworth-Heinemann, Oxford

Higgs J, Titchen A (eds) 2001 Practice knowledge and expertise. Butterworth-Heinemann, Oxford

H M Treasury 2001 Pre-budget report, a summary leaflet—building a stronger, fairer Britain in an uncertain world. H M Treasury, 2001–2002 figures, November. H M Treasury, London

Jowell R, Curtice J, Park A, Thomson K, Jarvis L, Bronley C, Stratford N 2000 British social attitudes: focusing on diversity. The 17th report: 2000–2001 edn. National Centre for Social Research, Sage Publications, London

McLuhan M 1967 The medium is the message. Routledge and Kegan Paul, London

McMeekin G 2000 The 12 secrets of highly creative women. Conari Press, Berkeley

Martin A C, Thornberg K, Shepard K F 1992 The professional development of expert clinicians in orthopedic and neurological practice. Physical Therapy 72:12–21

Miller N 1989 Personal experience, adult learning and social research: developing a sociological imagination in and beyond the T-group. Unpublished doctoral thesis, School of Education, University of Manchester

Mullavey-O'Byrne C 1994a Intercultural communication for health care professionals. In: Brislin R, Yoshida T (eds) Improving intercultural interactions. Modules for cross-cultural training programs. Sage Publications, Thousand Oaks, CA, p 171–220

Mullavey-O'Byrne C 1994b Intercultural interactions in welfare work. In: Brislin R, Yoshida T (eds) Improving intercultural interactions. Modules for cross-cultural training programs. Sage Publications, Thousand Oaks, CA, p 197–220

National Forum on Health 1995 The public and private financing of Canada's health system. National Forum on Health. Available: http://www.nfh.hc-sc.gc.ca/publicat/canada.htm 30 Dec 2001

National Health Service 2000 Meeting the challenge: a strategy for the allied health professions. NHS. Available: www.doh.gov.uk/meetingthechallenge 15 Nov 2001

Pearsall J (ed) 1998 New Oxford dictionary of English. Clarendon Press, Oxford

Pew Health Professions Commission 1995 Critical challenges: revitalizing the health professions for the twenty-first century. The third report. UCSF Center for the Health Professions, California

Reid M 2001 Noticeboard: from the director general—improvements in the NSW health system. Occupational Therapist 407:19–20

Ribbons R, Vance S 2001 Using e-mail to facilitate nursing scholarship. Computers in Nursing 19:105–110

Roberts G, Machon A 2000 Occupational therapy higher level practice and personal mastery. National Occupational Therapy Conference, Keele University, 2000

Ryan S 2001 Perspectives on widening university access: critical voices of newly qualified therapists. British Journal of Occupational Therapy 64:534–540

Salminen A-L 2000 Computer augmented communication in the daily life of severely disabled speech impaired children. Unpublished doctoral thesis. School of Health Sciences, University of East London, London

Schmoll B J 2000 Beyond parochialism and rhetoric: third annual Pauline Cersoli lecture. Journal of Physical Therapy Education 14:3–8

Smith K 2001 States' continuing competence. OT Practice 6:6

The Quality Assurance Agency for Higher Education 2001 Benchmark statement: health care programmes phase 1, occupational therapy subject bench marking group. QAA for Higher Education, Gloucester, UK

US Department of Health and Human Services 1999 Building the future of allied health: report of the implementation task force of the National Commission on Allied Health. US Department of Health and Human Services, Public Health Services and Administration, Bureau of Health Professions, Division of Associated, Dental, and Public Health Professions, Rockville, MD

von Zweck C 1999 The 1999 federal budget—time for a reinvestment in health. Occupational Therapy Now 1:5–6

Waters B 2001 Radical action for radical plans. British Journal of Occupational Therapy 64:577–578

Willey E L 1987 Acquiring and using power effectively. Journal of Continuing Education in Nursing 18:25–28

Other references and resources

Belanger A 1997 Can we aspire to power in physiotherapy? Physiotherapy Canada summer:164–166

Bennis W 1999 Managing people is like herding cats. Executive Excellence, Provo, UT

Bennis W 2000 Managing the dream. Reflections on leadership and change. Perseus, Cambridge, MA

Gilkeson G E 1997 Occupational therapy leadership. Marketing yourself, your profession and your organization. F A Davis, Philadelphia

Harvey D 1995 The condition of postmodernity. Blackwell, Oxford, UK

Katzenbach J R (ed) 1987 The work of teams. Harvard Business School Press, Cambridge, MA

Katzenbach J R 1998 Teams at the top. Unleashing the potential of both teams and individual leaders. Harvard Business School Press, Cambridge, MA

Martin A 1992 The professional development of expert clinicians in orthopedic and neurological practice. Physical Therapy 72:107–116

O'Malley J, Cummings S, King C S 1996 The politics of advanced practice. Nursing Administration Quarterly 41:78–81

Complementary healthcare

Publications from healthcare network at health canada website

Achiles R 2000 Defining complementary and alternative healthcare. Health Policy and Communications Branch of Health, Canada. Available: www.hc-sc.gc.ca/hppb/healthcare/cahc/index.html 27 May 2002

Advisory Group on Complementary and Alternative Health Care 2000 Towards an integrative health system. Available: www.hc-sc.gc.ca/http/healthcare/pdf/integrate.pdf 17 Oct 2002

Casey J, Picherack F 2000 The regulation of complementary and alternative healthcare practitioners. Health Policy and Communications Branch of Health, Canada. hc-sc.gc.ca/hppb/healthcare/pdf/regs.pdf 17 Oct 2002

Tartaryn D, Verhoef M 2001 Combining conventional, complementary and alternative healthcare: a vision of integration. Health Policy and Communications Branch of Health Canada. hc-sc.gc.ca/hppb/healthcare/pdf/combine.pdf 17 Oct 2002

Websites

American Occupational Therapy Association (AOTA)	www.aota.org
American Physical Therapy Association	www.apta.org
American Speech-Language-Hearing Association (ASHA)	www.asha.org
Australian Association of Occupational Therapists Inc.	www.ausot.com.au
Australian Physiotherapy Association	www.physiotherapy.asn.au
Canada's Health Care System	www.hc-sc.gc.ca/healthcare/cahc/index.html
Canadian Association of Occupational Therapists	www.caot.ca
Canadian Association of Speech-Language Pathologists and Audiologists	http://Speech-languagePathologist.org
Canadian Intergovernmental Conference Secretariat	www.scics.gc.ca/cinfo00/800038004_e.html
Canadian Physiotherapy Association	Physicaltherapist.com
Chartered Society of Physiotherapy	www.csp.org.uk
College of Occupational Therapy (UK)	www.cot.org.uk
Department of Health (UK)	www.doh.gov.uk
Evidence-based guidelines	http://www.sign.org.uk
National Committee of Inquiry into Higher Education: National Report	www.ncl.ac.uk/ncihe/nr_017.htm
National Health Service Plan	www.nhs.uk/nhsplan
Royal College of Speech Therapy	www.rcslt.org

Speech Pathology Australia	www.speechpathologyaustralia.org.au
The Times Higher Educational Supplement	www.thes.co.uk
World Health Organization	www.who.int
World Health Organization International Classification of Functioning, Disability and Health	www3.who.int/icf/icftemplate.cfm

2 Developing competencies for advanced practice: how do I get there from here?

Helen M. Madill and Vivien Hollis

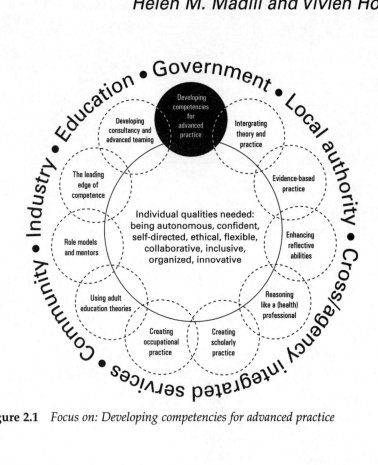

Figure 2.1 *Focus on: Developing competencies for advanced practice*

Chapter outline

In this chapter we explore the concepts and definitions of factors related to advanced practice in healthcare professions. We have focused on career-planning and decision-making in particular. In order to assist you to make informed decisions in the process of your career development, we have referred to different checklists and standardized assessments, which can be used to increase self-knowledge, and apply the insights to making decisions about further education and specialization. Different stages of career development are illustrated by examples from the career profiles of six fictitious health professionals: a dietician, an occupational therapist, a physical therapist, a pharmacist, a speech-language pathologist and a rehabilitation practitioner/manager/educator. These practitioners were created from interview data with health professionals from different fields of practice.

Key words: Career decision-making, self-knowledge, postgraduate education.

Anticipated   As a result of reading this chapter we anticipate that you will be able to:
outcomes
- define advanced practice
- apply knowledge of career-planning to your situation
- use knowledge of emotional intelligence, self-monitoring, learning styles, personality style and preferences, values, and locus of control in your career decision-making
- review graduate education opportunities in light of your self-knowledge and career planning.

Introduction   Whether you are starting your first job, changing your practice focus, or considering making a major career change, you will need to understand what constitutes advanced practice in your field. In this chapter we will explore several topics by providing some answers to the following questions:

- What constitutes advanced practice?
- What do I need to know about career-planning and decision-making to get there?
- What do I need to know about myself?
- How do I become an advanced practitioner?

To answer these questions we enlisted the help of several health practitioners from different countries and at various stages in their careers. Practitioners were asked what they understood was meant by the concept 'advanced practitioner'. They briefly described their careers and the decision-making points along the way. They commented on how they planned their careers and, if on looking back, they would have done anything differently. They reflected on changes they had made in their personal style to accomplish their career goals and what advice they would give recent graduates in their field. Through their experiences, and with their assistance, we have created six fictitious health practitioners whose situations may help you with your career decision-making.

- *Aden* is a rehabilitation practitioner with interests in management and education. He is finishing his doctorate and has recently been appointed as the curriculum director for a new educational program.
- *Robert* is an occupational therapist. He holds a graduate degree and owns a private practice where he employs a number of staff from a variety of healthcare fields.
- *Patricia* is a dietian. She has 15 years of practice experience and has recently taken time out to have children.
- *Diane* is a speech pathologist. After completing a graduate degree she moved from a focus on clinical service to corporate planning and quality assurance program development in the same health region.
- *Dorothy-Anne* is a physical therapist. After a short period as a clinician she completed her doctorate and embarked upon an academic career.

• *Erika* is a pharmacist. She has been working for a year. Already she can see that a graduate degree would be an asset, but she is unsure about which area to select.

You will find short career profiles for each of these fictitious practitioners at the end of this chapter. Summaries of reflections on their career development illustrate how they perceived their journey to this point. This resource material will be useful when you complete a series of exercises related to the concepts elaborated in this chapter.

What constitutes advanced practice?
Toward a definition

These practitioners defined the term 'advanced practitioner' in a variety of ways. They offered a number of alternatives. Here are several for you to consider before you write your version.

Aden described an advanced practitioner as 'a professional who has taken active steps to broaden and deepen knowledge of the practice arena in which he or she works. Also, someone who can demonstrate the ability to operate within the current political, economic, sociological and technological context at a high level of practice in one or more domains, such as education, management, research or clinical work'.

Robert saw an advanced practitioner as 'someone who knows what they are doing, is interested in understanding the reasons [behind] what they're doing. So they know one area or a couple of areas really well, but at the same time, someone who thinks critically and aims to continually develop their skills'.

Patricia stated: 'it would mean having several years of experience, and pretty intense experience dealing with patients . . . not just patients, but the whole healthcare team, being a vital member of that team and providing a vital service. It would be the quality of the time you've spent as well, and how much you've put into developing your career in terms of continuing education, those kinds of things. I do a lot of reading to keep up to date on the current developments in my field, attend conferences, teach . . . it's not just having 15 years of experience'.

Summary of points

Aden, *Robert*, and *Patricia* included a number of elements in their definitions. Some examples of the key elements they described include:

• breadth and depth of individual knowledge
• appreciation of the wider environmental context
• use of critical thinking and analysis
• extensive contribution to one or more areas of practice
• commitment to quality
• continually adding to personal knowledge
• continually striving to develop skills
• possessing advanced qualifications.

Activity box 2.1   Write a definition of advanced practice for your discipline. List the key skills that you need to develop together with an example of what constitutes evidence of your achievement of each skill.

What defines an 'expert' health practitioner?

Based on the perceptions of subjects in their study, Burke and DePoy (1991) described three outcomes of professional performance: mastery, excellence and leadership.

Mastery is a function of personal knowing characterized by experience, creative reasoning, commitment, knowledge, confidence and vision and is judged against an individual's internal standards, or personal knowing. *Robert* is an example of an advanced practitioner who has achieved mastery. He specializes in three areas of practice: rehabilitation technology, management of severe/multiple disabilities, and medical legal practice. He has creatively combined his knowledge and experience in a private practice venture that includes a staff of occupational and physical therapists, and speech-language pathologists. He established a private practice when his proposal for meeting clients' needs was not supported by middle management.

Excellence is a constant striving to become better than a previously established standard and is the recognition of ability by others when judged against external standards. These standards may be explicit or implicit. *Patricia* is an example of an advanced practitioner who has achieved excellence. She is one of only two dieticians in her state with specialized knowledge in her field of practice. She is recognized for her ability in providing an essential service and is a mentor to her colleagues.

Leadership is differentiated from excellence by having power and influence and is again recognized by others when judged against external standards. In essence, mastery and excellence are distinguished from leadership by the authority that is conferred by leadership. *Aden* is an example of an advanced practitioner who has demonstrated leadership. His peers quickly recognized his educational and managerial abilities. He has deliberately moved from one job opportunity to another to gain more responsibility. In each position he assumed more discretionary authority. *Aden* has received several professional awards.

Making the transition from 'novice' to 'expert'

Benner's (1984) major contribution to clinical practice and education in nursing is still referred to as a cardinal reference in the area of knowledge acquisition. Using Dreyfus and Dreyfus's (1986) original model of skill acquisition, she outlined five stages: novice, advanced beginner, competent, proficient, and expert.

Novice practitioners 'have had no experience of the situation in which they are expected to perform' (Benner 1984, p. 20). This level corresponds to students entering clinical practice or fieldwork situations that are part of their undergraduate programs.

Advanced beginners 'can demonstrate marginally acceptable performance, [they] have coped with enough real situations to identify the key elements in their current situation' (Benner 1984, p. 24). *Erika* is an example of an advanced beginner. As a recent graduate in pharmacy, her only practice experience has been through her residency and in her first position. Upon entering the field she was partnered with a peer and will require support from other practitioners who are functioning at the competent level or higher.

Competent practitioners 'have been on the job in the same or similar situations two or three years . . . [and have] a feeling of mastery and the ability to cope with and manage the many contingencies . . .' (Benner 1984, pp. 25, 27). They recognize salient elements, but lack complete comprehension of the whole picture.

Proficient practitioners have normally worked for 3–5 years and possess 'experience-based ability to recognize whole situations [they] can now recognize when the expected normal picture does not materialize' (Benner 1984, pp. 28, 29).

Expert performers combine extensive background and over 10 years' experience, with 'an intuitive grasp of each situation [that allows them to focus on the essential elements] of the problem without wasteful considerations of a large range of unfruitful alternative explanations' (Benner 1984, p. 32). Benner (1984) provided detailed descriptions of clinical nursing performance at each level, but it was not clear from her work how practitioners move from one level to the next. When we talked to *Patricia* she provided an example of moving from competency to proficiency to expert performance:

> When I first started, I was doing a combination of burns and neuro-surgery Intensive Care Unit and several other wards . . . about 3 years after that, I got an opportunity to take over from my colleague . . . I dropped all my other wards and I was just focusing on burns and the intensive care unit. That opened up a whole New World of learning potential and teaching potential. I slowly got the reputation of being a good educator for medical students, medical residents, nursing students [and others]. The metabolic work has been a real incentive [to do extensive reading and research] . . . I am the only clinician with this level of expertise in the city, there are only two of us in the province, it's a very good position that I have.

She has considerable experience in the direct patient service (helping role) and, she has extensive teaching experience, expertise in administering and monitoring functions and the lengthy organizational experience in the development of work-role competencies that denotes an expert. From these examples you can see that you have to be quite critical in your thinking about your work, and yourself, in order to move from one stage to the other. In the next section we discuss the role of critical thinking.

Role of critical thinking

There are as many definitions of critical thinking as there are academic papers on the subject and few of them are in agreement. A consensus study by the American Philosophical Association (1990, p. 3) provided a long list of desirable qualities:

> The ideal critical thinker is habitually inquisitive, well informed, trustful of reason, open-minded, flexible, fair minded in evaluation, honest in facing personal biases, prudent in making judgments, willing to reconsider, clear about issues, orderly in complex matters, diligent in seeking relevant information, reasonable in the selection of criteria, focused in inquiry, and persistent in seeing results which are as precise as the subject and the circumstances of enquiry permit.

Other authors relate critical thinking to reflective thinking and conclude that knowledge is the product of rational inquiry using evidence that is often uncertain, incomplete or inadequate (King & Kitchener 1994). What we do know is that critical thinking is a higher-order intellectual capability required of health and social care professionals who make judgments about client care.

So what is the difference between a thinker and a critical thinker? We believe thinkers know and understand the relevance of particular facts and can generalize those facts to other situations. But critical thinkers can take this to a higher level by recognizing connections between the components that make up the whole, bringing these together in different ways for the various circumstances they encounter and using the information gained through this process to make better judgments about practice (Bloom 1956). The difference between a thinker and a critical thinker has congruence with Benner's descriptions of the difference between the competent and the higher performance levels of proficient and expert.

Authors such as Browne and Keeley (1994) identified the importance of critical questions as a prerequisite to evaluating. One important factor for health and social care practitioners is the quality of the evidence. Thus, emphasis in undergraduate programs has focused on the critical analysis of research. However, critical thinking skills have wider application. For example, encouraging students to ask questions as a routine practice and regularly asking students to assess the implications of the answers that are provided helps foster this skill. Some practitioners have not learned such strategies during basic education, and they may now want to take responsibility for acquiring higher-order thinking skills. Mayer and Goodchild (1995) indicated that learning to become a critical thinker involves three levels of change: an affective change, a cognitive change and a behavioural change. So, those of you who aspire to advanced practitioner status should: learn to value critical thinking; learn strategies to master the process; and use critical thinking in the critical dimensions of your disciplines in order to facilitate your career-planning. See Chapters 5 and 6 for further discussion of thinking and reflection.

What do I need to know about career-planning and decision-making to get there?

There are many elements to consider as you plan your career. Here we describe several important ones:

- theoretical perspectives in career development
- career decision-making
- staying in place or moving on
- preparing to ladder up
- choosing to make a lateral shift
- health and social care trends.

Theoretical perspectives in career development

In his work as the international coordinator of the Work Importance Study, Super (1980, 1994, 1995a, b) introduced the concept of 'work salience' or the importance of work in relation to other roles. *Work* is one of our five major roles; the others are *studying*, *home/family*, *community service* and *leisure*. Super (1980) defined a career as 'the combination and sequence of roles played by a person during the course of a life-time' (p. 282). In keeping with Super's concept we view career development as a life-long process. It is a process in which you strive to implement your self-concept in roles that are consistent with your interests, values, personality, and opportunities (Herr 1996) and through the choices you make.

The process begins in childhood where you observe others, play, and explore roles. Through the process of growth and exploration you initially identify fields of interest, e.g. health sciences, business, or life sciences. Typically this takes place during your adolescence through young adulthood, a time when you are heavily involved in the student role, first through experiences in school and later through post-secondary education. Even after making a field choice and completing the necessary education to enter a particular career you are not completely committed to it; you are still checking the 'goodness of fit'.

For example, *Diane* questioned how well she was suited to her career choice of speech pathologist after she had only been working for 2 years. Her interests led her to work opportunities overseas where she found service-management provided the challenge she was looking for. Her experience is not unusual. New graduates often find they have to search for a 'good fit' between their skills and abilities and employment demands. As you gain experience you may select an area of specialization and undertake further education in that area. Your level of commitment to your chosen field has now moved to another level. You are establishing yourself in a career. You may also be entering a more stable period where you seek advancement or take on a leadership role and your level of responsibility may now go beyond direct service delivery. *Aden* and *Dorothy-Anne* both expanded their horizons, building on their undergraduate education. They made long-term professional commitments by establishing themselves in positions related to education and research and by completing graduate education. *Aden* deliberately sought advancement and is now in a leadership role.

Once established in your career you begin to pay attention to maintaining your position. During this period you will need to continue to develop, update your skills, and continue to learn, otherwise you will simply stagnate. You may also risk becoming unemployable. Some clinicians are very good at detecting when it is time to move on. Super's (1994) description of 'cycling and recycling of developmental tasks throughout the life span' (p. 70) can be applied to the health field and expanded to reflect a process of advanced practice.

Super (1994, p. 70) outlined his model of work-related and personal pursuits in terms of *declining*, *maintaining*, *establishing*, *exploring*, and *growing*, across four developmental levels of the life course: *adolescent* (14–25 years), *early adult* (25–45 years), *middle adult* (45–65 years) and *late adult* (65 years and over). Along the *declining* continuum, during adolescence there is less time for play (than during childhood), in early adulthood, there is less time for personal pursuits, during the middle adult years there is less time for non-essentials, and in later adulthood the working role is declining. The *maintaining* continuum proceeds along the four developmental stages from commitment to a career, securing a work role, acquiring recognized expertise, and in late adulthood remaining involved in areas of interest. The *establishment* continuum proceeds from getting started in a field of practice, developing areas of specialized knowledge, being involved in continuous learning within a field and, in later life, finding a balance between work and other roles. The *exploring* continuum starts with looking at alternatives, then proceeds to locating a position, next being involved in continuous learning related to the working role, and ends with finding a new balance between roles. Finally, the *growing* continuum includes the development of a realistic self-concept during adolescence, learning to relate to others in the work-place during early adulthood, accepting one's limitations during the middle adult years, and developing, as well as valuing, non-work-related roles during later adulthood.

This general overview of career development is simply a guide. The tasks listed within the various levels are examples and the age ranges should not be interpreted as deadlines by which certain career aspirations must be met. Opportunity, economic circumstances, and personal–social issues are three elements that will affect attainment of your career aspirations. For example, an individual who selects a health profession after several years of experience in another field will travel at a different pace, and need to acquire different practice experiences, than a younger individual who entered post-secondary education directly from high school and is about to undertake his or her first full time professional role. Individuals who complete their professional education and gain little practice experience before devoting several years to their home/family role can also expect to advance at a different pace.

Although their career experiences differ, it may still be realistic for the two people in the examples above to strive to become advanced practitioners. Giving priority to their working and studying roles, choosing to develop their skills, engaging in continuous learning, contributing to their profession, and acquiring higher qualifications were all ways in which the people we interviewed acquired that status. You may be viewed as an advanced practitioner because of your mastery, excellence, or leadership, but that status can be transitory if your skills are no longer needed or if you fail to update those skills. A practitioner may be growing in one aspect of his or her career, establishing in another and maintaining in another. How to maintain advanced practitioner status will become evident as you proceed through this chapter and other sections of this book.

Career decision-making   There have been many choices to make along the way and, no doubt, you have already made a number of important career-related decisions. Gouws (1995) described four levels of choice:

1. a choice in generic roles such as that of student or worker

2. evaluating the investment of time or the relative importance of a role that you currently occupy
3. adjusting one or more life roles to accommodate another that is of greater importance
4. making decisions about how to play a chosen role.

How might Gouws' concept of levels of choice be applied to your health-related practice situation? Before working in a professional capacity you had to choose whether to continue in your studying role by entering a health-related field of study or to begin working straight after high school. Once in your first professional position you had to consider the investment of time, or the relative importance of the role that you currently occupied. Next you had to adjust one or more life roles to accommodate another that is of greater importance. Many of you will have already had similar experiences, for example, if you held a part-time job while you were completing your professional qualification. You will find that as you gain professional experience you will be faced with decisions about how to play your chosen role. In another situation, remaining single may initially permit greater investment in tasks associated with your job responsibilities or permit greater participation in a leisure role. Involvement in leisure pursuits may also provide networking opportunities that facilitate your working role.

Everyone needs to strike a balance between roles. This means giving priority to one role over others as either a short-term or long-term arrangement. For example, if you have young children or ageing parents with health problems your home/family role may need to take priority over your working role. Your working role may have to be reduced to a part-time commitment, your studying role might have to be confined to reading professional literature, and more formal study may need to be put on hold for a period. Although it is a matter of personal choice, at times this may well be a forced choice. Embarking on an advanced degree will increase the time you spend in the studying role and likely limit extensive involvement in other roles over the short term.

Let us see how Gouws' levels of choice might be applied to *Aden's* career. *Aden* began working directly after he finished high school. He spent 12 years in law enforcement and during that time was able to evaluate the importance of his working role in relation to the investment of time and energy that it took and the manner in which it overlapped into his other roles. He wanted to be in education on a daily basis and in 1978 moved on to an adult education position. However, he was still looking for a career—one in which he could make a difference in people's lives, one that combined his interests in social service and education. Occupational therapy gave him that opportunity and 19 years later he is still in a related field. He made the choice to give both working and studying roles priority. His ultimate goal was to direct an educational program and he accepted an offer of such a position in 2001. As a new curriculum director he experienced a steep learning curve, but the principles he learned in his other positions were still applicable even though the culture in an educational institution was different. He needed to learn how to play his chosen role.

While salience, or the importance of a role, plays a part in your career development, so too do your values. Values 'are organized sets of general beliefs, opinions, and attitudes about what is preferable, right, or simply good in life . . . they form a certain organization of a person's needs, desires, and goals, hierarchically structured according to their relative importance and priorities' (Sverko and Vizek-Vidovic 1995, p. 5). We strive 'to attain a variety of goals or values' in our work, which may include 'economic security and material rewards, social interaction, social status, and self-fulfillment' (p. 5). These are examples of 'work values'.

Analyzing the level of importance you assign to various work-related values would enable you to seek out employment opportunities that permit you to implement those values. For example, Canadian students in occupational and physical therapy and speech-language pathology highly endorsed Personal Development and Ability Utilization, but student occupational therapists and speech-language pathologists placed greater importance on Social Relations and Social Interaction than student physical therapists. Both these work values are particularly important in the type of work that occupational therapists and speech-language pathologists perform and therefore are likely to play an important part in career choice (Madill et al 1989). Differences in the level of endorsement were also seen when Australian and Canadian student occupational therapists' values were compared with those that were characteristic of national value profiles.

Australian student occupational therapists endorsed Physical Activity and Lifestyle more highly than the Canadian participants in these studies (Casserly et al 1995, Esdaile et al 1997, Lokan and Shears 1995). Such differences are likely to have implications if you seek work in other countries. As discussed in Chapter 1, these differences will also influence the way in which you shape your own practice. Through the Work Importance Study, Super and colleagues (Sverko and Vizek-Vidovic 1995, p. 18) determined that: 'the importance or salience of work in individuals' lives depends mainly on their perception of the opportunities for realization of salient values within their work roles'. Our interviews with various health practitioners in several countries supported this perspective.

Staying in place or moving on

How do you determine whether to continue in your present position or move on? Many factors must be taken into consideration and, depending upon your personal–social situation, your choices may be constrained by the needs of others (e.g. home and family responsibilities, partner's employment situation, ageing and health concerns about parents and relatives). A partner's upcoming move, or a change in mandate, closures, or the sale of the agency may also force your choices where you are employed. If you are in the fortunate position of being able to make a move, or have received an offer, how do you determine what to do?

Activity box 2.2	You obviously have to assess the situation in terms of 'what's in it for me?' On one sheet of paper list the pluses and minuses that apply to your current position. Turn this page over. On a second piece do the same for the new position. Now turn over your first list and compare them. How many of the important elements you identified in your current position can you find in the new one? Are there important elements in the new job that are not mirrored in your current position? For example, would you have opportunities to learn more? Is financial support available for continuing education? Are there knowledgeable senior members of your new work team who would enhance your learning? Now look at the minus columns. Are there differences? For example, will you have longer to travel or will it be more expensive to get to the new position? Where would you be in 3–5 years in your current position as opposed to the new position?

If you are able to gain different experience by staying where you are and things are working well, it may be wise to stay. If it looks as though you will be marking time and it's going to be more of the same thing that is no longer challenging, it may be time to go. These are only a few of the questions that you need to ask yourself. The overall results of your personal investigation will give you a good idea of 'what's in it for you'.

Dorothy-Anne was very strategic in her career planning. She was ambitious and knew that she wanted to pursue an academic career. She had some teaching experience both before graduating and during her early work as a physical therapist, but she was anxious to develop her research skills and to make her mark as an expert in her field. She was careful to select the right doctoral thesis supervisor—someone who would support her area of interest and who had expertise to contribute from a related field. She requested a change of supervisor when she knew that the initial fit was not right. She took control of her educational program early and moved on when it was clear that she would not be able to reach her goal. (See Chapter 11, on individual tailoring of your continuing education.)

Robert held a series of related positions from 1986 to 1995. His interest was in rehabilitation technology and its application for individuals with severe disabilities and multiple handicaps. This interest continued when he moved to a management position in a community-based agency, but it was here that he saw many inequities in the social service programs available to his clients. He moved on when the bureaucracy no longer enabled him to develop the service as he saw fit. He took a risk and started a private practice. Moving into private practice and developing the medical legal aspect of the business proved to be the right choice for *Robert*.

Preparing to ladder up   When you are being interviewed for your chosen job, you also need to assess the agency in terms of its capacity to offer you an opportunity to continue to learn and develop as a professional. Having entered occupational therapy later than most of his colleagues, *Aden* set goals and took advantage of those opportunities that would further his aspirations. He said:

> I wanted to use the skills that I'd learned in different domains of practice. There's also the clinical education and management and research elements of my career that span different things, but there's a momentum to it where I haven't stayed very long in one particular post, setting my sights on the next one. The next position would be determined by my own confidence in progressing in a particular direction . . . sometimes that comes from my own realization and sometimes from others. For example, moving into the research post and the curriculum director post, I was actually headhunted for those. So someone somewhere had seen potential in me that I may or may not have seen in myself.

Choosing to make a lateral shift

When facing a forced career choice situation it may be preferable to make a lateral shift—a job change that does not take you to a more senior position, but one that allows you to continue to use your skills in a different context. This type of change can allow you to balance your roles more appropriately and thus afford you greater job satisfaction without further increasing your stress level. For example, *Diane* said:

> Security was a big factor in lots of career choices I've made. I've continually advanced. I was assistant director of rehabilitation services, and I really liked working in [this region], that's part of the reason that I moved here. But, when they did away with that position and opened one at the same level in corporate planning I knew I also had the skill set to do that job so I applied for it right away.

Health and social care trends

Funding levels for health and social services, coupled with new diagnostic procedures and treatment techniques, expensive new drugs, and a subsequent increase in client expectations all put pressure on healthcare systems worldwide. Health and social care organizations have been forced to review their efficiency and effectiveness in response to these economic pressures. You need to be aware of the socio-economic contexts of your practice that afford opportunities and also create constraints for practice and career development. These issues are discussed in detail in Chapter 1.

What do I need to know about myself?

Increasing our self-knowledge is an accepted aspect of personal and professional development in the 21st century. When we browse in any large bookstore, or visit websites, we are soon aware of the extensive and varied publications related to this field. These publications range from the scholarly to the populist. In this section we outline a number of ways you can learn more about yourself, using checklists and standardized tests, some of which are available electronically.

Emotional Intelligence

Emotional Intelligence (EI) is the social equivalent of IQ and is sometimes called maturity (Goleman 1999). EI refers to non-cognitive components of self-awareness, self-management, self-motivation, empathy and social skills that have a bearing on a person's ability to succeed in coping with environmental demands and pressures. Knowledge, technical skills and intelligence are the basics for jobs in health and social care. However EI has been shown to be positively related to all levels of job performance and is especially relevant in jobs that require a high degree of social interaction. As the construct of EI has become a popular topic in the general press and media, you may find over-simplified versions of Goleman's original ideas (1995, 1999). As understanding EI is useful in terms of working with others, as well as understanding ourselves, we suggest using the original texts. Goleman provides a clear explanation of the neurophysiological factors that may predispose some individuals to have less control of their emotions.

Self-monitoring skills

Self-monitoring is the ability to adjust your behaviour to specific external situational factors. It is an important part of being self-directed. People with high self-monitoring ability are more sensitive to social cues and can adjust their behaviour more quickly to suit different circumstances. People with low self-monitoring tend to be more consistent in their behavior (Lennox and Wolfe, 1984). Preliminary management and business research indicates that high self-monitors are better able to conform and those in management positions receive more promotion both within the organizations and from one organization to another. It may be surmised, therefore, that healthcare professionals who are adaptable may be more successful as organizations require them to participate in multiple roles.

Robert's career is an example of an individual with good self-monitoring skills, who responded to the social political trends that were internal and external to the organization he worked for. After working with the same organization for 5 years, one of his major projects was turned down at the middle management level. His understanding of the organization's vision and mission and the board's strategic plan reinforced his perspective, but he realized that he would not be able to carry out the project under the current management. He took his idea into private practice and his career has flourished.

Learning styles

Honey and Mumford (1995) developed a workbook titled *Capitalizing on Your Learning Style*. This provides a straightforward way of determining your learning style preferences. They described four general learning styles: *activists*, who enjoy new experiences, are open-minded and willing to try anything once; *reflectors*, who prefer to stand back and watch others first; *theorists*, who like to think things through using a step-by-step approach to problem-solving; and *pragmatists*, who enjoy experimenting with new ideas and testing them out in practice. Each of us prefers to use a combination of two, perhaps three styles, but we are likely to have strong preferences for some over others. Your preferred style can also change over time as you develop other abilities.

How might this information be useful to you as a health practitioner? In the practice setting, where you are likely to be working in a multidisciplinary team, knowledge of your learning style preferences may help you decide what type of role is best suited to you. In the search for the 'right' graduate program you may find that a Master's degree by course-work is the best complement if you have strong preferences for the activist and pragmatist learning styles. Similarly, those who wish to concentrate on clinical service rather than being groomed as independent researchers may find a professional/clinical doctorate a better fit than a Doctor or Master of Philosophy program. If you have strong preferences for the other end of these continua, the reflector and theorist learning styles, you may find that a Master's degree by research or a Doctoral program is more likely to put you in contact with others who share similar learning preferences. The wise person would not close any doors. Learning styles are preferences that can be altered when people are exposed to new and challenging learning opportunities and offer different perspectives on familiar problems or issues. While you might prefer to learn in a particular way, you can develop the capacity to adapt to the needs of your work environment. See Chapter 9 for more discussion of adult learning. You may wish to see the list of websites at the end of this chapter for the location of the on-line version of Honey and Mumford's Learning Styles Questionnaire (LSQ). In the following sections we describe two standardized assessment tools: one that can be used to examine personality style, and another to assess work values and salience (importance).

Personality style and preferences

Please note that, as with all personality assessments, a better way to look at the results would be to consult a vocational psychologist or a career guidance specialist who can administer, interpret, and discuss the results for you. Knowing more about your own personality style and that of others not only helps you to understand more about your own preferences, but also enables you to have better insights about other people's way of working.

Personality style and preferences play a part in the types of roles you may seek and your career preferences. The Myers-Briggs Type Indicator[R] (MBTI) was developed to test Jung's ideas (Myers and McCaulley 1985). Jung described four basic mental functions or processes used by all individuals. These comprised two types of perception: sensing (S) and intuition (N), and two types of judgment: thinking (T), and feeling (F). He identified two attitudes: extraversion (E) and introversion (I). Myers' and Briggs' contribution was in the development of facts about the judging and perceiving (JP) function and subsequently a JP scale (Myers and McCaulley 1985). Jung believed that we are born with distinct preferences that are shaped through our learning experiences and influenced by our environment. This implies that both functions and attitudes are developing throughout our lifetime and also suggests we may be able to modify the way we employ a preferred function or develop an attitude. We each have a preferred function, which we learn to rely upon, and the function at the other end of the same continuum does not develop to the same extent. For example, if you rely upon thinking (T), which is a preference for an objective, analytical approach, the other end of that continuum, feeling (F), will not be developed to the same degree and you will rely less on feeling and more on thinking. Katharine Briggs and her daughter Isabel Briggs Myers, observed that individuals differed in their perceptions (their awareness of things, people, ideas and events) and how they exercised judgment (the way they drew conclusions from their perceptions, made choices and arrived at decisions). The MBTI is the most widely used measure of 'normal personality differences' (Consulting Psychologists Press 2000).

Our personality style and preferences are important in relation to work expectations and choices. People's preferences are such that they 'are more likely to change their work environment to match their type than to change their type to match their work environment' (Myers and McCaulley 1985, p. 89). A summary of Myers' Type[R] descriptions (pp. 78–82) is provided below and applied to examples from healthcare practice. You can see that health practitioners are spread across the continua. There is no single Type[R] that is better than another. Myers and McCaulley (1985, p. 1) noted:

> The aim of the MBTI is to identify, from self-report of easily recognized reactions, the basic preferences of people in regard to perception and judgment, so that the effects of each preference, singly and in combination, can be established by research and put to practical use.

Extraversion and Introversion (E–I)

Extraverted Types[R] like variety and action. Their working with people (clients or team members) is important; short-term projects appeal to them, e.g. front-line service positions, home care, or sports medicine. Introverted Types[R] like to think and plan long-term projects. They work well alone, e.g. in curriculum development, service accreditation reviews, clinical research.

Sensing and Intuition (S–N)

Sensing Types[R] prefer using their established skills rather than acquiring new ones. They handle routine details efficiently and prefer an established, orderly approach, e.g. programs administration, wheelchair prescription, ordering equipment. Intuitive Types[R] like the variety of solving new problems, working enthusiastically in bursts of energy, and can be impatient with routine details, e.g. program development in community mental health, children with disabilities.

Thinking and Feeling (T–F)

Thinking Types[R] like to analyze and organize. Technical and scientific elements are important, e.g. program director, site coordinator, and researcher. Feeling Types[R] enjoy pleasing people. They seek harmony in their work settings; communication and interpersonal elements are important, e.g. front-line service in centers for children with disabilities, seniors' homes, and recreation for special populations.

Judging and Perception (J–P)

Judging Types[R] like environments that allow them to develop plans and carry them out. They like to use their abilities and once en route to a goal they like reach it, e.g. management, program evaluation, clinical research. Perceptive Types[R] like changing, evolving work environments where they can use their creativity and work with others, e.g. mental health services, counseling, adolescent programming. They are likely to have several projects on the go at once and may not finish all of them.

From the normative data presented by Myers and McCaulley (1985) of their sample of 765 'healthcare therapists', a little more than half were on the E side of the continuum and a little less than half were on the I side of the continuum. The distribution for S and N sides of the continuum was similar. For the T–F continuum, the balance was still relatively equal, but with an increase in favor of the F continuum. A similar pattern was seen for 'health technologists and technicians'. However, in terms of the J–P continuum, in a larger sample ($n = 1291$) of 'health technologists and technicians', the J function increased to 63.59% of the sample at the J end of this continuum.

Based on Myers and McCaulley's work, 16 types have been identified. For example, if your profile was INTJ, introversion, intuition, thinking, and judging would characterize your personality style. At the opposite end of those continua, extraversion, sensing, feeling and perceiving would characterize a person with an ESFP profile.

How might department heads with these profiles differ in their approach to personnel management? How might that affect your performance as a staff member? A department head with an INTJ profile will enjoy dealing with ideas; he or she will think systematically and need to understand why you wish to undertake a particular initiative and how you arrived at your decision. Your approach needs to be logical and well researched: outcome measures, cost–benefit ratios, and cost-effectiveness are likely to be important issues. The department head with an ESFP profile will enjoy the experience of implementing new initiatives: he or she will be more likely to try new programs, see how things unfold and problem-solve if and when necessary. Your approach needs to emphasize how the initiative will affect people's lives, the impact it will have upon individuals, and the hands-on role your head of department could play in making the initiative a success. Recognizing the personality-style preferences of members of your rehabilitation team will make it easier for you to work effectively together. If you would like to learn more about your personality style, you may wish to visit the websites listed at the end of this chapter.

The Values Scale and the Salience Inventory

Super and his colleagues (Super 1995a, b, Sverko and Super 1995) have conducted extensive studies internationally on work values and salience (importance). They developed the Work Importance instruments that can provide a useful basis for the study of career development and decision-making, and help you determine your career goals and make your career plans.

Values Scale

The Values Scale consists of 20 values. Each Value has five items. For each of these you indicate the degree of importance these have for you on a four-point Likert-type scale. For example, 'For each of the following statements, indicate how important it is for you: 1 = *little or no importance*; 2 = *some importance*; 3 = *important*; and 4 = *very important*, (Fitzsimmons et al 1985). The results of the Values Scale provide a measure of the priorities you place on each of the 20 values. These values are described in Table 2.1.

Table 2.1   *Content of the Work Importance Study cross-national Values Scale*

Value name	Definition
Ability use	Freedom to use and develop one's talents and skills and to find outlets for one's interests in the things one does
Achievement	Doing something well; the feeling one gets from doing or from having done something well
Advancement	Promotion, upward mobility in terms of progressing in one's career, to have a better standard of living, to live in a better environment, to have a better income
Aesthetics	Adding to and enjoying the beauty of processes, products or surroundings, both natural and artificial
Altruism	Helping others and being concerned for their welfare
Authority	Influence over others which requires others to follow a point of view or a policy, or which leads others to believe that they should accept these; the authority can be wielded through position, power, expertise, charisma or seniority
Autonomy	Making one's own decisions and carrying out one's own plans; independence of action within one's sphere
Creativity	Developing or making something original for the person concerned; the product may be an object, writing, painting or other artwork, an idea, a new method or an organizational procedure
Economic factors	Economic rewards such as salary, bonuses, possessions made possible by income; stability of income, assurance of being able to live in the desired way without threat to one's economic or social well-being
Lifestyle	Freedom to live as one wishes, according to one's own standards and values
Personal development	Opportunity to grow as a person, to develop one's senses of self-hood and personal integrity
Physical activity	Opportunity to obtain physical rather than mental exercise in one's work or leisure pursuits (the emphasis is on activity rather than on use of strength–see physical work, below)
Prestige	Social, economic or occupational status which arouses respect, esteem and admiration; the recognition of achievements or of personal qualities
Risk	The excitement of physical danger, financial gain or loss, and other risks incurred in projects either undertaken or proposed
Social interaction	The opportunity to be with others in a work, home or leisure setting; being part of a social organization; the social contact arising from group activities
Social relations	The opportunity for warmth, friendship, acceptance and understanding in one's relationships with people at work, in the home or in leisure and other pursuits
Variety	Change and diversity in what one does, whether of tasks, processes and methods, activity pattern, location or people with whom one associates
Work conditions	Physical aspects of the surroundings in which one works
Optional values	
Cultural identity	Freedom to conduct oneself, in public and private life, according to the mores of one's primary group or groups (e.g. the family, ethnic origin, religious membership); opportunity to identify with such personally important groups and to behave as they do
Physical work	Opportunity to use physical strength in one's work or leisure activities

Reproduced with permission from Esdaile SA, Lokan JJ and Madill HM 1997. A comparison of Australian and Canadian occupational therapy students' career choices. Occupational Therapy International 4:249–270.

Using this instrument, it is possible to determine the impact your values may have on your career decision-making. For example, Erika entered pharmacy after obtaining a general science degree, and with 2 years of volunteer experience that entailed setting up a women's cooperative organization. Her top seven values were *Ability Utilization, Altruism, Autonomy, Creativity, Personal Development, Prestige* and *Social Interaction*. Although *Economics, Working Conditions* and *Risk* were ranked much lower, her level of endorsement of *Risk* placed her in the 76th percentile when compared to other Canadians. Her values were consistent with her previous experience and entering a health-related profession. Knowing about your work-related values helps you to choose a compatible work environment, one that enables you to implement the values that you strongly endorse. For example, occupational therapists highly endorse *Ability Utilization, Social Relations* and *Social Interaction*. If your value endorsement pattern resembles that of people in business you might be better suited to clinic administration or private practice where your entrepreneurial work-related values could be implemented. Or you might be able to channel your business-related values into program evaluation and strategic planning in healthcare. Possessing a different set of work-related values from your peer group does not mean that you have to abandon your chosen health profession. But it does mean that you will have to seek opportunities to implement those values in a manner that differs from colleagues who fit the professional value pattern more closely than you do.

Salience Inventory

The Salience Inventory measures behavioural and affective components of five major life roles: *Studying, Working, Community Service, Home/Family* and *Leisure* on three dimensions: *Participation, Commitment,* and *Role Value Implementation*. Sample items for *Participation* begin with, 'I have spent time in or do spend time in . . .' or 'I have taken or do take advantage of opportunities in . . .'. Those for *Commitment* begin with: 'It is or will be important to me to be good in . . .' or 'I feel personally involved in . . .'. *Role Value* items begin with 'What opportunity do you see now or in the future to . . . use all my skills and knowledge in . . .' or 'be physically active as part of . . .' (Fitzsimmons et al 1985). These roles are described in Table 2.2.

It is possible to determine the impact that your *Participation, Commitment* and *Role Values* may have on your career decision-making. For example, *Erika* currently has high levels of *Role Value Implementations* in her working role. She is committed to *Home/Family* and *Studying* roles and sees implementing her values in these roles in the future. This picture is consistent with the demands upon her at this stage in her pharmacy career. She works long hours in a hospital pharmacy setting and enjoys a number of leisure pursuits. She has little time for *Community Service*, but given her international experience this role is of some importance in the future. By understanding that these roles continue to be of some importance to her, the desire to use her abilities in a creative and altruistic manner, the high value that she

Table 2.2   *Role descriptions for Work Importance Study Salience Inventory*

Role name	Definition
Studying	Taking courses, going to school, college or university (day or night classes, lectures or laboratory work); doing assignments or homework exercises, studying in a library or at home; also independent studying, formally or informally
Working	Working for pay or for profit, on a job or for yourself
Community service	Undertaking activities with community organizations such as recreational groups, Scouts, Red Cross, social service agencies, community associations, political parties
Home and family	Taking care of your room, flat or house; preparing or cleaning up after meals; shopping; caring for dependants such as children or elderly relatives
Leisure activities	Playing sports; watching television; pursuing hobbies; going to films, plays or concerts; reading; relaxing or loafing; being with your family or friends, doing nothing in particular

Reproduced with permission from Esdaile SA, Lokan JJ and Madill HM 1997. A comparison of Australian and Canadian occupational therapy students' career choices. Occupational Therapy International 4:249–270.

placed on *Social Interaction* in the Values Scale might be put aside until after her educational goal has been achieved. *Erika* understands her values profile and is trying to make decisions about her *Studying* and *Home/Family* priorities. If you are interested in learning more about your work values and career competencies, you may wish to visit the Psychometrics Canada website that is listed at the end of this chapter.

Locus of control

The Greek Stoic philosopher Epictetus said that people are not so much affected by events, as by the perceptions they bring to them. Our perceived locus of control is one of the factors that affect our ability to manage change. This is one of the crucial attributes of an advanced practitioner and was highlighted in Chapter 1. So, it is helpful to take this into consideration in relation to yourself. Locus of control refers to the perception that people have regarding control of their own fate. Some people see themselves as being governed by external influences, luck or chance, while others believe they are directly responsible for what happens to them. The research literature related to locus of control is extensive and takes into consideration that perceived locus of control is mediated by other perceived factors such as ability, task difficulty, effort and luck, and is also affected by health (Rotter 1990, Wallston 1992). Numerous studies have confirmed that individuals with an internal locus of control actively seek information before making a decision, are motivated to achieve and make a greater attempt to control their environment. Those with an internal locus of control may thus be more suited to jobs that require initiative and autonomy. Those with an external locus of control are more compliant and willing to follow directions, indicating that well-structured jobs requiring routine would help them to succeed. The wide spectrum of available job opportunities allows health and social care practitioners to choose one that is likely to help them succeed.

For example, *Patricia*, and *Robert* both referred to *luck* and being *in the right place at the right time*. However, what appeared to separate them from individuals with high external locus of control scores would be their ability to recognize an opportunity, analyze the advantages and disadvantages, and take action. For example, *Robert* stated 'when I left, I worked part-time at first and started doing a little bit of medical legal work in the area of specialized technology. That was another whole ballgame. I just fell into that'. *Robert* then pursued further study in medical legal work and is also a member of a special interest group in that area.

Your locus of control and your tolerance for ambiguity (the way you react to ambiguous, uncertain, dynamic situations) are important factors in coping successfully with change. To increase these factors, Whetton and Cameron (1998) suggested that you actively seek ways to broaden your perspective, including increasing your exposure to new information and engaging in different types of activities than you currently do. You should be aware that there is some debate about the concept of locus of control in relation to occupational therapy practice and education that also relates to other health professions. Similar arguments could be applied to career decision-making (Esdaile and Madill 1993).

Exercising internal locus of control is possible when choices can be made. However, there are times when there are only forced choices. While sometimes you have little choice, other times you can plan deliberately. *Aden*, who has a high internal locus of control score, was able to do this and his career appears to have been deliberately planned and self-driven. *Patricia* had worked for over 10 years and developed a reputation as an expert in her field before she negotiated a move to a part-time position to accommodate her home and family responsibilities. Through her initiative she demonstrated internal locus of control by using her level of expertise, investment and interest in such a way that her employer wanted to maintain the advanced practitioner in whom they had invested and have her continue to share her expertise within the health region.

How do I become an advanced practitioner?

In achieving advanced practitioner status you will need to consider whether it is mastery, excellence or leadership, or indeed some combination of these attributes for which you strive. Consider this in conjunction with what you know about yourself and your learning style. Then you can see what career-path best suits you at this time. Only then will you be able to decide how you might best utilize the resources available to you on your career-path, as you can see in the next section.

Career paths

Fisher et al (1999) identified four career patterns: *linear, expert, spiral* and *transitory*. These have particular relevance to the changing nature of employment within health and social care organizations. At one time most health and social care professionals worked in organizations offering the traditional *linear model*. Here people entered the organization and with advanced status slowly moved through a hierarchy of positions. While some professionals gained additional academic credentials, many used role models, mentors and on-the-job training to gain expertise. This model is still valued, although less so, as flatter organizational structures become more typical. This model was, and is, less acceptable to professionals who do not necessarily want to move into management positions for promotion. *Patricia's* career profile is an examples of a *linear* career-path.

The term 'advanced practitioner' has meant, for many, becoming a clinical expert in a particular specialty. Within universities or colleges becoming an *expert* means progressing from assistant professor/lecturer to associate professor/senior lecturer, associate professor/reader to professor, based on certain well-defined criteria. For clinical staff achieving *expert* status has been less easy because of the difficulty in identifying criteria of expertise. Increasingly, academic credentials are necessary for promotion as an expert and consequently there is an interest in pursuing Master's and Doctoral programs to gain advanced clinical skills. *Robert's* and *Stephanie's* career profiles are examples of clinical expert paths.

Another pathway was that of a *spiral*. According to Brousseau et al (1996), this affects many job opportunities, sometimes within the same organization. This career-path allows health practitioners to exercise creativity, to accumulate competencies in a range of areas and to broaden these experiences, thus enabling them to gain a deeper understanding of their organization, profession or occupation. Performance factors of people on a *spiral* path that are particularly valued by organizations are their people skills and their ability to work in teams. Lateral shifts often occur within the same organization. Those may result from interest in an emerging clinical area or aligning growing competence in other allied fields to a more suitable role.

A *transitory* career-path, according to Brousseau et al (1996), is a route that allows people to move in and out of organizations and posts, allowing them to search for better jobs and greater challenges. This best describes the contemporary health professional entrepreneur, consultant, independent practitioner and short-term locum staff. They have security and employability through their portfolio of competencies and breadth of experience in various organizations. Advanced practitioners may increasingly adopt this career-path as they gain confidence in their ability to invest in, and reap rewards from, learning opportunities and to capitalize on experience. In the future this entrepreneurial career-path may be the one of choice for those who want to remain in one location and who may be able to offer specific advanced skills to organizations on a temporary fee-for-service basis. *Aden* and *Dorothy-Anne's* career profiles are examples of *transitory* career-paths. You may wish to study examples of different career-paths by reviewing the career profiles at the end of this chapter, and comparing, and/or contrasting them with your own career-path.

How important is a graduate degree?

Graduate education is in-depth study in a discipline that increases candidates' research and evaluation skills with a view to preparing researchers who will add to the knowledge base of their own, and possibly that of other professions. In deciding to undertake a graduate degree or obtain advanced professional credentials, which are recognized or accredited, you need to know how this applies to your career goals. While Master's degrees are common in most health fields, professional Doctoral programs have been less evident. Professional or clinical Doctoral programs already exist in psychology, physical therapy, occupational therapy and pharmacy in the USA. There is growing interest in developing such programs, for example in Australia, Canada, and the UK.

We believe that it is appropriate to undertake an advanced degree once you have made a clear career choice. In doing so you are committing yourself to considerable expense in terms of time and money. You need to be sure. Advice from a mentor may be helpful here (for further information about role models and mentors, see Chapter 10). Possession of an advanced degree is a statement about your level of expertise: it implies that you have reached a certain standard of competency in relation to theory, research, practice or a combination of these elements. In our interviews, *Patricia* and *Aden* discussed the importance of mentors and professional support in their careers. *Patricia* benefited from collegial support and mentoring from within the teams in which she worked. However, she found her ability to continue to do so changed when she moved to a part-time appointment:

> So in that way, the support when you're working part-time is harder to get. Because you're not there every day of the week you miss out on certain things that are going on, and you feel that you can't participate in all the little extra-curricular activities like social events. Those are very important, I think, but I can't go to them all now because of my other obligations, and you just don't feel quite as integral a part as you'd like to be, or as you knew you once were.

Aden deliberately sought the support of colleagues who were at similar stages in their careers. He described himself as a late starter who knew that he had to make quick progress and some deliberate career moves. Regular contact with others in management positions and those completing graduate degrees on a part-time basis was particularly important. *Aden* described a group that functioned in a similar fashion to what Gail Howerton described as 'success circles ... a group of friends or colleagues getting together to assist each other in reaching their goals. They are more personal than a networking group ... more informal than a board meeting, and more synergy and success comes from them than any one person can generate alone'. Gail's own success circle eventually became an electronic group connected by e-mail. She recommends starting in person before developing a virtual circle. (See the list of websites at the end of this chapter for links to Gail Howerton's work).

Diane and *Aden* have been very involved in their professional organizations. They have each taken leadership roles of some kind, either serving as an officer or chairing major committees, working parties or task forces. In both cases involvement with their professional organization was a source of collegial support. It provided a networking opportunity and in *Aden* and *Diane's* case led to more than one job offer.

While graduate work requires additional commitment, studying and learning are stimulating and empowering and lead to mastery. The time investment will certainly be rewarded by dividends such as a broadening of opportunities, the esteem that comes from being in demand and the financial rewards that result from being successful in a competitive world.

Reflecting multiple interests in a career path

It is not unusual to possess more than one area of interest that could form the basis for a career. For example, there were probably several people in your professional classes who possessed undergraduate degrees in science or arts. A liberal arts background exposes students to a broad range of subject matter and the possibility of entering many fields. For example, you may have done well in English and be interested in creative writing and as a health practitioner you may use that interest and skill to prepare educational material for client groups and families. Or you might exercise your creative writing through your leisure role by writing short articles for magazines, as distinct from professional journals. One of the ways that health practitioners have satisfied their interest in other fields is to combine their fields by completing their graduate work in other areas. For example, the combination of occupational therapy and educational psychology has proved to be successful for numerous therapists in North America. This combination allows therapists to practice with greater expertise in schools, facilitates their understanding of educators' roles, and may enhance their credibility in the eyes of their educational colleagues. However, if you do this you need to be clear about your primary role, whether you are an educational psychologist with an occupational therapy background, or whether your graduate work in educational psychology supports your work as a therapist. Depending on the country in which you work, an additional degree may not automatically provide you with credentials to practice.

Broadening areas of competency

To broaden your area of competency you may undertake continuing education in a particular area to become a clinical specialist. Refer to Chapter 11 for detailed information about Continuing Professional Education. From short courses in areas such as musculo-skeletal disorders, sports medicine, or hand therapy you can expect to expand your practical or applied knowledge. Your credentials will have been gained through a professional program and will be recognized by others in your field. Your credibility will come from working in a specialized area and this may lead to advanced practice in your field. *Robert* described his situation: 'So we got two or three more services funded and a new one started up over that year. I was now a manager of a large and diverse department. That was really good. It was fantastic, but I felt I needed more skills in management, so during that time I went off and did a management course'. *Robert's* decision to broaden his areas of expertise developed out of a deficiency he detected in his level of knowledge.

Another alternative would be to complete a graduate degree in a program where you can specialize in one of these areas by completing a Master's thesis. Expect to expand your theoretical knowledge through such programs and this may lead to advanced practice in your field. For a detailed review of continuing professional education, refer to Chapter 11.

Conclusion

By now you will have realized that there is no single route to becoming an advanced practitioner. This whole concept is explored further in different perspectives in subsequent chapters of this text. The six practitioners you 'met' at the beginning of this chapter ranged from novice to expert; the length of their careers ranged from a recent pharmacy graduate to a dietician with 15 years of experience. Most went directly from high school to post secondary education in a health-related field, but in the one instance where an individual had significant experience in two fields before entering a health profession this did not hamper his career progress. A brief summary of the key issues outlined in this chapter follows.

What constitutes advanced practice?

At this point you may want to review the section '*What constitutes advanced practice?*' at the beginning of this chapter, where the six characters give their initial definitions of advanced practice. Some of the key elements included the breadth and depth of individual knowledge, continually adding to personal knowledge, appreciation of the wider environmental context, continually striving to develop skills, extensive contributions to an area or areas of practice, using critical thinking and analysis, possession of advanced qualifications and commitment to quality. An expert was described as a practitioner who demonstrated mastery or excellence or leadership or some combination. The ability to think critically is one of the essentials of advanced practice. It is the de-marker between those who reach technical proficiency and those who are truly considered to be experts in their discipline.

What do you need to know about career-planning and decision-making to get there?

Career development theories provide a basis for individual career decision-making. Career-planning is advisable, but not always possible when external circumstances only present forced choices. Practitioners are likely to move through four levels: growing, exploring, establishing, and maintaining. Research shows that individuals cycle and re-cycle through these levels when they change careers. It is likely that practitioners have similar experiences when they change jobs, undertake new projects, or take on a graduate student role. Career decision-making involves making choices and striking a workable balance between various roles. The level of importance you assign to a role and the work-related values you endorse both play an important part.

What do I need to know about myself?

The advanced practitioners you 'met' in this chapter clearly possessed high levels of self-knowledge. They obtained some of their knowledge from experience, from reviewing the results of measures designed to enhance self-knowledge, e.g. emotional intelligence, self-monitoring skills, learning styles, personality style and preferences, values and salience (priorities), and locus of control, and through reflection.

How do I become an advanced practitioner?

The breadth and depth of their knowledge characterize advanced practitioners. This means embarking upon Continuing Professional Education, as outlined in Chapter 11. This is now becoming a requirement to maintain registration or licensure by most healthcare professions. Completing a graduate degree potentially increases your chances of advancement. It is clear that we believe, and the people we interviewed agree, that continuous learning through an appropriate mechanism is necessary in order to reach advanced practitioner status.

Discussion topics

- You now have a lot of resources at your fingertips. Suppose *Erika* or *Patricia* came to you for career advice, how would you approach the task? What can you tell about each of them from their career profile? What more would you want to know?

- Compile your own career profile and compare your employment history with that of a colleague. Describe your career plans to each other. Take an on-line inventory, or do the tests listed at the end of this chapter; look over the results. Has your instructor, a mentor, or a person with expertise in vocational testing analyzed and interpreted the results with you? Write a set of career goals, with timelines based on what you now know about your interests, values, and personal style.

Career profiles

Aden

Educator—rehabilitation science

Qualifications

2001	Doctorate of Education
1992	Master of Philosophy
1987	Bachelor of Arts
1981	Diploma of Occupational Therapy

Memberships

Maintains memberships in state, national, and world occupational therapy organizations as well as a national health management institute.

Work experience

2001 to present	Curriculum director health sciences program
1998	Manager continuing education for regional health authority
1992	Head occupational therapist for major health facility
1989	Research occupational therapist
1987	Regional occupational therapy consultant
1986	Senior occupational therapist (regional mental health service)
1984	Senior occupational therapist (mental health program)

1982	Occupational therapist (physical disabilities)
1978	Instructor, adult education program
1966	Law enforcement officer

Consultancies

2001	Chair defining competency project for mental health services
1998	Consultant program accreditation educational setting
1997	Consultant career mentoring scheme for regional health authority
1992	Chair strategic planning initiative for mental health services

Publications and presentations

Aden has an extensive publication record. He has presented numerous papers at national and international conferences and delivered several keynote addresses in his area of specialization. He has received several professional awards and scholarships.

Contribution to professional organizations

Aden has been an active participant in professional affairs since he graduated in 1981. He has served as a member of the editorial review board for a major occupational therapy publication since 1985. He has participated in planning groups, task forces developing and revising educational standards, and served as the national association's representative on state health education initiatives.

Reflections on career success

Aden maintains a broad interest in health and social policy. He sees engaging in and contributing to his profession as essential and through this he has developed a strong professional network. He has set goals and taken advantage of employment opportunities that would further his aspirations. His has used his experience in related fields to advance in areas such as management. Aden sought out challenging positions: when he found that he was not continuing to learn in a position he took advantage of other opportunities. He has sought supervision and mentoring along the way, and benefited from those opportunities. He considers it important that he now also provides mentoring for younger members in his profession.

Robert   Private practitioner—occupational therapy

Qualifications

| 2000 | Master of Science in Occupational Therapy |

| 1995 | Postgraduate Diploma in Business—Organizational Change and Development |
| 1984 | Bachelor of Applied Science in Occupational Therapy |

Continuing professional education

Qualified Assessor, Functional Independence Measure (FIM)

Qualified Assessor, Assessment of Motor and Processing Skills (AMPS)

Administration of the Canadian Occupational Performance Measure (COPM)

Memberships

Maintains memberships in state, national and world occupational therapy organizations as well as several societies dedicated to assisting various client groups with which he works.

Work experience

1995 to present	Private practice focusing on clients with severe/multiple disabilities and medical legal work
1990	Manager outreach services for community-based agency working with major disability group
1987 to present	Clinical specialist, guest lecturer, State University
1986	Occupational therapist—school based program
1984	Occupational therapist (basic grade)—acute care setting

Consultancies

2000 to present	National disability group
1999	Program evaluation of community-based agency
1998	Chair, Policy Development Task Force, State Government housing plan for persons with severe disabilities
1995 to present	Various initiatives, including: strategic planning, ad hoc committees, task forces, review committees, feasibility studies

Publications and presentations

Robert has given numerous presentations to community and professional groups. He has had several publications in conference proceedings at national and international levels, professional newsletters, and a chapter in an edited book. He has received several professional awards and scholarships.

Reflections on career success

Robert attributes his success to networking and making connections within the wider community. He also believes in making the most of professional opportunities. This includes learning from colleagues in allied fields, pursuing learning opportunities where they were available, giving and receiving professional support—then, moving on when challenge or ability to learn is no longer available.

Patricia

Clinical dietician—specialist in burns, critical care and metabolic monitoring

Qualifications

1985	Bachelor of Science Nutrition
1986	Dietetic Internship

Continuing Professional Education

American Burn Association Annual Meeting
American Society for Parenteral and Enteral Nutrition Conference
Western Canada Nutrition Day
Local professional continuing education programs (regional/state levels)
Attendance at Nutrition Rounds and Journal Club

Memberships

Maintains memberships in state and national dietetic organizations

Work experience

2000 to present	Coordinator metabolic monitoring and clinical dietetic specialist responsible for burns (half-time position)
1986	Clinical dietician (burns and critical care) with teaching responsibilities for dietetic and medical interns, residents, fellows, nursing and allied health staff

Publications and presentations

During the period in which Patricia was a full-time clinical dietician she regularly gave presentations at regional, national, and international conferences. She is a co-author of two published papers.

Reflections on career success

Patricia did not have a clear idea about an area of specialization until she finished her dietetic internship. After 3 years of general clinical work she got an opportunity to focus on burns and intensive care, which 'opened up a whole new world of learning and teaching potential'. Patricia is one of only two dieticians with these areas of specialization in the state and has no desire to look beyond this position. She developed a reputation as an excellent teacher and enjoys working as a vital member of a team, providing an essential service to patients. The support and mentoring of colleagues played an important part in her development as a specialist, particularly from a senior dietician who served as a significant role model. Patricia believes her career interests contribute to her overall effectiveness in her combined working and home/family roles. Although this requires a high degree of organization, she believes that it contributes to her overall satisfaction.

Diane   Corporate Planning and Support—Regional Health

Qualifications

1996	Master of Speech Language Pathology
1983	Bachelor of Science in Speech Pathology

Memberships

Maintains memberships in state and national speech pathology organizations. Has served on the board of directors of the state organization and on advisory committees for non-profit organizations and self-help groups dedicated to assisting various client groups with which she works.

Work experience

2000 to present	Assistant director corporate planning and support. Coordinator quality improvement and regional accreditation initiatives
1997	Assistant director rehabilitation
1996	Seconded to state health department as project consultant—community rehabilitation programming
1995	Acting program manager—gerontology services
1994	Supervisor speech pathology
1990	Coordinator speech pathology services (overseas appointment)
1986	Case coordinator—home care program
1984	Speech pathologist—gerontology

Publications and presentations

Diane has given numerous presentations to community and professional groups. She has published her Master's thesis research and has co-authored three publications related to her specialty area (assessment of functional performance in neurological conditions). She has received a professional practice award from her state organization.

Reflections on career success

Diane attributes her success to not being afraid to take risks. She practiced for a relatively short time and quickly became disenchanted with front-line service demands. However, before deciding to change careers, she took advantage of an opportunity in the same field, working in another country. She reasoned that pursuing an advanced degree would be required at some point, but that option would still be there upon her return. She was right. Working in another culture and the management experience that she received there was invaluable. It broadened her horizons and increased her confidence in her abilities. The graduate degree she completed on her return and the management opportunities she has sought since then have taken her into broader policy-related areas that are more compatible with her interests.

Dorothy-Anne

Educator—physical therapy

Qualifications

1993	Doctorate of Philosophy
1988	Bachelor of Applied Science in Physical Therapy

Memberships

Maintains memberships in state, national and international physical therapy organizations as well as membership in other professional organizations related to her area of specialty.

Work experience

1999 to present	Associate professor, physical therapy, State University
1995	Assistant professor, physical therapy, State University
1993	Assistant professor, physical therapy (overseas appointment)
1992	Physical therapy consultant and clinical specialist
1990	Sessional lecturer, physical therapy (part-time)
1988	Physical therapist (basic grade) (rehabilitation)

Continuing professional education

1995	Registration with American Physical Therapy Association
1994	Certified A-ONE Assessor Administrator
1991	Accredited Trainer Functional Independence Measure (FIM), re-accredited 1999

Publications and presentations

Dorothy-Anne already has an impressive publication record. She has presented numerous papers at national and international conferences and has held several research grants in her area of specialty. She was one of six people in 2001 to receive a young researcher award from her university.

Contribution to professional organizations

Dorothy-Anne has been active in her professional organization since 1991 and now serves on major faculty committees. She is a member of the editorial review board for five major physical therapy publications.

Reflections on career success

Dorothy-Anne has been very strategic in her career-planning. She was careful not to undertake responsibilities, or accept employment opportunities that she considered beyond her level of ability. Although she knew immediately following graduation that she would like to embark on an academic career, she did not accept an appointment until she had obtained some experience at a leading overseas university. Dorothy-Anne did not hesitate to consult widely and change supervisors when necessary so that she could pursue the PhD topic of her choice. She is confident, and has a good understanding of what she needs to do to progress through the ranks. She has made a point of understanding the academic culture and is well aware of the reward system and how it works. She benefited early from mentors within physical therapy and now relies upon academic colleagues outside the profession for support and advice.

Erika

Hospital Pharmacist

Qualifications

1997	Bachelor of Science (Pharmacy)

Continuing Professional Education

2001	Attendance at Pharmacy Rounds (required to maintain 15 continuing education unit credits per annum to retain her license)
1999	Intersectoral Action for Health

Memberships

Maintains memberships in state and national organizations relevant to pharmacy practice and public health.

Work experience

2001 to present	Pharmacist (large teaching hospital)
1999–2000	Volunteer work (accompanied husband on Canadian Inter-

national Development Agency project)

1998	Hospital Residency (pharmacy)
1997	Pharmacy Assistant (community pharmacy setting, part-time position)

Publications and presentations

Erika has made two presentations at the local level. She is a co-author of one article in a professional journal that was based on work she did as a research assistant in her senior undergraduate year.

Reflections on career success

Work experience, volunteer work and networking proved to be critical in Erika's career decision-making. Her progress has been by trial and error. She knew little about health professions when she completed high school and entered pharmacy along with a couple of friends with similar interests. From her first part-time job in a community pharmacy setting she knew she wanted a more challenging position. After graduation she accompanied her husband overseas when he coordinated an international development project. While there, she did some part-time volunteer work and was struck by the poverty and needs of women and children where they were posted. With 3 years' experience in hospital-based pharmacy practice and a continuing interest in community-based service delivery, she is now looking into possibilities for graduate work in clinical pharmacy, health promotion studies, or community development. Starting a family is also a priority.

References

American Philosophical Association 1990 Critical thinking: a statement of expert consensus for purposes of educational assessment and instruction. The Delphi report: research findings and recommendations prepared for the committee on pre-college philosophy. ERIC document ED 315 423. American Philosophical Association, Newark.

Benner P 1984 From novice to expert: excellence and power in clinical nursing practice. Addison-Wesley, Boston

Bloom B S 1956 Taxonomy of educational objectives: the classification of educational goals. Longmans, New York

Brousseau K R, Driver K, Eneroth K, Larsson R 1996 Career pandemonium: realigning organizations and individuals. Academy of Management Executives 10:52–66

Browne M N, Keeley S M 1994 Asking the right question: a guide to critical thinking. Prentice-Hall, New Jersey

Burke J P, DePoy E 1991 An emerging view of mastery, excellence and leadership in occupational therapy practice. American Journal of Occupational Therapy 45:1027–1032

Casserly C, Fitzsimmons G W, Macnab D 1995 The Canadian study of life roles and values. In: Life roles, values, and careers. Super D E, Sverko B (eds) Jossey-Bass, San Francisco, p 117–146

Consulting Psychologists Press 2000 Know your type: personality testing for teams and individuals. Marylebone Holdings, UK

Dreyfus H, Dreyfus S 1986 Mind over matter. MacMillan, New York

Esdaile S A, Madill H M 1993 Causal attributions: theoretical considerations and their relevance to occupational therapy practice and education. British Journal of

Occupational Therapy 56:330–334 (an earlier, shorter version was published in ACTA Ergotheraputica Belgica 4:133–136)

Esdaile S A, Lokan J J, Madill H M 1997 A comparison of Australian and Canadian occupational therapy students' career choices. Occupational Therapy International 4:249–270

Fisher C D, Schoenfeldt L F, Shaw J B 1999 Human resource management. Houghton Mifflin, Boston

Fitzsimmons G W, Macnab D, Casserly C 1985 Technical manual for the life roles inventory: values and salience. Psychometrics Canada, Edmonton

Goleman D 1995 Emotional intelligence. Why it can matter more than IQ. Bantam, New York

Goleman D 1999 Working with emotional intelligence. Bantam, New York

Gouws D J 1995 The role concept in career development. In: Super D E, Sverko B (eds) Life roles, values, and careers. Jossey-Bass, San Francisco, p 22–53

Herr E L 1996 Toward the convergence of career theory and practice. In: Savikas M L, Walsh W B (eds) Handbook of counseling theory and practice. Davies-Black, Palo Alto, p 13–44

Honey P, Mumford A 1995 Capitalizing on your learning style. Organization Design and Development, King of Prussia, PA

King P M, Kitchener K S 1994 Developing reflective judgment: understanding and promoting intellectual growth and critical thinking. In: Super D E, Sverko B (eds) Adolescents and Adults, Jossey-Bass, San Francisco

Lennox RD, Wolfe RN 1984 Revision of Self-Monitoring Scale. Journal of Personality and Social Psychology 6:1361

Lokan J J, Shears M 1995 Studies of work importance in Australia. In: Super D E, Sverko B (eds) Life roles, values, and careers. Jossey-Bass, San Francisco, p 77–99

Madill H M, Macnab D, Brintnell E S G 1989 Student value preferences: what do they tell us about program selection? Canadian Journal of Occupational Therapy 56:171–178

Mayer R, Goodchild F 1995 The critical thinker, 2nd edn. Brown and Benchmark, Madison

Myers B I, McCaulley M H 1985 Manual: a guide to the development and use of the Myers-Briggs Type Indicator. Consulting Psychologists Press, Palo Alto, CA

Rotter J B 1990 Internal versus external control reinforcement. A case history of a variable. American Psychologist 45:489–493

Super D E 1980 A life-span, life-space, approach to career development. Journal of Vocational Behavior 16:282–298

Super D E 1994 A life span, life space perspective on convergence. In: Savikas M L, Lent R W (eds) Convergence in career development theories: implications for science and practice. Consulting Psychologists Press, Palo-Alto, p 63–74

Super D E 1995a Values: their nature, assessment, and practical use. In: Super D E, Sverko B (eds) Life roles, values, and careers. Jossey-Bass, San Francisco, p 54–61

Super D E 1995b Tests of the work importance study model of role salience. In: Super D E, Sverko B (eds) Life roles, values, and careers. Jossey-Bass, San Francisco, p 321–324

Sverko B, Super D E 1995 The findings of the work importance study. In: Super D E, Sverko B (eds) Life roles, values, and careers. Jossey-Bass, San Francisco, p 349–358

Sverko B, Vizek-Vidovic V 1995 Studies of the meaning of work: approaches, models and some of the findings. In: Super D E, Sverko B (eds) Life roles, values, and career. Jossey-Bass, San Francisco, p 3–21

Wallston K 1992 Hocus-pocus, the focus isn't strictly on locus: Rotter's social learning theory modified for health. Cognitive Therapy and Research 16:183–199

Whetton D A, Cameron K S 1998 Developing management skills, 4th edn. Addison-Wesley, Boston

Websites

Consulting Psychologists Press 2000	www.knowyourtype.com
Emotional Intelligence	www.eqi.org www.cjwolfe.com
Foundation for Critical Thinking	www.criticalthinking.org
Gail Howerton's work	www.funcilitators.com
Honey & Mumford's Learning Styles Questionnaire (LSQ)	www.psi-press.co.uk/LSS-I/ LSS_Admin.htm
MBTI: cost of taking the test and type of report:	www.knowyourtype.com www.serve.com/douglass/myersbriggs www.psychometrics.com
Psychometrics Canada: offers online testing of career values and career competencies and provides comparative normative data, updated at appropriate intervals.	www.psychometrics.com

3

Integrating theory and practice: using theory creatively to enhance professional practice

Maralynne D. Mitcham

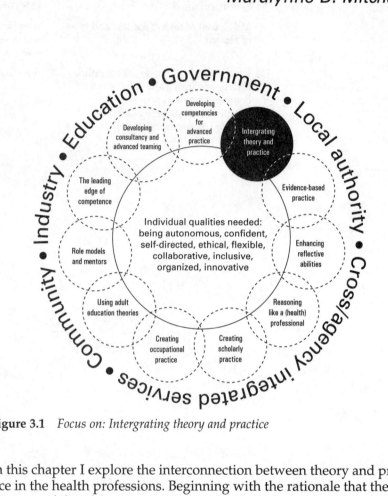

Figure 3.1 *Focus on: Intergrating theory and practice*

Chapter outline

In this chapter I explore the interconnection between theory and practice in the health professions. Beginning with the rationale that theory is a powerful tool for practice, I trace the evolution of theory and practice in the health professions. Next, I try to demystify theory by examining the nature of theory and its component parts. I propose a progression of skills that will help practitioners become good consumers of theory. Then I look at a variety of ways in which the theory–practice connection is manifest in different health professions through top-down approaches and theory-driven practice guidelines. I propose my own framework for integrating theory and practice, which I offer as a tool for practitioners who wish to advance their practice. I conclude the chapter with two examples of integrating theory into practice—one of my own from the educational domain and one from the published literature in the clinical domain.

Key words

Theory, consumer of theory, theory–practice connection

Anticipated outcomes

As a result of reading this chapter, I anticipate you will be able to:

- appreciate theory as a tool for professional enhancement
- understand how theory and practice
  evolved in the health professions
- recognize theory, its component parts and related terminology
- hone your skills as a consumer of theory
- recognize different strategies for linking theory and practice
- appreciate the ways different authors integrate theory into their practice
- use examples in the chapter as a guide for designing programs relevant to areas of professional practice.

Introduction

For every complex problem, there is one solution that is neat, simple, and wrong (H. L. Mencken 1880–1956).

Theory is one of those words we use happily and colloquially in everyday conversation. At a superficial level, theory is not a word that causes us much concern. We say things such as 'theoretically speaking, I agree with you', meaning, I agree with you in principle, but I'm not sure if I agree with you in practice. We dismiss it lightly and move on to the next task that requires our attention. However, we panic when a keen, bright-eyed student asks us in the clinic one day, 'Which theoretical approach guides your practice?' We stumble, and mumble a response along the lines of, 'Oh, I haven't touched that theory stuff since I graduated', or 'I'm eclectic, I use a little of everything'. Again, we try to dismiss theory lightly but there is a nagging feeling that perhaps we should know more. When we were students, theory always seemed vague and abstract, something slightly mysterious that we thought was less pressing than the real world of practice. Now we are in practice, theory still retains that mystique. How, then, can we come to grips with theory in a way that frees us to use theory creatively and, in turn, enhances our professional practice?

In the health professions, theory provides a way to organize our thinking and to frame our actions. Theory gives us a foundation for solving problems, and you can depend on theory to give you a strong rationale for what you are doing. Theory is an ever-present transportable gift; you can take it anywhere and use it anytime; it's always there. If you select wisely, theory will do a lot of the work for you because someone else has done the hard part. Someone else has spent years organizing and testing the theory; all you have to do is use it in a way that makes sense in your situation. Theory makes your life easier.

Selecting one or more theories to use in a given situation depends on your values, beliefs, and preferences. When you are faced with a problem to solve, certain solutions will have more appeal to you than others. Beneath all the trappings, there are basic tenets that drive your thinking. Throughout life, your family, community, teachers, and peers influence your thinking, and to some degree their thoughts and ideas rub off on you. In fact, some of your early thoughts and ideas probably influenced your choice of health profession. Now, in your selected field, you are in a position to make choices about how to solve the problems that present themselves on a daily basis. Stop and think for a minute about the underlying values and orientation of the theories you typically use in your practice. Why are the theories appealing to you? What little piece of you is reflected in the theories? I'm aware that I often select theories that help me take a new journey and feed my pioneer spirit. For example, when I am designing a new curriculum or a new course, I find theories of adult learning appealing. I like theories that offer suggestions about how adults learn or theories that suggest alternatives for sequencing learning. Adult learning theories speak to developmental issues experienced by adult learners and these issues are important to me, because my major responsibilities in higher education involve designing and directing university degree programs. Chapter 9 will give you ideas for using and developing theory in this area.

Once you've selected a theory, then you have to put the theory to work. Using theory requires you to think deductively. Deductive thinking means you start with existing general principles that you wish to apply to a specific context. The theoretical principles are already established but you have to decide how you want to apply them. For example, if you are a physical therapist, you know the principles of physics that govern how levers work. Consequently, when you are working with a patient who demonstrates limited joint range of motion, you select an intervention to increase your patient's range of motion. If the intervention is successful and the patient shows improvement, you judge your choice of theoretical principles to have been successfully applied in practice. Your knowledge of well-established principles allows you to select an intervention that is clearly appropriate and effective for the specific patient's problem. You do not have to spend unnecessary time engaging in a process of trial and error to see what might work for your patient. Your ability to provide the necessary intervention efficiently makes your life easier, your patient's life more comfortable and your administrator's life much happier.

Theory gives us a foundation, something that is tried and true. It gives us internal confidence to be persuasive in the context of our practice. For example, we can use theory to strengthen our case with administrators when we are seeking approval and funding for a new program, or we can use theory to explain what we are doing when we give a presentation to a group of colleagues at a staff development meeting. When our reasoning is grounded in theory we come across as poised, polished and professional. Often, after taking a theory course with me, I hear post-graduate students say that finally they have the language to communicate with their colleagues, particularly those in super-ordinate positions. As practitioners they feel more credible, and now perceive that their superiors hold them in high regard.

There are, however, people for whom theory is neither attractive nor appealing because they can't see it, smell it, or touch it. For people who prefer to do their thinking in more concrete ways, I recommend using diagrams and flow charts to summarize the key points you want to make. Visually representing major stages in your argument is a powerful tool for making your case. To help concrete thinkers become more comfortable with theories and principles, I use more tangible examples when explaining theoretical information. For example, in the paragraph above I indicated that theory gives us a foundation, something that is tried and true. What can you think of in your life that serves as a foundation? What would you classify as something that is tried and true? In response, I might say that my little black dress is the foundation of my wardrobe. Whenever I put it on, I have confidence it will work for the occasion; my little black dress will never let me down. I can dress it up for a night on the town, or I can play it down for a meeting with the dean. I add to the little black dress those accessories that communicate my intent. Changing the accessories changes my intent, and so it is with theory. Once we select a theoretical foundation in which we have confidence, we can go on to select additional principles that make the most sense for each occasion or each type of client with whom we work.

Theory, then, is an important tool that helps us recognize what we know and organize what we do. Theory provides the clarity and necessary guidance for solving complex problems in a fast-paced and increasingly complex world. In health care, theory helps us as practitioners to validate our practice and influence our future. Theory gives us the energy to create new possibilities for the individuals, groups, and communities we serve. As one who teaches theory, it has helped me tremendously to understand the history of knowledge and the way in which theory and practice have evolved over time. Several authors (Depoy and Gitlin 1994, 1998, Mosey 1992, 1996, Portney and Watkins 1993, 2001) address the way in which knowledge in the health professions has developed through the ages. Based on their work, let's take a quick hop, skip, and a jump through time and look at the evolution of theory and practice in the health professions.

The evolution of theory and practice in the health professions

Our ancestors were practical people who paid attention to the world around them and used trial and error as their modus operandi. They paid attention to fortuitous happenings, respected the supernatural, and realized that they were not in control of their universe. They handed on their knowledge by word of mouth to subsequent generations, but by the time the Greeks emerged, discussion about the nature and organization of the universe took place in the guise of broad principles. The Greeks called themselves philosophers and judged theoretical knowledge to be far superior to practical knowledge. For the first time in history, knowledge was valued for its own sake and not for any practical purpose. The philosophers and their disciples waxed eloquent while others carried out the practical tasks, and schism appeared between practical and theoretical knowledge.

The dichotomy of practical and theoretical knowledge continued as we moved into the first century. Craftsmen and artisans still relied on trial and error for the development of practical knowledge and superstition prevailed. In contrast, physicians were still influenced by the general principles or medical tenets of Greek philosophers such as Galen. During the dark Middle Ages knowledge was considered a dangerous thing and new knowledge was well hidden for fear of reprisal. As the Renaissance dawned bright and clear, light shone on new knowledge and the world was turned upside down. A new breed of scholars calling themselves natural philosophers was born. These natural philosophers were attracted to a combination of practical and theoretical knowledge. They relied less on the past, and introduced a new way of looking more objectively at problems, even verifying their observations by experiment. For example, the Polish astronomer Copernicus (1473–1543) was the first to suggest that the earth moved round the sun and not vice versa. Galileo (1564–1642), an Italian astronomer, mathematician, and physicist, constructed the first telescope and upheld the views of Copernicus. The early explorers began to realize that the world was round and no longer feared falling off the face of the earth. The development of scientific thought and knowledge had reached a major turning point and the foundation for the development of scientific thinking as we know it today was laid down.

It was the English philosopher John Locke (1632–1704) who first promoted the idea that we are born with a blank slate (tabula rasa). Locke, the founder of British empiricism, reasoned that knowledge comes from our human experiences and so our ideas must reflect our reality; thus, science is possible. David Hume (1711–1776), a Scottish philosopher and historian, carried empiricism to a radical form of scepticism. He demanded concrete evidence from experiments; if he couldn't see it, he didn't believe it. Hume posited the view that we can know the world as a single reality, and he set the scene for the traditional theory of science known as logical positivism. Eventually, around the end of the nineteenth century, theorists became known as scientists and their major purpose was to develop valid theories. They used agreed-upon methods of inquiry and research designs to explain the physical universe. The basic science disciplines were born and basic scientists dedicated themselves to developing and testing valid theories of science.

Meanwhile, the practitioners became more sophisticated in applying their practical knowledge. Although they still focused on solving the practical problems at hand, practitioners accumulated their own bodies of knowledge, which they handed down from generation to generation. Tradition prevailed and practitioners carried out their work based on the authority of their predecessors. Society recognized the value of solving practical problems and professions emerged to respond to the practical needs of society. However, it was not until the middle of the nineteenth century that practitioners recognized the potential of using theoretical information as a basis for solving practical problems. The social sciences emerged to provide new theories and new knowledge. Over the next hundred years or so, practical inquiry gradually became known as applied science. Applied scientists helped professions such as engineering, medicine, education and the health professions solve specific, practical and social problems using a variety of research approaches and designs.

Today, at the beginning of the twenty-first century, we are still grappling with theory and the ways in which the health professions can best serve society. Not everyone agrees that the relationship between theory and practice has to be quite so dichotomous, and some authors (Creek and Ormston 1996, Kielhofner 1997) argue for a more integrated approach between philosophy, theory, and practice. My personal view is that any tension still remaining between practical and theoretical knowledge can be a healthy tension. We don't have to take sides. It's not a matter of either/or but a matter of what/when. The ability to recognize the differences between theoretical and applied knowledge, to accept what each has to offer, marks our progress as reflective practitioners. Strengthened with skills in critical thinking and clinical reasoning, neither the setting in which we work nor the complexity of the presenting problem prevents us from thoughtfully responding and providing efficacious service to our patients and clients.

Taking the mystique out of theory

Now that we have a broad sense of how theory evolved through the ages, perhaps we can better appreciate how theory can be friend rather than foe. When we were students, we learned much from the basic and social sciences, and we also learned theoretical information that underpins the basis for our diagnostic and intervention activities. Think back to your days as a student. When, where, and how were you introduced to theory? Did you learn the names of theories and their content, or did you learn about general principles and different evaluation and treatment approaches? Who taught you theory and was it fun? I suspect that few of us learned what goes into making a theory or how it is constructed and tested. At best, we probably learned an overview of important points—enough to pass our exams, conduct an evaluation, write a treatment plan, or carry out a procedure.

What do we really mean by theory? Reed (1998, p. 521), writing for the health professions, offers us the following definition of theory:

> Theory is an organized way of thinking about given phenomena . . .
> Theory attempts to:
> 1) define and explain the relationships between concepts or ideas related to phenomena of interest,
> 2) explain how these relationships can predict behaviour or events, and
> 3) suggest ways that the phenomena can be changed or controlled.

From this definition you can see that a theory is not a mass of isolated facts that takes our fancy, nor does theory answer the question 'why'? Theories cannot control events or phenomena, nor can they provide an answer to what is right and good.

Although different health professions may organize their knowledge in different ways and different authors may use different terms to discuss theory, theories have many characteristics in common. The literature is replete with a broad array of language and terms that may be judged as either complementary or confusing. Perhaps this is why we think theory is so mysterious. Let us take a little time now to demystify theory. In this section of the chapter we will examine characteristics of theory, the building blocks that make up a theory, different types of theories, and a selection of theory-related terms. When we increase our understanding of theory, we will be less intimidated and gain confidence in using theory more creatively in the future.

Characteristics of theory

Reynolds (1971), a social psychologist, describes three characteristics of theory: abstractness, inter-subjectivity, and empirical relevance. First, and most importantly, theories of necessity must be *abstract*; they cannot have conditions placed upon them. For example, if you are looking at a particular theory of behaviour, it must take into account all possible conditions under which the behaviour can take place. The particular behavioural theory must be developed and tested in a way that allows you to use it in future times and in many different places. A theory is not much good to you if it is tied down to a specific point in time or to a particular place in the universe. When theories are independent of time and space, their abstractness is a blessing, not a curse. It means you can use a theory at any time and in any place, and thus you are relieved of any constraints that might inhibit your sense of freedom and creativity.

Second, a theory must have *intersubjective agreement* about its phenomena of interest and the relationship of the phenomena to each other. Inter-subjective agreement comes about when scholars explicitly define the phenomena within their theory and other scholars understand and agree with their definitions. Likewise, there must be shared agreement for understanding the relationships between phenomena. There has to be some agreed-upon system of logic that supports the way in which relationships are understood. To use the example of a behavioural theory again, scholars must agree upon the definition of the behaviours and how the behaviours in the theory relate to each other.

Third, for theories to become more than philosophical whim, they must have *empirical relevance*, that is, they must be testable and compared with objective, observable data. In this way, others can verify findings for themselves and, in turn, have more confidence in the utility of the theory. So, the behavioural theory in our earlier example must be tested with many different people at many different times in many different places.

Building blocks of theory

Theories are made up of concepts or constructs and the propositions that link them together. Concepts and constructs are important to us because they represent phenomena of interest; they are the building blocks of theory. A *concept* is made up of an array of characteristics that have been organized and classified to create a new whole. Therapist, technologist and patient are examples of human concepts, and wheelchair, X-ray and computer are examples of non-human concepts. If we want to be sure that everyone interprets the concept of patient in the same way, we create an operational definition that describes all aspects of the concept. In this way, each concept is distinguishable from all other concepts. Sometimes we specify the context of the concept, for example, in-patient or outpatient. When the concept is not tangible or observable, we call it a *construct*. Anxiety and intelligence are examples of constructs because we cannot directly see them, but we infer their presence by tallying the scores on a self-report anxiety scale and by administering a standardized intelligence test (Portney and Watkins 1993, 2001).

Propositions describe the nature of the relationship between the concepts or constructs. Mosey (1996) describes seven different categories of propositions. *Spatial* propositions describe how concepts are arranged in space; for example, the arrangement of bones in the human skeleton. *Temporal* propositions describe the timing of how concepts unfold; for example, the typical sequence of developmental milestones of childhood.

Quantitative propositions describe a numeric relationship between concepts, such as the number of repetitions and accompanying weight needed for a program of strength training. In contrast, *qualitative* propositions describe the special characteristics between concepts; for example, the quality of caring between a daughter and her mother with Alzheimer's disease. *Causal* propositions describe cause-and-effect relationships; for example, when the outside temperature falls to zero, water in the pond will freeze. *Correlative* postulates describe how two concepts vary together. Take the old adage, 'an apple a day keeps the doctor away'. A correlative proposition would say that the more apples you eat, the fewer doctors' visits you will need. In this instance, when the apple concept increases, the doctor's visit concept decreases. Finally, *hierarchical* propositions describe the position of concepts in relation to each other. For example, Maslow's (1970) hierarchy of needs is a well-known psychological theory that describes several stages through which a person must move before attaining self-actualization. Basic physiological needs must be met before higher-level needs such as love and belongingness are addressed.

Understanding the building blocks (concepts or constructs and propositions) of theory is important if we are going to use theory creatively in our practice. Perhaps a good analogy for the building blocks of theory is to think about your wardrobe of clothes. In your wardrobe there are several tangible *concepts* such as suits, dresses, skirts, trousers, jackets, shirts, sweaters, hats, coats, and gloves. When you get dressed in the morning, you select clothing concepts that reflect the nature of the day ahead, be it formal or informal. You select items that go together well and have a relationship with each other.

The relationship between clothing concepts is mainly spatial—you wear your jacket on top of your shirt or your socks inside your shoes. Organizing clothing concepts in relationship to each other brings about a desired outcome—you look ready for work or for that weekend getaway to the mountains. Sometimes you accessorize and sometimes you keep it simple. Or think about packing your suitcase with clothes to go away for the weekend. Your itinerary influences what you pack for the journey, and you select items from your wardrobe that are flexible and go with many other items. Your weekend activities require certain kinds of clothing, and if you are not sure what to wear, you usually fall back on your favorite suit or sports coat that never lets you down.

And so it is with our practice, we select theoretical concepts that make sense for the occasion. Speech-language pathologists are interested in theories of language development and theories of motor control and their relationship to speech apraxia. In contrast, medical technologists explore theories of science that affect the immune system when searching for an explanation of test results that do not match the physician's expectation of a particular disease state. If we can think about the building blocks of theory in the same way as our wardrobe of clothes, then our imagination is the only limit to using theory creatively in our practice.

Types of theory

There are several different types of theories in the health professions. Reed (1998) suggests four types of theories that range from the most abstract to the most specific. *Meta theories* typically define the uniqueness and viability of a profession, and are the most abstract and overarching of all theories. For example, theories that describe the meaning of 'occupation' in occupational therapy or 'speech' and 'language' in speech-language pathology are considered meta theories. *Grand theories* are general, and focus on the broad goals of a profession; for example, in physical therapy theories that describe motor control and motor learning form a large part of the profession's knowledge base (Shumway-Cook and Woollacott 2001). *Middle-range theories* focus on some of the unique phenomena of interest in a profession; for example, relevance theory may be used by speech-language pathologists when they explore impairment of pragmatic comprehension in children (Leinonen and Kerbel 1999). *Practice theories* provide goals and action for the practitioner. For example, neurophysiological approaches to treatment such as those proposed by Rood (discussed by Metcalfe and Lawes 1998) and Brunnstrom (discussed by Smith and Sharpe 1994) are often used by physical and occupational therapists when they are working with patients who have sustained central nervous system damage. Understanding these different types of theory makes it easier for us to select theories that best meet our needs in a given situation. When we want to start a new service for elders, we may select a middle-range theory, or if we are designing a new protocol for a group of patients with schizophrenia, we will more likely select a practice theory.

Theory-related terms

If theory still seems a little complicated, the terms related to theory may be even more confusing. To minimize some of the confusion, I want to look at three theory-related terms that frequently appear in the literature: paradigms, models and frames of reference.

In the 1960s Thomas Kuhn, a philosopher of science, first started writing about *paradigms*. He noticed that members in each of the scientific disciplines shared a common vision or unique perspective, which he named a paradigm. When applied to professions, the word paradigm has come to mean the accepted or prevailing way of looking at the scope of practice. Paradigms help keep professions focused and unified and allow practitioners to feel part of the same corpus. According to Kuhn (1996, p. 23), 'paradigms gain their status because they are more successful than their competitors in solving a few problems that the group of practitioners has come to recognize as acute'. A new paradigm usually emerges when the usual way of doing business is not successful and fails to solve the problems at hand. For example, in the USA when healthcare practitioners started moving into community-based practice, they discovered that the reductionistic orientation of the medical model was not particularly useful for solving problems related to the health of a community and its residents. Consequently, a new paradigm emerged, which focused more on the holistic nature of humans and their readiness to embrace life style changes that would promote their health and well-being. The new paradigm subsequently influenced development of new theoretical perspectives, which, in turn, led to the development of new theoretical frameworks such as the Transtheoretical Model of Behaviour Change (Prochaska and DiClemente 1983) and the Health Belief Model (Rosenstock et al 1994). These models reflected the new way of thinking and offered guidance to practitioners planning community-based health programs.

Models are helpful for defining the uniqueness of a profession and are predicated on the status of a profession's paradigm. Their development and evolution come from a variety of sources, including clinical practice, emergence of new knowledge, reexamination of old models, interest in exploring new disciplines, consolidation of existing models and the future direction of healthcare (Reed 1984). When the term *conceptual model* is used in the health professions, it generally refers to the *what* and the *why* of the profession. A conceptual model is often the way a profession perceives itself and presents itself to other professions and society. Krefting (1985) calls a conceptual model a 'theory in training', because it is more tentative and less well formulated than theory. Kielhofner (1997) argues that a conceptual model provides practitioners with a viable link between theory and practice. Conceptual models serve as a collection of theoretical concepts related to a specific area of concern. Once organized, the theoretical concepts help practitioners identify areas for assessment and intervention, and provide direction for testing how well the model works in practice. Conceptual models emerge in the health professions because practitioners are busy solving a plethora of practical problems on a daily basis. If practitioners can reach for organizing structures that help them 'name and frame' the problems at hand (Schön 1983), then they are better able to retain a central focus for their work.

Models are usually dynamic and they change when new knowledge develops in response to solving the problem at hand. Because healthcare practitioners are concerned with solving problems, they want to understand better the nature and extent of problems. Models often provide a useful way of encapsulating the scope and magnitude of a problem, and they provide a schema for examining the relationship between interconnected parts. For example, in dental hygiene,

Williams et al (1998) propose use of an oral health-related quality-of-life model, and contend that models provide a common language and infrastructure for defining the process of care (assessing, planning, implementing, and evaluating outcomes). Much like an architect's blueprint, you might say that a model is a two-dimensional representation of what becomes three-dimensional action in the real world.

Frame of reference is a term used more in occupational therapy than other health professions, and closely resembles the conceptual model described by Kielhofner (1997). Frames of reference are the tools that let us focus on a particular area of practice. Mosey (1992, 1996) suggests that frames of reference are the link between theory and practice. She argues strongly that the business of the science-based professions is to develop frames of reference that describe the treatment techniques specific to problems encountered in practice. Occupational therapists often use the term 'frame of reference' when talking about the specific parameters that guide their particular areas of practice. According to Young and Quinn (1992), frames of reference describe the nature, aims, and procedures that distinguish the application of theory by one profession from another, and thus they are helpful in differentiating what each profession will do when working in an interdisciplinary context.

Although theory-related terminology may be confusing at times, the intent is clear to me. Writers are searching for words to express the connection between theory and practice in ways that make sense and, ultimately, in ways that will improve the quality of service we provide as healthcare practitioners. If you can get beyond troubling semantics, deepening your level of understanding of the theoretical underpinnings of your profession not only strengthens the work you do but also enhances your career progress.

Developing skills as a consumer of theory

A good strategy for deepening your understanding of theory is to become a good consumer of theory. In a previous work (Mitcham 1985) I wrote about developing skills as a consumer of research and suggested strategies to help students come to grips with the research literature. I argued that you did not have to be a researcher to be a good consumer of research, and suggested many instances in which we behave as consumers without having the skills to develop the original product. We do not have to be a classical composer to enjoy listening to a symphony or a mechanic to know that something is wrong with our car. I compared the activities of a researcher with those of a research consumer, and developed a hierarchy of 10 skills necessary for becoming a research consumer. I now propose developing a similar set of skills to help us become good consumers of theory and strengthen our ability to link theory with our practice. Most of us will not participate in the time-consuming process of generating new theory, but all of us have the opportunity to evaluate what we read and carefully select what we wish to incorporate into our practice.

In Table 3.1, I delineate a progression of active consumer of theory skills for use in the health professions. The progression of skills begins with understanding the evolution of theory in the health professions

Table 3.1   *Becoming a consumer of theory: progression skills for use in the health professions*

1. Understanding the nature of theory in the health professions and its place in the evolution of scientific knowledge
2. Recognizing that theory has a set of parameters that influence its utility for practice
3. Recognizing the difference between theory and other theory-related terms such as paradigms, models and frames of reference
4. Recognizing that theory development follows an orderly and cyclical process which includes a series of sequential steps as follows:
- Observation of phenomena of interest over time
- Recognition that phenomena present themselves in certain ways and form patterns
- Organization of phenomena into a conceptual framework
- Empirical testing of propositions that hold the conceptual framework together
- Refinement and retesting of propositions and the concepts they organize and integrate
- Acceptance of newly developed theory
5. Evaluating theories and their component parts (concepts/constructs and propositions) to determine relevance for practice
6. Evaluating the results of how others have used theory in their work
7. Confidently selecting theories that have potential to inform our own practice:
- Congruence with personal and professional beliefs
- Suitability for practice environment
- Alignment with practice milieu

Adapted with permission from Mitcham (1985) Integrating research into occupational therapy. A teaching guide for academic and clinical educators. Rockville, MD. American Occupational Therapy Foundation.

and the nature of theory and its component parts, as described in the beginning of the chapter. The next steps involve recognizing the sequence of theory development and evaluating existing theory and its component parts. The final steps in the progression require us to evaluate how others have used theory to guide their practice and to feel confident in selecting theories that may be useful for us in practice. With this progression of skills in mind, let us look at ways in which we can increase our comfort as consumers of theory.

Increasing our comfort in the supermarket of theory

We are consummate consumers. We peruse mail-order catalogs, browse on-line, and saunter through shopping malls; no doubt, in some countries, shopping has become a national pastime. Our consumer behavior is greatly influenced by cognition and affect, and market researchers know how to tap into our knowledge and emotion. The behavior of consumers in general is discussed in the marketing literature which is helpful in understanding the differences between active and passive consumers. Assael (1981) suggests that *active consumers* seek and process information, evaluate before accepting and make comparisons to gain the most benefit and ensure maximum levels of satisfaction. Active consumers are weakly affected by advertising. Their identities and beliefs are closely tied to their consumer behavior, and reference group norms and values influence their consumer behaviors. In contrast, *passive consumers* gather and learn information at random, accept before evaluating, accept familiar items least likely to give them problems, and tolerate minimal levels of satisfaction. Passive consumers are strongly affected by advertising. Their identities are not closely tied to their consumer behaviors, nor are their consumer behaviors likely to be influenced by group norms and values. Understanding the differences between active and passive consumers may help us as we consider our approach to shopping for theory. If we can identify situations in our own lives in which we have behaved as either passive or active consumers, we can turn our passive approach into a more active one, and become more comfortable shopping in the supermarket of theory. But, how do we maneuvre our way down the aisles of theory, shop for conceptual bargains, wheel out the best propositions, or shelve phenomena for future consumption?

Buying concepts and propositions

We must be sure that *concepts* of interest are understandable and well defined before we decide which ones to buy and determine how best to use them. Do we need to buy concepts for an overarching framework for a new program or do we wish to incorporate new concepts into a specific treatment context? Sometimes we want concepts to serve as inclusion or exclusion criteria for a new project, and, in this way, concepts act as a boundary for what we do. In other instances, new concepts may broaden our horizons and extend existing or traditional boundaries in our practice. Later in this chapter I will give you a detailed example of using broad and specific concepts for developing a post-graduate degree program and modifying courses for distance delivery. You will see how I selected broad concepts from adult learning theories for the foundation of the degree program, and how I selected specific concepts from a particular theory of motivation as a guide for making instructional decisions when I was faced with adapting courses for distance delivery.

When we buy *propositions*, we must buy those that are representative of our profession because we want to show that what we do makes a difference. Propositions serve as principles for action, so if we want to build an early intervention program to minimize future deterioration, or design a program to limit subsequent loss of function, we will buy temporal propositions that describe when the timing of our intervention is important.

The interconnection between theory and practice

So far in this chapter we have looked at theory as a way of informing and potentially improving our practice. In searching the literature about the theory–practice connection, it became evident to me that each health profession looks at this relationship somewhat differently. The diagnostic-based health professions such as medical technology, radiography, or radiation therapy technology rely heavily on theories from the traditional basic sciences such as chemistry, physics, immunology, anatomy, and physiology. In contrast, the therapy-based professions such as occupational therapy, physical therapy, and speech-language pathology use a broader range of theories from both the basic and social sciences because of the strong interpersonal component to their practice. In addition, the therapy-based professions have developed their own theories to guide their practice with different groups of patients and clients. Consequently, there is more discussion in the literature from the therapy-based professions about ways in which theory and practice are interconnected.

Top-down approaches for connecting theory with practice

One way to connect theory with practice is to use a top-down approach. By top-down approach, I mean that your thinking is moving in a direction from abstract to concrete or from broad principles to specific instances. When you take a top-down approach you are engaging in deductive thinking. Let me give you three examples of top-down approaches for connecting theory with practice.

British author Hagedorn (1995) suggests that some practitioners use theory-driven patterns of practice, which she calls a 'theory first–then practice' approach. These theory-driven patterns of practice are top-down, deductive sequences of clinical reasoning, which begin with the profession's core values, purposes, principles and processes. Depending on the nature of the presenting problem, practitioners select one or more theoretical frameworks to solve the problem at hand. Within the parameters of the selected frameworks, the needs, priorities and preferences of the person receiving service are considered. Practitioners then select compatible treatment approaches for a particular person with a particular problem at a particular time.

Canadian authors McColl et al (1993) undertook a major project for the profession of occupational therapy by producing an annotated bibliography of theory-based articles published in North American journals from 1900 to 1990. These authors simplified the confusion surrounding theory-related terminology by dividing theory into two major camps: theoretical information that helps us understand what we know and theoretical information that helps us know what to do. McColl et al (1993) organized their bibliography by creating a three-tier taxonomy, which moves from the broadest to the most specific of theoretical information.

The first tier of the taxonomy includes only theories that define and describe the central construct of occupation—occupational nature of humans, need for meaningful occupation and the essence of balanced occupational functioning for health. The second tier of the taxonomy focuses on six areas of theory that describe occupational function and dysfunction. For each of these areas, McColl et al (1993, pp. 7–16) describe theories directly related to occupation and indicate the scientific basis and disciplines from which the theories have their origin. For example, here is their description related to socio-adaptive theories:

> The socioadaptive approach refers to the process of successfully organizing one's occupation into social patterns or habits that conform to the social and cultural roles one fulfils. According to this approach, occupation is analysed in terms of the roles and responsibilities one expects or is expected to fulfil, and dysfunction occurs when performance and expectations diverge. Remediation is generally aimed at rationalizing

expectations, demands, and capabilities and structuring social roles and occupational activities to enhance success. This approach has its foundations in the social sciences, such as sociology and anthropology.

The third tier of the taxonomy contains theories that address specific components of occupation but do not address occupation per se. Often these theories come from other disciplines and provide the underpinnings for theories at the second level of the taxonomy. For example, McColl et al (1993) include role theory, group theory, feminist theory, and theories from anthropology and sociology as components of the socioadaptive approach described in the second tier of their taxonomy.

Users of the annotated bibliography can find articles at their level of interest or need. Academicians and researchers may select articles related to the first or second levels of the taxonomy to gain better understanding of theories that address overarching constructs in the profession (what we know). Practitioners will find articles about theories at the third level (what to do) immediately relevant and applicable to their professional work. The utility of McColl et al's (1993) work for occupational therapy is not that it provides a definitive theoretical classification to which everyone is encouraged to subscribe. Rather, the authors demonstrate their ability, a priori, to see the big picture and to produce it in a way that is understandable and easy for others to follow.

Australian author Kortman (1994) identifies four levels of theoretical information used in occupational therapy. He, too, proposes a top-down, broad-to-specific arrangement and progression of theory. At the broadest level he puts what he calls professional models that widely describe the role and practice of the profession across many client groups and practice settings; for example, the Model of Human Occupation (Kielhofner 1997). Next, Kortman identifies delineation models that provide guidelines for assessment and principles for interventions for particular client groups; for example, biomechanical models that help therapists remediate physical dysfunction of musculo-skeletal origin. Then Kortman proposes application models that describe specific actions for assessment and techniques for intervention. Application models tell you which protocol to use or how to carry out a procedure; for example, using specific neurodevelopmental techniques such as proprioceptive neuromuscular facilitation for clients who have sustained damage to their central nervous system. Finally, Kortman (1994) suggests that practitioners use personal models that reflect their personal values and preferences. It is through personal models that practitioners select from and interpret theoretical information from the three preceding types of models to use in their particular practice environments. Like McColl et al (1993), Kortman organizes his thinking in a way that progresses from 'what we know' in general to 'what to do' in a particular setting with a specific client. Top-down approaches are useful when we are trying to organize a large project with many component parts, or to provide service for a broad range of clients, yet portray a unified approach.

Theory-driven practice guidelines

Another way to connect theory with practice is to look at how some professional organizations have developed theory-driven practice guidelines. A professional association representing its practitioners usually undertakes the preparation of a set of practice guidelines, and volunteer members of the profession participate by serving on committees and review panels. Members' input assures that the practice guidelines reflect all aspects of the profession's domain of interest. The purpose of a set of practice guidelines is to help practitioners identify the problems they can solve. Once produced, practice guidelines are usually updated at regular intervals to reflect new developments in the profession and society, along with new knowledge generated by research. Sometimes, people other than practitioners, for example, policy makers, government agencies, and third-party payers, use practice guidelines. I often wonder what people outside our professions think about the way we articulate our theoretical base in an official document and describe what we do in practice. I found three North American examples of professional practice guidelines that made a clear connection between theory and practice. These examples come from the Canadian Association of Occupational Therapists, the American Physical Therapy Association, and the American Occupational Therapy Association.

Canadian Association of Occupational Therapists

During the 1980s and early 1990s, the Canadian Association of Occupational Therapists produced five guideline documents and an outcome measure that focused on occupational performance and advocated client-centred practice (Canadian Association of Occupational Therapists 1997). Following an impact study, a new set of guidelines was developed as a leadership document to take occupational therapy's major concepts and processes into the twenty-first century. The new guidelines, published as *Enabling Occupation: An Occupational Therapy Perspective* (Canadian Association of Occupational Therapists 1997), are unique in that they emanate from a generic conceptual model, the Canadian Model of Occupational Performance, that defines and describes the profession of occupational therapy in Canada.

The Canadian Model of Occupational Performance is based on a set of occupational therapy values and beliefs, which guides the practice of occupational therapy in Canada. Of particular interest is the seven-stage process of practice. The first stage involves naming, validating, and prioritizing occupational performance issues, and the second stage requires selection of a theoretical approach to guide the remaining stages of the process. Here we see the 'theory first–then practice' sequence at work again. When selecting theoretical approaches, the authors recommend using one or more specific theoretical approaches depending on the complexity of the situation. Theoretical approaches may be changed or added as the client progresses through the therapeutic action plan. The Canadian Model of Occupational Performance is a powerful tool for helping practitioners articulate and organize their approach to treatment. The Canadian occupational therapy practice guidelines clearly show the profession's decision to let theory directly guide practice.

American Physical Therapy Association

The *Guide to Physical Therapist Practice* (American Physical Therapy Association 2001) is now in its second edition. The authors of the document acknowledge that the guide is very much evolutionary on nature. The major purposes of the guide are as follows:

1. to describe physical therapist practice in general, using the *disablement model* as the basis
2. to describe the roles of physical therapists in primary, secondary and tertiary care; in prevention; and in the promotion of health, wellness and fitness
3. to describe the settings in which physical therapists practise
4. to standardize terminology used in and related to physical therapist practice
5. to delineate the tests and measures and interventions that are used in physical therapist practice
6. to delineate preferred practice patterns that will help physical therapists: (a) improve quality of care; (b) enhance positive outcomes of physical therapy services; (c) enhance patient/client satisfaction; (d) promote appropriate utilization of healthcare services; (e) increase efficiency and reduce unwarranted variation in the provision of services; (f) diminish the economic burden of disablement through prevention and promotion of health, wellness, and fitness initiatives.

Following this list of purposes is a very strong statement that says, 'The Guide does not provide specific protocols for treatments, nor are the practice patterns contained in the Guide intended to serve as clinical guidelines'. Clearly, the profession expects its practitioners to engage in clinical reasoning and make informed judgments in each and every individual treatment situation. The Guide uses and expands upon the disablement model first introduced by Nagi (1965, 1969) as one of three concepts that provides 'the theoretical framework and classification scheme by which physical therapists make diagnoses' (American Physical Therapy Association 2001). The *Guide to Physical Therapist Practice* demonstrates how practice guidelines are organized around the theoretical perspective provided by Nagi's disablement model.

American Occupational Therapy Association

The Guide to Occupational Therapy Practice was published in 1999 and is accompanied by 16 sets of practice guidelines for specific clinical conditions. The Guide itself:

• provides guidance but does not preclude professional judgment
• represents an overview of the scope of occupational therapy
• includes only general methods of care
• requires supplemental information in regard to specific conditions
• does not represent specific circumstances of persons served (Moyers 1999, p. 252).

The guide defines occupational therapy and its outcomes, discusses terminology, and describes the scope and the process of delivering occupational therapy service. The Guide itemizes nine theoretical principles for using occupation as intervention. Each principle is substantiated by an extensive literature review that includes case series, correlational studies, meta-analyses, non-randomized trials, outcome studies, qualitative research, randomized trials, and retrospective designs (Moyers 1999). The *Guide to Occupational Therapy Practice* demonstrates how practice generated from a research and evidence-based practice perspective is based on the theoretical underpinnings of the profession.

Integrating the connections between theory and practice

Even though the preceding discussion has shown strong evidence for top-down approaches for connecting theory with practice and theory-driven practice guidelines, I am not convinced that the connection between theory and practice is entirely linear. In Figure 3.2 I have created a framework to represent the way in which I think we integrate theory and practice. Let me explain my reasoning to you. Although I first drew a vertical axis to represent the connection between what we know (theory) and what to do (practice), I quickly added a horizontal axis representing the connection between who we are (practitioner) and who we serve (recipient). Something very important happens at the point where the vertical and horizontal axes intersect. I think a process of reflective reasoning is at work mediating our behind the scenes thinking with our day-to-day actions. I believe it is reflective reasoning that helps us integrate the connections between theory and practice, and in my diagram I use a diamond shape with dotted lines to represent the mediating effect of reflective reasoning. Next, I selected thin, black arrows to show the dynamic relationship between the vertical and horizontal axes and reflective reasoning. I hope the black arrows represent the give and take or tension between the different parts of the diagram, and suggest the possibility of integrating theory and practice from any one of the four different vantage points: what we know, what to do, who we are, and who we serve.

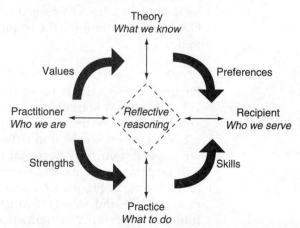

Figure 3.2   *A framework for integrating theory and practice from a practitioner's perspective*

Although I was pleased with my emerging diagram, I felt something else was needed to integrate fully the connection between theory and practice. Finally, I realized that four personal factors—*values, preferences, strengths* and *skills*—play an important part in the way we each integrate the connection between theory and practice, and I linked the four personal factors with strong, black arrows. Let me now explain the relationship between the four personal factors and the other parts of the diagram.

Values

Our personal and professional values link who we are as practitioners with what we know (theory). Our values influence the type of theoretical information to which we are drawn. Some of us are inherently drawn to detailed, mechanistic aspects of our professional knowledge whilst others prefer more global, intuitive concepts. Our values reflect our basic philosophy of the world, and consequently we select theories that are compatible with our values.

Preferences

Based on what we know, most of us have strong preferences for working with different kinds of clients and patients. Some of us are passionate about working with children and others are moved to work with elders. If we are to experience cohesion between what we know and who we serve, we must honour our personal and professional preferences. Theories that have little correspondence between the *what* we know and *who* we serve will not work well for us. We will be faced with a forced-fit dilemma, the death knell for creativity.

Strengths

Our personal and professional strengths lead us to operate in some practice settings better than others. Some of us are much more suited to fast-paced acute care settings, others to the more unpredictable rhythms of community-based practice. Some of us like variety and seek settings where there is a lot of diversity in the practice milieu. Our strengths reinforce the connection between who we are and what to do.

Skills

Finally, what to do is often influenced by our areas of expertise. When we know something works, we have confidence in our skills, and therefore contribute to the quality aspect of our practice. If we are to experience cohesion between what to do and who we serve, we must honour our personal and professional skills. These skills will lead us to practice environments that provide the just right challenge for us. In Figure 3.2, the outer circle created by our *values, preferences, skills* and *strengths* must be sufficiently taut to support the inner core of reflective practice. With this overall framework in place, we are in a position to integrate theory and practice creatively. Whenever we have an opportunity to reflect on our practice, we can use Figure 3.2 to help us look at what we are doing from many different perspectives.

Integrating theory and practice in a variety of professional domains

In this section I bring the chapter to a close by describing examples that demonstrate ways in which theory and practice are integrated in two different professional domains. The first example is one from my own domain of educational practice and the second example is taken from a published journal article that describes an area of clinical practice.

Education

As a university professor, I am frequently required to integrate theory and practice in many of the classes I teach, hence my interest in writing this chapter. One example that vividly stands out in my mind was my first attempt at distance education, an experience that more aptly might be named 'Fools rush in'!

Back in 1985, I launched a new post graduate degree program for occupational therapists who worked full-time and wished to take courses on a part-time, evening-hours basis. A year later, Barbara O'Shea, then Director of the School of Occupational Therapy at Dalhousie University in Halifax, Nova Scotia, Canada, invited me to consider combining forces with her in offering post-graduate courses via distance education. Dalhousie University was very experienced in using distance technology to deliver degree programs to students at a distance but did not yet have a post-graduate program in occupational therapy. Occupational therapists in Atlantic, Canada, were keen to participate in post-graduate education, and based on the relative strengths of each university, we decided to collaborate and offer one of my existing courses on a trial basis. The challenge before me, then, was to redesign one of my courses for delivery using distance technology. Could I use theory as a friend or foe? Let me tell you about the way I responded to the challenge.

First, I went shopping in the literature for theory about distance education. I behaved as a consumer of theory while I read journal articles (consumer reports) that described the effectiveness of different distance delivery methods. I learned that two-way audio teleconferencing was the least expensive of the teleconferencing methods and well suited to interaction, especially if visual material was not an essential element. Two-way audio teleconferencing had immediate appeal to me because I valued interaction as a key ingredient in my post-graduate classes. Consequently, based on my reading, I 'bought' the *concept* of using two-way audio teleconferencing as the major medium of delivery. This purchase was an act of faith on my part because I had neither previous practical experience with, nor training in, distance education.

Next, I had to envision how my existing course would fit into a new delivery medium, one that would keep me apart from the students. Again, I shopped for theory, this time educational theory. The design of my post-graduate degree program was heavily influenced by Malcolm Knowle's (1980) theory of adult learning which included *constructs* such as self-directedness, problem-centred learning, immediate relevance, life experience, and internal motivation. I had embraced these constructs and used them in the design of my existing courses. I had firsthand experience linking theory to practice and directly saw the results of my theory-based decisions. I had every confidence that these principles would hold up in a new context. What I did not know, though, was how to orchestrate the learning for the students under the conditions of distance delivery. Another theorist came to my rescue.

I had recently come across the work of Raymond Wlodkowski (1985) and his Time Continuum Model of Motivation. Wlodkowski's work suggested that timing (a temporal *proposition*) the application of motivational strategies was critical for their success. He proposed that existing theories of motivation had six major factors in common: attitude, need, stimulation, affect, competence, and reinforcement. Wlodkowski linked these six factors to three critical stages in the learning cycle: motivational strategies that addressed learner attitudes and needs are required at the beginning of the learning cycle; motivational strategies needed for stimulation and affect are needed during the cycle of learning; and motivational strategies that support competence and reinforcement are best used at the end of the learning cycle (Table 3.2). I 'bought' these temporal propositions and made the sequencing decisions that moved the course along (Mitcham 1989).

Table 3.2   *Linking theory and practice: using Wlodkowski's Time Continuum Model of Motivation to redesign a post-graduate course for delivery via distance education*

Three stages of the learning cycle	Six motivational factors	Examples of instructional strategies used in post-graduate courses offered via distance education
Beginning	*Attitude:* learner's positive or negative predisposition to people, ideas, events	Created a positive attitude by making an initial visit at the central distance site to get to know students and for students to get to know each other
	Need: internal force that moves learner in the direction of a goal	Met instructional safety needs by developing a structured *Learning guide* to provide support for students while the professor was distant from them
During	*Stimulation:* change in perception or environment that makes learner active	Maintained learner attention from a distance by using multiple learning modalities throughout course
	Affect: emotional experiences that influence learner	Maintained emotional climate by conducting a midterm visit to central distance site to meet with students individually and to give formative feedback on drafts of term papers
Ending	*Competence:* learner's awareness of personal mastery	Enhanced learner confidence via feedback from peers and professor after final oral presentations via audio teleconference
	Reinforcement: learner's response to events that support and maintain learning	Affirmed learner desire to continue with distance learning by providing summative feedback from professor on term papers and requiring learners to engage in self-evaluation to reflect on their progress

Figure 3.3 shows you some examples of how I went about linking theory and practice. Wlodkowski's six major motivational factors gave me a set of parameters for adapting my course. Without such parameters, my first foray into distance education would have been a disaster. The time I spent grappling with the theoretical concepts and propositions prior to teaching the course was critical to its success. I had confidence in the a priori decisions I made and felt I had a firm foundation on which to build my course. Within my chosen set of parameters, I had freedom to make changes as the course progressed. The unfamiliar became more familiar, and the course came alive, paving the way for several more distance courses between 1987 and 1993 (Mitcham and O'Shea 1994).

In the spirit of holding my own feet to the fire, let me superimpose my educational example on to the framework I drew earlier in Figure 3.2 as a way to explore further the integration of theory and practice. Look now at Figure 3.3 and you will see that the axis what we know–what to do links the educational theories of Knowles (1980) and Wlodkowski (1985) with the educational practice environment of redesigning courses for distance delivery. The who we are–who we serve axis clearly links the professor with the post-graduate students, and reflective instructional reasoning is now required to mediate behind-the scenes thinking with day-to-day instructional actions.

On the outer circle, you can see that my instructional *values* of inter-action and life experience influenced the choice of educational theo-ries. Likewise, my instructional *preferences* for working with small groups using the discussion method is well suited to work with post-graduate students and compatible with the selected educational theo-ries. My instructional *strengths* include teaching adults rather than children and a strong set of interpersonal traits that provide an active learning environment for the students. Finally, my instructional *skills*

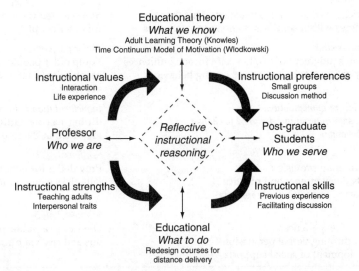

Figure 3.3 *Integrating theory and practice from an educator's perspective*

made it possible to redesign a course for distance delivery because of the depth and breadth of my previous instructional experience and my expert ability to facilitate discussion, a skill needed for engaging with post-graduate students. With all these elements in place, I was able to create the desired outcome and offer a quality learning experience for the students. Why am I telling you about my course in such painstaking detail? Mainly because the process I went through is analogous to the context of clinical practice.

Practice

Having scrutinized my own work, I wanted an opportunity to look at someone else's work, and examine it in the context of this chapter. I selected a journal article from the published literature that clearly articulated the theoretical basis for the development of a clinical program. Cheal and Clemson (2001), two Australian occupational therapists, adapted an existing falls prevention program based on the work of Albert Bandura, a social psychologist. When Cheal and Clemson (2001) shopped for theory, they 'bought' Bandura's self-efficacy theory for three reasons. First, they perceived the theory as having relevance for their profession. Second, the *concept* of self-efficacy was being used in studies and programs that focused on helping people initiate and maintain changes in health behavior. Third, the concept of self-efficacy had the potential to form the basis for the learning and teaching approaches used in the program. What is self-efficacy? In this article, self-efficacy is operationally defined as 'a person's perception of their capabilities within specific situations and activities'.

Table 3.3 *Linking theory and practice: using Bandura's Self-Efficacy Theory for the development of a falls prevention program*

Bandura's Self-Efficacy Theory	Occupational therapy practice
Major concept Self-efficacy is a person's perception of his/her capabilities within specific situations and activities	*Program description* Steady as You Go — a 6 week falls prevention program for older people
Major proposition A person's judgment of his/her self-efficacy influences activity choice, environment and coping behaviors	*Major purpose* Equip older people with skills and beliefs in their capabilities in fall-risk situations, specifically outdoor activities
Theoretical recommendations *for inclusion in programs designed to change* *health behaviors*	*Implementation of theoretical recommendations* during six consecutive weekly sessions with content identified in the research literature
● Information provision ● Skills development and practice ● Exposure to positive role models	*Sessions 1, 2, 6* Provided information and demonstration on modifying falls-risks using multidisciplinary and peer presenters
● Mastery experiences ● Self-affirming verbal persuasion ● Development of social supports	*Sessions 3, 4, 5* Outings to a public park, local shopping center via public bus and city via train

In Table 3.3, I have extrapolated from the journal article to show you how the major *concepts, propositions* and theoretical recommendations of Bandura's self-efficacy theory (1995) were linked to practice, in this case to a falls prevention program. The major concept of self-efficacy was reflected in the title of the program, 'Steady As You Go', and the major proposition of the theory directed the purpose of the program. Six theoretical recommendations were implemented into the 6-week program. In reading the article, it was clear to me how Cheal and Clemson (2001) had put theory to work for them. When they described the study they conducted to evaluate their program, they discussed the utility of using theory to guide their practice, and I quote directly (p. 89):

> This study found that Bandura's theory (1982) was easily translated into practice and was readily applicable to the issue of falls prevention among older people. It was useful as it provided specific recommendations for enhancing self-efficacy which can lead to health behaviour change, and, in particular, an emphasis on developing mastery in daily activities.

Bandura's theory is appropriate for health promotion programs due to its emphasis on multiple strategies for producing change in health behaviors.

In this example, we see how pleased the authors were with their success, and how they recommend using self-efficacy theory as the basis for other health promotion programs.

As you progress in your career, you will have many opportunities to develop new programs similar to mine and that of Cheal and Clemson (2001). You will strengthen your professional credibility when you can describe your work from a theoretical basis, and you will be perceived as thoughtful, logical, rational, methodical, knowledgeable, innovative, and creative. When you present your work in a way that can be replicated, and in a way that lends itself to analysis and evaluation, your work will become the stimulus for generating new knowledge, modifying existing knowledge, and strengthening the ties that integrate theory and practice.

Activity box 3.1

1. Personal Reflections

Take some time to think about how you make the connection between theory and practice. How would you describe the way you connect theory and practice? Do you operate in the *theory first–then practice* sequence? Are there examples in this chapter that are analogous to your practice situation?

2. Professional Reflections

How does your profession address the role of theory in practice? Does your profession have a set of theory-driven practice guidelines? Do you have a copy of them? Where would you find the latest theoretical information in your profession?

Continued

Activity box 3.1 *cont'd*

3. Application
Look at Figure 3.2 and think about a specific context in which you provide service. Try to embellish this figure with your information, the way I did in Figure 3.3. Do your embellishments capture the essence of what you do?
Look at Table 3.1 and evaluate your progress as a consumer of theory. How far along the progression of skills are you? How well can you shop for concepts and propositions?
Look at Tables 3.2 and 3.3. Next time you have to design a new program, use these formats to help you select and transpose theoretical information. Look for ways to get theory to work for you.

References

American Physical Therapy Association 2001 Guide to physical therapist practice, 2nd edn. American Physical Therapy Association, Alexandria, VA

Assael H 1981 Consumer behaviour and marketing action. Wadsworth, Belmont, CA

Bandura A 1982 Self-efficacy mechanisms in human agency. American Psychologist 37:122–147

Bandura A 1995 Self-efficacy in changing societies. Cambridge University Press, Cambridge

Canadian Association of Occupational Therapists 1997 Enabling occupation: an occupational therapy perspective. Canadian Association of Occupational Therapists, Ottawa, Ontario

Cheal B, Clemson L 2001 Older people enhancing self-efficacy in fall-risk situations. Australian Occupational Therapy Journal 48:80–91

Creek J, Ormston C 1996 The essential elements of professional motivation. British Journal of Occupational Therapy 59:7–10

Depoy E, Gitlin L N 1994 Introduction to research. Understanding and applying multiple strategies 1st edn. Mosby, St Louis

Depoy E, Gitlin L N 1998 Introduction to research. Understanding and applying multiple strategies, 2nd edn. Mosby, St Louis

Hagedorn R 1995 Occupational therapy: perspectives and processes. Churchill Livingstone, Edinburgh

Kielhofner G 1997 Conceptual foundations of occupational therapy 2nd edn. F A Davis, Philadelphia

Knowles M S 1980 The modern practice of adult education: from pedagogy to andragogy, 2nd edn. Association Press, New York

Kortman B 1994 The eye of the beholder: models in occupational therapy. Australian Occupational Therapy Journal 41:115–122

Krefting L H 1985 The use of conceptual models in clinical practice. Canadian Journal of Occupational Therapy 52:173–178

Kuhn T S 1996 The structure of scientific revolutions 3rd edn. University of Chicago Press, Chicago

Leinonen E, Kerbel D 1999 Relevance theory and pragmatic impairment. International Journal of Language and Communication Disorders 34:367–390

McColl M A, Law M, Stewart D 1993 Theoretical basis of occupational therapy: an annotated bibliography of applied theory in the professional literature. Slack, Thorofare, NJ

Maslow A H 1970 Motivation and personality 2nd edn. Harper & Row, New York

Metcalfe A B, Lawes N 1998 A modern interpretation of the Rood approach. Physical Therapy Reviews 3:195–212

Mitcham M D 1985 Integrating research into occupational therapy. A teaching guide for academic and clinical educators. American Occupational Therapy Foundation, Rockville, MD

Mitcham M D 1989 Bridging the gap: building a sense of community for graduate students at a distance. Paper presented at the 5th Annual Conference on Teaching at a Distance, Madison, Wisconsin

Mitcham M D, O'Shea B J 1994 Using audio teleconferencing to link occupational therapy graduate students in the United States and Canada. American Journal of Occupational Therapy 48:619–625

Mosey A C 1992 Applied scientific inquiry in the health professions: an epistemological orientation, 1st edn. American Occupational Therapy Association, Rockville, MD

Mosey A C 1996 Applied scientific inquiry in the health professions: an epistemological orientation, 2nd edn. American Occupational Therapy Association, Bethesda, MD

Moyers P A 1999 The guide to occupational therapy practice. American Journal of Occupational Therapy 53:247–322

Nagi S 1965 Some conceptual issues in disability and rehabilitation. In: Sussman M (ed) Sociology and rehabilitation. Institute of Medicine, National Academy Press, Washington, DC, p 100–113

Nagi S 1969 Disability and rehabilitation. Ohio State University Press, Columbus, OH

Portney L G, Watkins M P 1993 Foundations of clinical research. Applications to practice, 1st edn. Appleton & Lange, Norwalk, CT

Portney L G, Watkins M P 2001 Foundations of clinical research. Applications to practice, 2nd edn. Prentice Hall Health, Upper Saddle River, NJ

Prochaska J O, DiClemente C C 1983 Stages and processes of self-change of smoking: towards an integrative model of change. Journal of Counseling and Clinical Psychology 51:390–395

Reed K L 1984 Models of practice in occupational therapy. Williams & Wilkins, Baltimore, MD

Reed K L 1997 Theory and frame of reference. In: Neistadt M E, Crepeau E B (eds). Willard and Spackman's occupational therapy 9th edn. Lippincott, Philadelphia

Reynolds P D 1971 A primer in theory construction. Macmillan, New York

Rosenstock I M, Stretcher V J, Becker M H 1994 The health belief model and HIV risk behaviour change. In: DiClemente R J, Peterson J L (eds) Preventing AIDS: theories and methods for behavioural interventions. Plenum, New York

Schön D A 1983 The reflective practitioner. Basic Books, New York

Shumway-Cook A, Woollacott M H 2001 Motor control: theory and practical applications 2nd edn. Lippincott, Williams & Wilkins: Philadelphia

Smith R H, Sharpe M 1994 Brunstromm therapy: is it still relevant to stroke rehabilitation? Physiotherapy Theory and Practice 10:87–94

Williams K B, Gadbury-Amyot C C, Bray K K, Manne D, Collins P 1998 Oral health-related quality of life: a model for dental hygiene. Journal of Dental Hygiene 72:19–26

Wlodkowski R J 1985 Enhancing adult motivation. Jossey-Bass, San Francisco

Young M, Quinn E 1991 Theories and practice of occupational therapy. Churchill Livingstone, Edinburgh

4

Evidence-based practice: informing practice and critically evaluating related research

M. Clare Taylor

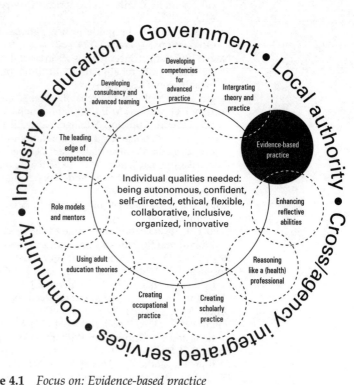

Figure 4.1 *Focus on: Evidence-based practice*

Chapter outline

In this chapter I will explore the nature of evidence-based practice (EBP) and how it has evolved from evidence-based medicine (EBM) into not only EBP, but also evidence-based occupational therapy (EB OT), evidence-based nursing (EBN) and evidence-based physiotherapy (EB PT), amongst others. The chapter then outlines and explores the processes and skills required of the evidence-based practitioner. The nature of evidence will then be explored, with a broad definition of evidence being adopted. The critical use of evidence will be discussed as well as ways of developing an evidence-based culture within the workplace. The chapter will conclude by giving an overview of the range of evidence-based resources available to the advanced practitioner.

Key words

Clinical effectiveness, clinical governance, quantitative research, qualitative research

Anticipated outcomes   As a result of reading this chapter, I anticipate that you will be able to:

- identify what EBP means for you and your area of practice
- identify the EBP skills that you already possess and those that you need to develop, and be able to outline strategies that will allow you to develop these skills
- explore the nature of 'evidence' and the breadth of material that might be used as evidence to explore your practice
- develop a clinical scenario into an evidence-based question and explore a diverse range of evidence relevant to this scenario
- identify activities that will help you to develop an evidence-based culture within your workplace.

Introduction   EBP was seen as one of the buzzwords of the 1990s. However, unlike other fashions, EBP remains one of the underpinning concepts of health and social care of the century and is enshrined in policy such as *The New NHS: Modern, Dependable* (Department of Health 1997) and National Service Frameworks (Department of Health 2000, 2001). The critical use of evidence will be an essential tool as health professionals argue the case for the practice of their specific skills and interventions to Primary Care Trusts and other purchasers. Advanced practitioners will be involved in, and leaders of, practice developments that are evidence-based and they will be involved in developing an evidence-based culture.

EBP is developing. It has grown beyond the rigidly scientific approach of EBM. This chapter offers a personal perspective of the ways in which EBP might develop and the ways that advanced practitioners might be at the forefront of the development not just of EBP and interventions but also of EBP itself.

The aim of this chapter is to provide practical examples and activities to help readers to develop their understanding and application of EBP. The activity boxes throughout the chapter can be used by the reader as an individual, or as a group as a way of developing practice and skills within the staff team. Whilst many examples are drawn from the author's experience as an occupational therapist, it is hoped that this approach does not exclude colleagues from other professional groups from finding relevance for their own practice areas.

Setting the scene   Before exploring how we can become evidence-based practitioners, it is worth exploring both the nature and the origins of EBP. This will provide us with a stepping stone for a discussion of EB OT, EB PT and the other variants of EBP.

EBP has its roots in EBM and so we should begin our exploration of the nature of EBP with a definition of EBM. Sackett et al (1997, p. 71) have defined EBM as:

> The conscientious, explicit and judicious use of current best evidence in making decisions about the care of individual patients, based on skills which allow the doctor to evaluate both personal experiences and external evidence in a systematic and objective manner.

While this definition can be seen as a starting point for an exploration of EBP, it immediately raises a number of dilemmas for the evidence-based therapist. Firstly, how can this use of evidence to inform practice be linked to client-centred practice? The emphasis is on the practitioner to evaluate the evidence. However, if the decision-making process is explicit, as outlined in the definition, this implies that the client is involved in the process, although s/he might not be seen as the driving force behind the decision-making process, as would be expected in true client-centred practice. This dilemma will be explored further as we discuss the process of EBP. Secondly, basing decisions on evidence might mean that a rigid, cookbook, approach is applied, with research evidence being indiscriminately applied to all similar clients. However, if evidence is critically appraised and judiciously applied, the narrow cookbook approach can be avoided. The third dilemma is probably the major stumbling block for the development of EBP into EB OT/EB PT, namely, the nature of 'evidence' and what exactly is accepted as 'best' evidence. This dilemma will be explored in some depth later on in this chapter, as the nature of evidence is crucial to the successful development of EBP and evidence-based cultures within health professions.

EBP is about 'doing the right things right' (Gray 1997, p. 20), about 'asking the right questions' (Cusick 2001, p. 104), about ensuring that practice is based on up-to-date, valid and reliable (or trustworthy) evidence of the effectiveness of the interventions being used. Surely this is self-evident. Any self-respecting health or social care professional would always ensure that her/his practice was based on up-to-date, valid and reliable (or trustworthy) evidence that what s/he was doing was effective? Refer to Activity Box 4.1 to help you reflect on how evidence-based your practice is.

Activity box 4.1	How evidence-based are you?
	Briefly describe a client you have worked with recently:
	■ What problems did s/he have?
	■ What interventions did you use?
	Briefly outline your clinical reasoning:
	■ Why did you identify those particular issues as problems?
	■ How did you identify those problems?
	■ Why did you decide to use those interventions?
	What evidence did you base your decisions on?
	Which of the following influenced your decisions?
	■ Past experience
	■ Custom and practice/always do things that way
	■ Things taught during preregistration education and training
	■ Discussion with colleagues
	■ Clinical guidelines

Activity box 4.1 *cont'd*	■ Care pathways ■ Departmental policy ■ Government policy ■ Attendance at a short course/workshop ■ Presentation by an expert ■ Information from a professional special-interest group ■ Professional reading ■ Research evidence ■ Critical appraised research evidence ■ Evidence-based clinical guidelines Do you have any evidence that your interventions were effective? ■ Does this evidence come from the client? ■ Is this evidence based on your observations? ■ Is this evidence based on your opinions? ■ Is this evidence based on any form of standardized outcome measure?

Do not be surprised if your main source of evidence/influence is your own past experience and information that you learnt during preregistration training: you will not be alone. Previous research studies with occupational therapists, physiotherapists and speech and language therapists (Pringle 1999, Upton 1999a, b) and physiotherapists (Turner and Whitfield, 1997, 1999), amongst others, have found that most health professionals rely mainly on their previous experience for decision-making. Not only does this research finding highlight the need for advanced practitioners to become champions of EBP and an evidence-based culture, it also highlights some of the reasons why EBP should be high on the agenda for advanced practitioners.

One of the commonly cited (Trinder 2000) driving forces for the development of EBP has been the research–practice gap. Other drivers have been the fact that research evidence is often not high-quality and so must be used with caution, and the fact that so many research papers are being published that it is impossible to keep up with the latest evidence. These factors mean that the interventions being used might not be effective and that interventions based on 'custom and practice' are not challenged. However, challenging and changing well-established practice is uncomfortable. EBP is as much about developing a culture, which is questioning, as it is about finding specific pieces of research evidence to underpin practice. The issue of change management and research utilization will be discussed later in this chapter.

EBP, with its roots in medical practice, is underpinned by a philosophy that does not always sit comfortably with the philosophies underpinning all the health professions. This has led to a reluctance to incorporate EBP and a lack of consensus about the meaning of EBP for different professional groups (Dubouloz et al 1999, Egan et al 1998), which has led, in turn, to the redefinition of EBP by different professional groups. These re-definitions of EBP should be viewed positively. They demonstrate a willingness, by these different professional groups, to engage with the debates about EBP and to own and develop it so that it can be used to demonstrate the effectiveness of interventions and the evidence underpinning professional practice. EBP is evolving to become EB OT and EB PT, amongst others. How do these variations differ from each other and from the original EBM?

Evidence-based occupational therapy

EBP has been advocated within occupational therapy for some years, with special issues of various occupational therapy journals dedicated to EBP (*British Journal of Occupational Therapy* 1997 vol. 60 (11), 2001 vol. 64 (5), *Canadian Journal of Occupational Therapy* 1998 vol. 65 (3)), books and articles on implementing EBP (Brown and Rodgers 1999, Taylor 2000). However, as Dubouloz et al (1999) pointed out, occupational therapists have been slow to integrate research evidence into their clinical decision-making processes. One of the barriers to EBP within occupational therapy has been the need to reconcile a client-centred approach to practice with a medical model approach to EBP. Client-centred evidence and research evidence were seen as incompatible. In order to recognize the range of evidence available to the occupational therapist, evidence-based occupational therapy has been defined as:

> Client-centred enablement of occupation, based on client information and a critical review of relevant research, expert consensus and past experience (Canadian Association of Occupational Therapists et al, 1999, p. 267).

Evidence-based physiotherapy

Physiotherapists have chosen not to redefine EBP into a more specific form of evidence-based physiotherapy; they appear to have accepted the Sackett et al (1997) definition cited earlier in this chapter (Bithell 2000). There has, however, been debate about the nature of evidence used in physiotherapy and in the appropriateness of the medically based hierarchy of evidence (Bithell 2000, Straker 1999). Physiotherapists appear to draw on three types of evidence to underpin their clinical reasoning. These three forms of evidence are clinical experience (as highlighted earlier), a biological rationale for why an intervention should work and explicit tests of the effects of interventions (Research Committee (Victorian branch) of the Australian Physiotherapy Association 1999). The hierarchy of evidence will be discussed in detail later on in the chapter, when the hierarchy proposed by Australian physiotherapist Leon Straker (1999) will be compared with medically based hierarchies of evidence. A major contribution to EBP that has been developed by physiotherapists is PEDro and the Centre for Evidence-based Physiotherapy (Herbert et al 1998/9). PEDro is a database of clinical research, mainly randomized controlled trials (RCTs) and systematic reviews of RCTs, which have been scored on the basis of methodological quality (for more details about PEDro, see the further reading and resources section at the end of this chapter).

Evidence-based everything else

Many disciplines and professional groups have developed and evolved their own approaches to EBP. These groups are as diverse as nursing, social work, human resource management, psychology and education. Indeed, Trinder (2000) provided an interesting and insightful critique of the EBP explosion.

EBN has, perhaps, the most to contribute to the current exploration of EBP, with definitions and developmental initiatives. DiCenso et al (1998, p. 38) have defined EBN as:

> The process by which nurses make clinical decisions using the best available research evidence, their clinical expertise and patient preferences, in the context of available resources.

The reader will note that this definition has many similarities both with Sackett et al's (1997) original definition of EBM and with the definition of EB OT.

Two other major contributions from EBN are the EBN Centres:

- Centre for Evidence-based Nursing at the University of York
- Joanna Briggs Institute of Evidence-based Nursing and Midwifery

and the international journal *Evidence-based Nursing*, published quarterly as a joint initiative between the BMJ Publishing Group and the Royal College of Nursing. This journal publishes structured summaries with clinical commentaries of nursing-related research.

As the discussion above highlights, EBP is developing and becoming 'owned' by different professional groups. Part of this ownership process is the re-definition of EBP. However, what is interesting to note is that the essential components of any of these re-definitions of EBP remain faithful to Sackett et al's (1997) original definition. Evidence-based *medicine* has tended to concentrate on the 'current, best *research* evidence'; however, as the discussion of the nature of evidence later in this chapter will demonstrate, EBP has developed ways of utilizing evidence from research, from practitioner expertise and from the client's perspective.

The process and skills of EBP

This section will remind readers of the process of EBP; however, it will concentrate on ways of developing the skills required for the first stages of the EBP process. Ways of implementing and utilizing EBP will be discussed later in the chapter.

The process of EBP appears simple and straightforward. It mirrors the problem-solving and research processes. It is only when the process is broken down into its component parts that the complexity of becoming an evidence-based practitioner emerges. The process of EBP consists of the following five stages:

- identifying a problem and clinical question
- finding the appropriate evidence to address the question
- appraising the evidence
- utilizing the evidence in practice
- evaluating the impact of the evidence on practice.

The process of EBP should not be viewed as a one-off event: it should run parallel to the process of clinical reasoning. At each stage of the intervention process it should be possible to explore and review the appropriate evidence.

The skills of EBP

In order to develop as an evidence-based practitioner it is important to identify the skills required for each stage of the process. Table 4.1 gives an overview of the skills of EBP.

Identify a problem and clinical question

The first stage in the EBP process is to identify the problem and question for which you wish to explore the evidence base. This is the stage at which you ask what Cusick (2001) described as the 'right' questions. These questions can cover the whole of the intervention process and can be as diverse as:

- Is this the right assessment to use?
- Is this the best frame of reference?
- Is daily activity/treatment/intervention the right amount?
- Am I the right type of therapist?
  - Should it be an occupational therapist or a physiotherapist?
  - What are the right skills needed for this intervention?
- Is this the right intervention?
- Is home/hospital the right location for intervention?

Table 4.1   *The skills of evidence-based practice*

Identifying a problem and clinical question
- Understanding and articulating practice
- Developing a clinical scenario
- Developing a question using the PICO structure (see Activity Box 4.3 for an explanation of PICO)

Finding the appropriate evidence to address the question
- Identifying available resources
- Developing key words
- Database searching
- Understanding the meaning and variety of 'evidence'
- Articulating qualitative evidence

Appraising the evidence
- Critical reading and appraisal skills
- Identifying the strengths and weaknesses of different types of evidence
- Understanding the concepts of rigour, trustworthiness, validity
- Understanding data analysis and interpretation
- Reflection and synthesis of the range of evidence

Utilizing the evidence in practice
- Using evidence to evaluate and change practice
- Application of evidence to practice
- Critical reflection on current practice
- Clinical reasoning
- Change management

Evaluating the impact of the evidence on practice
- Critical review of practice
- Objective setting
- Audit

- Is this the right client? Will s/he improve without any intervention?
- What are the right factors to consider when planning a new intervention?

Activity box 4.2	Developing a scenario Identify an incident or client from your current practice for which you would like to explore the evidence base. Briefly describe the key aspects of the incident or client.
	Example 1 ■ 32-year-old unmarried female ■ Diagnosed with chronic fatigue syndrome ■ Difficulty completing household tasks ■ Unable to work for the last 7 months ■ On medication for depression ■ Referred to occupational therapy for energy conservation and relaxation training ■ She has heard about cognitive behaviour therapy and wants to know if 'it would help her be able to feel better and look after herself more'
	Example 2 ■ Physiotherapist as a member of a dedicated Stroke Therapy team ■ The team is interested in developing the long-term and community aspects of the service ■ The team is interested in establishing a Stroke Club ■ You are interested in locating information that might guide the development of such a group, particularly information from the perspective of group members about what they might want from a Stroke Club

The initial stimulus for a question will be a particular incident or practice scenario. Articulating this scenario will help to develop the final question. The clearer you are with your question, the more likely you are to be successful in searching for suitable evidence. For help with formulating this scenario, see Activity Box 4.2.

It might be helpful to try to identify a group of like-minded colleagues who would be interested in exploring the evidence base of their practice. This could be a uni-professional or a multiprofessional group. Establish a time for regular meetings. At your 1st meeting spend time developing clinical scenarios and deciding which ones to explore in more detail.

Having articulated the scenario, it is possible to refine this further to create an EBP question. Evidence-based questions are usually articulated in terms of:

What is the evidence for the effectiveness of x (the intervention) for y (the outcome) in a patient with z (the problem or diagnosis)?

Whilst this approach to structuring questions is derived from the EBM approach, it can quite easily be adapted to include a wide range of problems, interventions and outcomes. Richardson et al (1995) proposed the notion of a 'well-built' question which includes:

- *Problem*—how would you describe the client/group of clients or the issue being considered?
- *Intervention*—what main intervention or activity is being considered?
- *Comparison or alternative intervention* (if appropriate)—what is the main alternative to be compared with the intervention?
- *Outcome*—what outcomes would you like to measure/improve/affect?

This is often referred to as the PICO model of clinical question. See Activity Box 4.3 about developing an EBP question.

Activity box 4.3	Developing an evidence-based practice (EBP) question
	Review the scenario you developed earlier. Using the PICO structure, identify the:
	■ Problem
	■ Intervention
	■ Comparison or alternative intervention (if appropriate)
	■ Outcome
	and write your EBP question
	Example 1
	Problem — Patient with chronic fatigue syndrome
	Intervention — Cognitive behaviour therapy
	Comparison intervention — Conventional medical intervention
	Outcomes — Reduction in fatigue; improvement in level of function
	Question — For patients with chronic fatigue syndrome, does cognitive behaviour therapy reduce fatigue and improve level of function in comparison with standard medical intervention?
	Example 2
	Problem — Patients who have had strokes
	Intervention — Stroke Clubs and/or group intervention
	Comparison outcome — Not appropriate for this question
	Outcomes — Successful planning of intervention group
	Question — What are the important issues to be aware of when considering establishing a Stroke Club or group for people who have had strokes?

Finding the appropriate evidence to address the question

Having identified a suitable scenario and used the information from the scenario to identify the components of the EBP question, you then have the information to move on to the next stage of the process—

finding some evidence which might provide the evidence base for your chosen intervention. However, you should not begin to search for evidence just yet. Before setting foot in the library or logging on to the Internet you should spend some time developing a clear search strategy and identifying the resources at your disposal. Searching without a clear search strategy will result in frustration and wasted time with little or no useful evidence at the end of the search.

The potential range of resources available to the evidence-based practitioner is vast. Table 4.2 identifies the key resources for EBP.

Further details of these resources can be found at the end of the chapter or in Taylor (2000). However, please note that you may not have access to all of these resources.

Table 4.2 *Evidence-based practice resources*

Specialist databases	*General databases*
■ Cochrane Library	■ MEDLINE/ PubMed
■ PEDro	■ CINAHL
■ OTDBASE	■ AMED
■ DHSS-DATA	■ EMBASE
	■ ERIC
	■ ASSIA
	■ HealthSTAR
	■ PsychLIT

Web-based resources
■ Netting the evidence
■ OMNI

Human resources
■ librarians

Having identified the potential resources at your disposal (see Activity Box 4.4) you can now begin to develop your search strategy. A good search strategy should consist of:

● a clear question
● type of research evidence required
● database(s) to be searched
● search terms
● estimated budget available for photocopying and Inter Library Loans
● a time scale for completion of search and evidence gathering.

Activity box 4.4	Identifying ways of accessing evidence-based practice resources
	Have you made friends with your librarian?
	● Do you know what databases your library has access to?
	Do you have access to the internet?
	● Do you have access to a local intranet facility?
	● What databases and other resources are available on the intranet?
	What resources and search facilities does your professional association provide?

Different types of EBP questions will require different types of research to provide the 'best' evidence; the nature of evidence will be discussed later in the chapter. Any database will have a specific focus, whether it is biomedical (MEDLINE), RCTs and systematic reviews (the Cochrane Library) or social sciences (ASSIA). Many topics of interest to the advanced practitioner will draw on a variety of disciplines for evidence. It is therefore useful to identify more than one database for searching. Although using multiple databases will result in some repetition of information, it will also provide a greater breadth of resources and diversity of evidence. Searching for evidence is costly, both in terms of time and in terms of the financial costs of photocopying and Inter Library Loans. It is worth setting clear time and financial limits before beginning the search. Table 4.3 on page 101, gives some tips for successful searching.

Space in this chapter does not permit me to explore the intricacies of searching in any detail (see Activity Box 4.5). More information is available in a variety of EBP sources, e.g. Taylor (2000) and Palmer and Brice (1999).

Activity box 4.5	Developing a search strategy
	Using the scenario and question you developed earlier:
	■ Clarify your question
	■ Can you be more specific about the:
	■ problem?
	■ intervention?
	■ outcome?
	■ What type of evidence would best answer your question?
	■ What databases do you want to search?
	■ What key words/terms can you identify from your question? (start with the problem and the intervention)
	■ Can any of these terms be usefully combined by the use of Boolean operators (AND or OR), truncated or enclosed in " "?
	■ Do you want to set limits for your search, in terms of publication date or language?

Example 1		
	Question	What is the evidence for the effectiveness of cognitive behaviour therapy in reducing fatigue and improving function in a client with chronic fatigue syndrome?
	Type of research	Question about the effectiveness of treatment/interventions—need to look for systematic reviews and randomized controlled trials (RCTs)
	Database(s)	Cochrane Library/MEDLINE
	Key words	"chronic fatigue syndrome" AND "cognitive behaviour therapy"
	Limits	None

Activity box 4.5 *cont'd*	Search outcome	Two completed reviews and five RCTs, including: Price J R, Couper J 2001 Cognitive behaviour therapy for adults with chronic fatigue syndrome (Cochrane review). In: The Cochrane Library, Issue 1. Update Software, Oxford Sharpe M, Hawton K, Simkin S et al 1996 Cognitive behaviour therapy for chronic fatigue syndrome: a randomised controlled trial. British Medical Journal, 312: 22–26
Example 2	Question	What are the important issues to be aware of when considering establishing a Stroke Club or group for people who have had strokes?
	Type of research	Question about the insider perspective—need to look for qualitative research
	Database(s)	PubMed (http:// www.ncbi.nlm.nih.gov/PubMed/) and CINAHL
	Key words	"stroke" AND "qualitative research"
	Limits	English language only
	Search outcome	Six hits, including: Sabari J J, Meisler J, Silver E 2000 Reflections upon rehabilitation by members of a community based stroke club. Disability and Rehabilitation 22:330–336

Table 4.3   *Tips for successful searching*

Improving the search terms
■ Use synonyms and both English and American terminology, e.g. learning difficulty/learning disability/mental retardation
■ Use English and American spellings e.g. paediatrics/pediatrics
■ Use " " for collections of words which together mean something, e.g. "occupational therapy"
■ Use * (the truncation symbol) to find all terms beginning with . . . e.g. disab* will retrieve articles related to both disability and disabled
■ Use Boolean operators (AND and OR) to expand or limit the search, e.g. "occupational therapy" OR physiotherapy will retrieve all articles related to occupational therapy and physiotherapy individually, whereas "occupational therapy" AND physiotherapy will retrieve only those articles that relate to combinations of occupational therapy and physiotherapy

Setting limits
■ Limiting your search to English-language-only references means that you won't identify a potentially useful reference only to find that you need a translator as the original paper is in German or Japanese
■ Limiting your search to papers published in the last 5 years will mean that you only access 'current' evidence and not something that was published in 1960, which may have since been refuted, although sometimes historical evidence may be of value

Appraising the evidence

One of the most important things for the evidence-based practitioner to remember is that not all evidence is good evidence, let alone 'best' evidence. Although many journals have a rigorous process of peer review and critique, it does not mean that the research that is published is flawless. Research is often carried out in highly controlled environments, which bear little true comparison with the complex working environment of many practitioners.

Having found some evidence, the next stage of the EBP process is critically to appraise the evidence. Critical appraisal can be defined as the ability to read original and summarized research, to make judgements on its scientific value and to consider how its results can be applied in practice. Chapter 7 gives ideas for becoming critical and scholarly.

The skills the advanced practitioner must develop are the ability to read a piece of research critically, weigh up the impact of any flaws in the research without becoming too negative, judge the power or strength of the findings and judge how well the research setting matches the practice setting, in order to assess the strength of the research findings in the light of both client preferences and expectations and local resource issues.

In order to appraise any research critically, the advanced practitioner must ask the following three questions:

● Is the research trustworthy/rigorous/valid and reliable?
● What are the results?
● How will these results help me to work more effectively with my clients?

Each of these questions can be further broken down to address specific types of research. One of the mistakes that novice practitioners often make is to attempt to appraise a piece of research using inappropriate criteria. It is important to use the appropriate criteria for particular research approaches and methodologies. Thus, a qualitative study should not be appraised using quantitative criteria and questions, nor should a systematic review be appraised using criteria and questions suitable for the appraisal of an RCT.

It is not within the scope of this chapter to present detailed accounts of appraisal of individual research approaches and methodologies. Appraisal is usually best facilitated by using a specific checklist of questions as a focus for discussion within a journal club. There are over 70 different checklists available; some of the most useful checklists are outlined in Table 4.4.

The nature of evidence

The aspect of EBP that has been the focus of much discussion and development is the debate around what actually counts as 'evidence', and particularly the nature of 'best evidence'. The traditional approach, drawing on the EBM model, has been to adopt the accepted view of a hierarchy, or levels, of evidence. Table 4.5 gives an overview of the hierarchy of evidence.

The reader will note that this hierarchy appears to value quantitative research (systematic reviews and RCTs) above more qualitative approaches to research (non-experimental studies). There also appears to be no place for evidence from experience or from the client's perspective. The hierarchy of evidence outlined in Table 4.5 does not seem to acknowledge the breadth of potential evidence available to the evidence-based practitioner.

Table 4.4 *Finding the right appraisal checklist*

Taylor (2000) gives worked examples of appraisal using separate checklists for:
- Randomized controlled trials (RCTs)
- Systematic reviews
- Qualitative studies

CASP: www.casp.org.uk/critical appraisal checklists can be downloaded from their site for:
- RCTs
- Qualitative research
- Systematic reviews
- Cohort studies
- Economic evaluation studies

McMaster: www-fhs.mcmaster.ca/rehab/ebp/appraisal checklists can be downloaded from their site for:
- Quantitative research
- Qualitative research

Humphris (1999) gives a brief overview of the questions that might be used to appraise:
- RCTs
- Case-controlled studies
- Cohort studies
- Surveys
- Qualitative studies
- Guidelines
- Consensus studies

Benton & Cormack (1996) give general guidelines for critical reading of research papers

Greenhalgh (1997) outlines the types of questions to ask of a range of medical research approaches, including:
- RCTs
- Systematic reviews
- Economic analyses
- Diagnostic and screening tests
- Qualitative research

Helewa & Walker (2000) give a basic overview of the questions to ask when evaluating a variety of articles:
- Outcome measures and diagnostic tests
- Treatment efficacy and effectiveness studies
- Economic evaluations
- Review articles and meta-analysis

Information on evaluating web-based resources and information can be found on the following websites:
www2.widener.edu/Wolfgram-Memorial-Library/webevaluation/inform.html
http://ils.unc.edu~fents/MLA/

Table 4.5 *Hierarchy of evidence*

- Systematic reviews and meta-analysis of randomized controlled trials (RCTs)
- RCTs
- Non-randomized experimental studies
- Non-experimental studies
- Respected opinion, expert discussion

Reproduced with permission from Taylor MC 2000 Evidence-based practice for occupational therapists. Blackwell Science, Oxford.

This evidence can include:
- systematic reviews of RCTs
- RCTS
- non-randomized experimental studies

- single case design studies
- cohort studies
- practice guidelines
- qualitative research studies
- systematic reviews of qualitative research
- surveys
- case studies
- expert consensus
- experience
- client views and preferences.

The advanced practitioner might find her/himself wondering how to make sense of all of this research in terms of a hierarchy of evidence as s/he searches to find the 'best evidence' with which to answer her/his evidence-based question. Straker (1999), drawing on his experience of teaching physiotherapy students, proposed an alternative hierarchy of evidence, which is outlined in Table 4.6. This hierarchy can be used to give a star rating to any evidence, with the best evidence being given a five-star rating, thus allowing a variety of evidence to be compared and the 'best evidence' to be identified. Straker (1999) suggested that his hierarchy attempts to unify both quantitative and qualitative research evidence into one hierarchy. However, whilst acknowledging the place of both qualitative research and evidence based on reflection and personal experience, Straker's (1999) hierarchy does not value these types of evidence very highly.

Both the hierarchy in Table 4.5 and Straker's (1999) hierarchy were originally designed as ways of valuing and weighing evidence for the effectiveness and efficacy of therapeutic interventions. The reader is encouraged to visit the Centre for Evidence-based Medicine's (CEBM) web-site, where the work of developing and updating the levels of

Table 4.6   *Straker's (1999) hierarchy of evidence for clinical decision-making*

*****	*Excellent* evidence is provided by complementary evidence from rigorous studies replicated across the population of interest, thus demonstrating wide generalizability
****	*Very good* evidence is provided by either:
	■ a very high-quality study, with strong design (e.g. randomized controlled trial, sequential clinical trial, factorial or repeated measures study, single case studies with replication), using measures with demonstrated reliability and validity, rigorous data collection and appropriate analysis
	or
	■ multiple-level *** studies using different approaches (i.e. not sharing the same errors)
***	*Good* evidence is provided by a moderate-quality study which is basically sound but with possible caveats (e.g. presumed reliability and validity of measures or weaker 'cause–effect' evidence due to design (survey, AB single case design, phenomenology))
**	*Some* evidence is provided by reflective practice case study
*	*Minimal* evidence is provided by expert opinion, reasoning, case description
—	*No* evidence is provided by traditional, novice opinion, poor-quality study (e.g. one with serious design flaws (finding no effect due to insufficient power), one where dependent variable measurement was not reliable and valid, one where data collection was sloppy)

evidence is presented (see further reading and resources, at the end of this chapter). The CEBM has acknowledged the usefulness of the levels of evidence as ways of providing a means of highlighting when evidence may be flawed. It has also acknowledged the need for other levels of evidence for a variety of evidence-based questions, and developed levels of evidence for:

● therapy/prevention/aetiology/harm questions
● prognosis questions
● diagnosis questions
● differential diagnosis/symptoms questions
● economic questions (Phillips et al 2001).

You will be beginning to realize the complexity of evidence and the process of identifying the 'best evidence' with which to address any evidence-based question. One approach to deciding which type of evidence might be seen to provide the 'best evidence' is to identify the type of evidence that is appropriate for a particular type of evidence-based question. Table 4.7 gives an overview of types of research linked to types of evidence-based questions. However, this approach also marginalizes both experiential evidence and evidence based on the client's needs and preferences.

Using specific types of evidence to address particular evidence-based questions may seem the most useful approach as it may lead to the development of further specific hierarchies of evidence. However, it may also act as a constraint, if not a straightjacket, to the development of a broad perspective on the 'best evidence' with which to answer evidence-based questions. Certainly an RCT or a systematic review will provide powerful evidence for the effectiveness of a particular intervention. It should not, however, be the only evidence required for clinical reasoning and decision-making. The client's needs and preferences must be taken into account. The economic and resource climate should also be considered. Qualitative research and the practitioner's own knowledge and experience will give further insights into the perceived effectiveness of the chosen intervention. Evidence should not be seen in terms of a hierarchy but in terms of pieces of a complex jigsaw (Figure 4.2) which together provides the 'best evidence' to answer any evidence-based question.

Table 4.7   *Appropriate evidence for particular types of evidence-based questions*

Effectiveness of interventions and therapeutic activities:
■ Systematic reviews, randomized controlled trials, single-case experimental studies
■ Qualitative studies might also give an insight into clients' perceptions of effectiveness
Client experiences/concerns:
■ Qualitative studies
■ Likely course of disease/disability
■ Cohort/follow-up studies
Cost-effectiveness of any intervention or action:
■ Economic studies comparing all outcomes against costs
■ Guidance about the types of interventions being used currently in practice
■ Clinical guidelines, expert consensus studies/Delphi studies, surveys

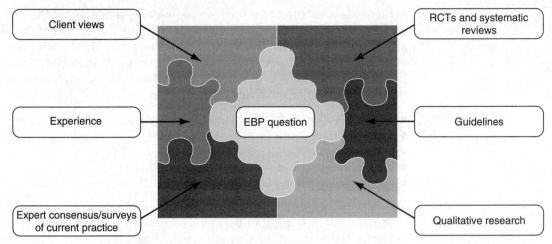

Figure 4.2   *The jigsaw of 'evidence' EBP, evidence-based practice; RCTs, randomized controlled trials*

However, it must be remembered that this emphasis on a jigsaw of evidence does not mean that levels of evidence can be ignored. Any evidence must be looked at critically and, where a hierarchy exists, must be viewed within the context of the appropriate hierarchy and the level of evidence established. This will ensure that any evidence is given suitable weight and that weaker evidence is not given undue importance. It is also acknowledged that, for some forms of evidence, such as qualitative research evidence, the whole notion of a hierarchy is a complex and contentious topic. The jigsaw of evidence should, however, allow the evidence-based practitioner to develop a broader perspective on the evidence suitable for her/his particular evidence-based question.

Rather than discuss the whole variety of types of evidence, which is beyond the scope of this chapter and has been done elsewhere (Helewa and Walker 2000, Sackett et al 2000, Taylor 2000), this section will now explore two particular approaches to evidence: the use of reflection and experience as evidence; and evidence-based case studies.

Using experience and reflection as evidence

A key theme within all the definitions of EBP/EBM, outlined at the beginning of the chapter, was the use of experience and experiential knowledge as part of EBP. The research discussed at the beginning of the chapter also demonstrated that experience is the most frequent source of information and evidence used by therapists when making clinical decisions. However, nowhere in any text on EBP is the use of this form of personal experiential knowledge discussed. Although Enkin and Jadad (1998) put forward a sound and coherent argument for the use of experiential, or, as they term it, 'anecdotal', evidence within EBP, they do not give any practical suggestions. The evidence-based practitioner is left wondering how experience can be brought explicitly into the process of EBP.

Experiential evidence is useful for any healthcare decision-making. It is particularly useful in the following circumstances:

- when there is no formal research evidence readily available, or where the research evidence is of poor quality
- when there is a balance between the evidence in favour and against the chosen intervention or action
- when there are equal strengths and weaknesses/flaws in the formal research evidence
- when the formal research evidence has to be weighed against economic/resource or environmental factors or client preferences.

The question that remains is exactly how to articulate and use evidence based on experience and reflection. Reflection and experiential knowledge can be articulated as a part of the 'finding the evidence' stage of the EBP process. This activity should occur in parallel with the search for formal research evidence. Activity Box 4.6 outlines questions that might be helpful when attempting to articulate experiential knowledge and evidence. This evidence can be used to assist the debate when the formal research evidence is appraised and when the practicalities of using the evidence to inform or change practice are discussed and explored.

Activity box 4.6	Questions to ask when articulating experiential knowledge and evidence

Using the scenario you developed earlier, or another suitable intervention or action from your practice, think about a previous occasion when you have used that intervention or action. Use the questions below to help you to articulate your experiential knowledge and evidence for the usefulness of that intervention or action.

- What did you do?
- Why did you use the intervention or action?
- What were your goals?
- What were the expected outcomes?
- How were these outcomes measured?
- What effect did the intervention or action have?
- How do you know whether the intervention or action was effective?
- Do you have any quantitative or qualitative evidence of effectiveness (e.g. formal outcome measurements, comments from the client)?

Evidence-based case studies

Much of the evidence the evidence-based practitioner may find as s/he searches and appraises the literature may not directly relate to the specific needs of her/his client. The skill of the evidence-based practitioner is in the practical application of the evidence. Two tools can help with this task and it is, perhaps, the role of the advanced practitioner to develop these tools and to disseminate them to other professional colleagues. The two tools are: critically appraised papers and evidence-based case studies.

A number of journals are now including critically appraised papers (e.g. *Australian Journal of Physiotherapy*), whilst journals such as *Evidence-based Nursing* contain nothing but critically appraised papers. The importance of these papers is that they include not just a summary of a previously published piece of research but they also include a commentary, by a practitioner, outlining the usefulness of the research as evidence for practice. Advanced practitioners should be involved in producing critically appraised papers and in encouraging wider publication of critically appraised papers within professional journals.

Evidence-based case studies can provide another way of synthesizing and disseminating practice based on sound reasoning and evidence. Examples of evidence-based case studies are beginning to be published (Dorling and Salt 2001). The evidence-based practitioner should consider preparing and sharing evidence-based case studies with colleagues at local, regional and national levels. Activity Box 4.7 outlines one way of developing an evidence-based case study. Ideally, any evidence-based activity should be prospective (as in Dorling and Salt 2001); however, evidence-based activity should also form part of continuing reflection and professional development and could, therefore, be retrospective.

Activity box 4.7	Developing evidence-based case studies

- Identify and describe a suitable case study
- Be concise—identify the key features of the person and her/his problems/needs
- Reflection on action
- Reflect on your decision-making and interventions. Why did you do what you did? What were your feelings about the intervention? What went well/less well? On what knowledge and assumptions did you base your actions?
- Articulate any experiential evidence of effectiveness
- What evidence do you have that your interventions were successful? What outcomes were achieved? How were these outcomes measured? How do these outcomes compare with other similar cases?
- Explore and appraise the research evidence
- Articulate your case study in terms of an evidence-based practice question; search for any research evidence; appraise the research evidence; is there any research evidence to support your actions?
- Synthesis
- Draw together the above sections to give an overview of what you have learnt as a result of this analysis; identify alternatives/options/ ways forward; explore how your practice might change as a result of this analysis

Putting EBP into practice

Asking the questions and, finding and appraising the evidence are the beginning stages of EBP. The most important stage of the EBP process is actually using the evidence to review and change practice. While the vast topic of change management is beyond the scope of this chapter, it is within the remit of this chapter to highlight some activities that the advanced practitioner might use and to provide her/him with some tools to facilitate the development of an evidence-based culture and the development of practice that is truly evidence-based.

Developing an evidence-based culture

Fundamental to the development of EBP is the development of a departmental culture that supports an evidence-based approach to practice. Gray (1997, p. 36) suggests that an organization, or department, with an evidence-based culture has 'an obsession with finding, appraising and using research-based knowledge in decision making'. To draw on Cusick's (2001) notion of asking the 'right' questions, we could develop Gray's definition and suggest that an evidence-based culture facilitates practitioners to ask the 'right' questions about their practice and to answer these questions with the 'right' evidence. Departments with evidence-based cultures should be challenging places to work; they should expect practitioners to evaluate their practice and to be able to support and justify their actions using suitable evidence. To do this, however, requires support, evidence-based skills and evidence-based activities.

Support

The main obstacles to the development of EBP have been identified as:

- lack of time
- lack of access to resources
- lack of skills
- lack of available evidence (Close and Lewin 1998, Humphris et al 2000, Pringle 1999, Richardson and Jerosch-Herold 1998).

Although Walsh (1997) identified resistance to change within the clinical environment as the major barrier to research utilization and EBP, the advanced practitioner needs to work creatively with management colleagues to ensure that time and funding are available for EBP activities. The government's agenda, clearly set out in the White Paper *The New NHS: Modern, Dependable* (Department of Health 1997), gives trusts a responsibility for ensuring quality, accountability and clinical effectiveness.

Changing to an evidence-based culture can be a challenging process and support will be needed to maintain motivation. One source of support can be through links with higher education establishments. These links can be used to develop programs of skill development as well as providing expertise and guidance. Joint projects can be developed, which might not only develop an evidence-based culture but might also extend into research projects. What support mechanisms are available to you within your organization? How can these mechanisms be utilized to ensure that time and resources are available for EBP activities?

A particular strategy, adopted by the author, has been to develop undergraduate projects that focus on a real evidence-based question developed by practitioner colleagues. The findings of these projects can then be disseminated through student conferences. Try to identify any links with higher education establishments. How can these links be developed further to facilitate the development of an evidence-based culture in your work setting?

Skills

Even if time and resources are not a barrier to the development of an evidence-based culture, lack of skills and lack of confidence in the skills of EBP may still prove to be a barrier. Within any group of practitioners or team there will be a range of levels of skill and confidence. Newly qualified practitioners should, by virtue of the type of pre-registration education they experience, have skills in finding and appraising evidence. They may not, however, have the confidence to use these skills in practice. More senior practitioners may, on the other hand, feel threatened by their lack of skill.

Research skills have been a recent focus for the curricula of some professional groups. Lack of skills and lack of confidence in skills will be one of the first challenges the advanced practitioner has to address when s/he attempts to establish an evidence-based culture. What research skills do the staff already have? The first task should be to conduct an audit of the evidence-based skills within the staff team. The skills of EBP were reviewed earlier in this chapter and this information might be used to help structure an audit tool. How confident are they with these skills? What skills need to be developed?

Once the audit has been completed you can then develop a strategy for EBP skills development within the staff team. The skills of newly qualified staff can be utilized to help more senior colleagues to develop their skills. Library colleagues should be contacted to help develop search skills. Trust Research and Development units and local higher education contacts can be approached for more specialist appraisal and research interpretation training.

Activities

Many therapists wonder how to become involved in EBP without realizing that they are already working within an evidence-based perspective. The processes of reflection, supervision and discussion with a mentor are all opportunities to review one's practice from an evidence-based perspective. EBP, as we have seen, is not about *doing* research; it is about *using* research very explicitly to underpin the intervention decisions we make on a daily basis as practitioners (Taylor 2000).

The questions and activity boxes earlier in the chapter should have provided you with tools to guide your evidence-based reflections. These reflections can form the basis of supervision or mentoring discussions. By thinking through and articulating the reasoning processes we use, unconsciously, every day we can strengthen, rather then weaken, our practice. Outdated and redundant interventions can be stopped and effective interventions can be reinforced. Reasons can be articulated to management.

Journal Clubs

In Taylor (2000) I discussed the use of journal clubs, as one way of ensuring focused reading, and developing an evidence-based climate. Journal clubs:

- consist of three to 10 group members who meet regularly (every month or 2 months) to review and discuss one or more articles of relevance to their practice
- provide useful opportunities to practice the critical appraisal skills discussed in the previous chapters
- can be uni-professional or multi-disciplinary depending on the local setting.

Sackett et al (1997) advocated a journal club based on a critical appraisal format. A much more successful, and useful, format for journal clubs is when a group of colleagues meet together to share a discussion and appraisal of one of more papers, probably using an appraisal checklist as a way of structuring the discussion (Taylor 2000).

Journal clubs have been a part of 'medical practice' for many years. These journal clubs often consisted of one person presenting a critical review of an article to her/his colleagues. However, as Sackett et al (1997) point out, this type of journal club is becoming extinct. Journal clubs, using an appraisal format to review and reflect upon current practice are seen as the most appropriate approach for the development of critical skills. See Chapters 7 and 9 for further ideas.

Before setting off to establish a journal club it might be helpful to think about some of the practical issues. Each meeting can look at single articles or a number of articles. Single articles can be useful to start with, as everyone develops their appraisal skills. However, although looking at a number of papers may take longer, it will give a broader and more interesting perspective on any given topic or evidence-based question (Taylor 2000). Searching for relevant articles may feel like an onerous responsibility, but if searching and session leadership is divided among the group members it should not prove too difficult and time-consuming a task. Journal clubs do require time and an element of commitment. Given the current climate of clinical effectiveness and continuing professional development, managers should encourage and facilitate the establishment of journal clubs.

The outcome of a journal club provides a forum for practising appraisal skills, but can also provide an opportunity for club discussion about changing current interventions or practice. The journal club, provides a valuable opportunity for colleagues to explore issues, share ideas, consider differing perspectives and participate in the shaping and developing of departmental practice and policy (Taylor 2000). Membership of, and commitment to, a journal club could provide useful evidence of continuing professional development for an individual's professional portfolio and appraisal. Chapter 11 will give you ideas for this aspect of your professional development.

Try to identify a group of like-minded colleagues who would be interested in establishing a journal club. Establish a time for regular meetings. Decide on a number of evidence-based questions and allocate the planning of each session (Taylor 2000). Hold your first journal club meeting. Record the discussion and include this evidence in your portfolio of continuing professional development. In addition, do not forget to include how you implemented this evidence into your practice.

Developing practice that is evidence-based

Using a questioning and critical approach to practice is at the heart of the philosophy and skills of the advanced practitioner. An evidence-based approach to the development of practice has benefits, as Rosenberg and Donald (1995) pointed out, not just for the individual practitioner but also for the multi-disciplinary team and for the client. These benefits include the following.

For individual practitioners it:

- enables practitioners to upgrade their knowledge base routinely
- improves practitioners' understanding of research methods and makes them more critical in using data
- improves confidence in intervention decisions
- improves computer literacy and data-searching techniques
- improves reading habits.

For teams it:

- gives the team a framework for group problem-solving and for teaching
- enables juniors to contribute usefully to team.

For patients and clients it gives:

- more effective use of resources
- better communication with clients about the rationale behind management decisions.

An evidence-based approach to practice development ensures that outdated and ineffective practices are challenged and change is facilitated. Practice can be developed using a variety of methods such as audit and review, guidelines and action learning.

The use of evidence-based audit and guidelines has been discussed extensively elsewhere (Buttery 1998, Joyce 1999, Taylor 2000). Both Conroy's (1997) and McAuley's (1999) articles provide useful models for evidence-based service reviews. Conroy (1997) used the conventional EBP approach of asking a series of questions and finding and appraising research evidence. McAuley's (1999) approach was more creative and wide-ranging. In her evidence-based review of weekend physiotherapy services her strategy was to use brainstorming to develop a range of answerable questions. She then used a wide range of evidence to answer these questions. The types of evidence she used included published research and other more descriptive literature;

however, she also surveyed other facilities to discover consensus on practice, she carried out internal polls to identify problems and needs of the service and she reviewed departmental records. This approach provided evidence to support the continued use of physiotherapy weekend services, and demonstrated the value of using a broad perspective on evidence rather than relying on a narrow quantitative research evidence perspective. These two papers also demonstrate the value of disseminating not just research findings, but the process and findings of evidence-based service reviews and developments. Chapter 1 gives a table outlining these processes (Table 1.2).

Audit and service reviews are major exercises. However, practice can become evidence-based through smaller, more on-going activities. Journal clubs and the use of supervision have already been discussed. Another form of group activity, which can be used as a tool for developing practice based on evidence, is the use of action learning sets.

Action learning has been defined as:

> . . . a continuous process of learning and reflection, supported by colleagues, with an intention of getting things done. Through action learning individuals learn with and from each other by working on real problems and reflecting on their own experiences. The process helps us to take an active stance towards life and helps to overcome the tendency (merely) to think, feel and be passive towards the pressures of life (McGill and Beaty 1995, p. 27).

Action learning, thus, provides an opportunity for peer group reflection. However, action learning requires time and commitment and so must be supported within the work environment. The group should not work alone; action learning requires experienced facilitation. Without a facilitator action learning sets can descend into a 'whine and moan' session and will lose the focus of evaluation and development of practice. Facilitation might be offered by an academic from a local higher education establishment. This can then help to develop the theoretical aspects of discussion and might help to close the theory–practice gap. The key components for action learning are:

- a group of individuals meeting regularly together to review and develop practice
- time for regular meetings must be negotiated and approved
- confidentiality and trust are essential
- each individual brings a real issue or project and is allowed time to present the issue to the group
- the whole group works on each individual's issue in turn to refine, challenge and develop ideas and solutions
- a challenging, creative and supportive environment is facilitated
- action plans are developed and reviewed during subsequent meetings.

Action learning sets can be seen as useful tools for continuing professional development and the action plans can be included as evidence in portfolios of professional development. Consider how you would

Table 4.8   *Factors essential for the development of practice that is evidence-based*

- Creative approach to problem-solving
- A challenging and questioning attitude
- The use of a broad range of evidence, from quantitative studies to experiential and reflective evidence
- Education and skills development, e.g. critical appraisal skills, search skills
- Commitment and support from managers
- Commitment from team members
- Time
- Economic resources
- Access to information technology and sources of evidence
- An evidence-based culture
- Empowerment and accountability
- Dissemination of evidence and evidence-based initiatives

set up your own action learning set. Think about the practicalities first. Who would be involved? Where would you meet? What topics might be included? What ground rules would be needed? What problems might you encounter and how might you overcome them?

In conclusion, in this chapter I have attempted to outline ways in which the advanced practitioner can use evidence to develop practice.

Joyce (1999) has outlined a number of factors, which are essential to the process of practice development. These factors, within the context of EBP, are developed in Table 4.8. What activities can you undertake to ensure that practice is evidence-based? What resources will you need? What barriers might you need to overcome? What are your time scales? Review what you have learnt from this chapter and make use of the strategies to support being an evidence-based practitioner.

References

Benton D, Cormack D 1996 Reviewing and evaluating the literature. In: Cormack D (ed) The research process in nursing, 3rd edn. Blackwell Science, Oxford, p 78–87

Bithell C 2000 Evidence-based physiotherapy. Physiotherapy 86:58–60

Brown G T, Rodgers S 1999 Research utilization models: frameworks for implementing evidence-based occupational therapy practice. Occupational Therapy International 6:1–23

Buttery Y 1998 Implementing evidence through clinical audit. In: Bury T, Mead J (eds) Evidence-based healthcare. Butterworth-Heinemann, Oxford, p 182–207

Canadian Association of Occupational Therapists, Association of Canadian Occupational Therapy University Programs, Association of Canadian Occupational Therapy Regulatory Organizations and the Presidents' Advisory Committee 1999 Joint position statement on evidence-based practice. Canadian Journal of Occupational Therapy 66:267–269

Closs S J, Lewin B J P 1998 Perceived barriers to research utilisation: a survey of four therapies. British Journal of Therapy and Rehabilitation 5:151–155

Conroy M C 1997 'Why are you doing that?' A project to look for evidence of efficacy within occupational therapy. British Journal of Occupational Therapy 60:487–490

Cusick A 2001 OZ OT EBP 21c: Australian occupational therapy, evidence-based practice and the 21st century. Australian Occupational Therapy Journal 48:102–117

Department of Health 1997 The new NHS: modern, dependable. London, HMSO

Department of Health (2000) www.doh.gov.uk/nsf/coronary.htm. Accessed 25 May 2002

Department of Health (2001) www.doh.gov.uk/nsf/mentalhealth/htm. Accessed 25 May 2002

DiCenso A, Cullum N, Ciliska D 1998 Implementing evidence-based nursing: some misconceptions (editorial). Evidence-based Nursing 1:38–40

Dorling J, Salt A 2001 Assessing developmental delay. British Medical Journal 323:148–149

Dubouloz C J, Egan M, Vallerand J, Von Zweck C 1999 Occupational therapists' perceptions of evidence-based practice. American Journal of Occupational Therapy 53:445–453

Egan M, Dubouloz C, von Zweck C, Vallerand J 1998 The client-centred evidence-based practice of occupational therapy. Canadian Journal of Occupational Therapy, 65:136–143.

Enkin M W, Jadad A R 1998 Using anecdotal information in evidence-based healthcare: heresay or necessity? Annals of Oncology 9:963–966

Gray J A M 1997 Evidence-based healthcare. Churchill-Livingstone, Edinburgh

Greenhalgh T 1997 How to read a paper: the basics of evidence based medicine. London, BMJ Publishing

Helewa A, Walker J M 2000 Critical evaluation of research in physical rehabilitation. W B Saunders, Philadelphia

Herbert R, Moseley A, Sherrington C 1998/9 PEDro: a database of randomised controlled trials in physiotherapy. Health Information Management 28:186–188

Humphris D 1999 Types of evidence. In: Hamer S, Collinson G (eds) Achieving evidence-based practice. Baillière Tindall, Edinburgh, p 13–40

Humphris D, Littlejohns P, Victor C, O'Halloran P, Peacock J 2000 Implementing evidence-based practice: factors that influence the use of research evidence by occupational therapists. British Journal of Occupational Therapy 63:516–522

Joyce L 1999 Development of practice. In: Hamer S, Collinson G (eds) Achieving evidence-based practice. Baillière Tindall, Edinburgh, p 109–127

McAuley C 1999 Evidence-based care: determining the appropriateness of weekend physiotherapy services in an acute care tertiary hospital. Physiotherapy Canada., 51:126–132

McGill I, Beaty L 1995 Action learning: a guide for professional, management and educational development 2nd edn. Kogan Page, London

Palmer J, Brice A 1999 Information sourcing. In: Hamer S, Collinson G (eds) Achieving evidence-based practice. Baillière Tindall, Edinburgh, p 61–83

Phillips B, Ball C, Sackett D 2001 Oxford Centre for Evidence-based Medicine levels of evidence (May 2001). Online. Available: http://cebm.jr2.ox.ac.uk/docs/levels.html 15 Oct 2001

Pringle E 1999 EBP: is it for me? Therapy Weekly 25:12

Research Committee (Victorian branch) of the Australian Physiotherapy Association and invited contributors 1999 Evidence-based practice. Australian Journal of Physiotherapy 45:167–171

Richardson B, Jerosch-Herold C 1998 Appraisal of clinical effectiveness—an ACE approach to providing evidence-based therapy. Journal of Clinical Effectiveness 3:146–150

Richardson W S, Wilson M C, Nishikawa J, Hayward RS 1995 The well-built clinical question: a key to evidence-based decisions (editorial). ACP Journal Club 123:A12–A13

Rosenberg W, Donald A 1995 Evidence based medicine: an approach to clinical problem-solving. British Medical Journal 310: 1122–1126

Sackett D L, Richardson W S, Rosenberg W M C, Hayes R B 1997 Evidence-based medicine: how to practise and teach EBM. Churchill Livingstone, New York

Sackett D L, Straus S E, Richardson W S, Rosenberg W, Haynes R B 2000 Evidence-based medicine: how to practise and teach EBM, 2nd edn. Churchill Livingstone, Edinburgh

Straker L 1999 A hierarchy of evidence for informing physiotherapy practice. Australian Journal of Physiotherapy 45:231–233

Taylor M C 2000 Evidence-based practice for occupational therapists. Blackwell Science, Oxford

Trinder L 2000 A critical appraisal of evidence-based practice. In: Trinder L, Reynolds S (eds) Evidence-based practice: a critical appraisal. Blackwell Science, Oxford, p 212–241

Turner P, Whitfield T W A 1997 Physiotherapists' use of evidence-based practice: a cross-national study. Physiotherapy Research International 12:17–29

Turner P, Whitfield T W A 1999 Physiotherapists' reasons for selection of treatment techniques: a cross-national survey. Physiotherapy Theory and Practice 15:235–246

Upton D 1999a Clinical effectiveness and EBP 2: attitudes of health-care professionals. British Journal of Therapy and Rehabilitation 6:26–30

Upton D 1999b Clinical effectiveness and EBP 2: application by health-care professionals. British Journal of Therapy and Rehabilitation 6:86–90

Walsh M 1997 How nurses perceive barriers to research implementation. Nursing Standard 11:34–39

Further reading and resources

It is not intended for this list of resources to be exhaustive. It should, however, provide the reader with a variety of resources to facilitate her/his exploration of the breadth of evidence-based practice. The author takes no responsibility for the current accuracy of any URLs, as web sites change and evolve very rapidly.

Books

Bury T, Mead J 1998 Evidence-based healthcare: a practical guide for therapists. Butterworth-Heinemann, Oxford

Gray J A M 1997 Evidence-based healthcare. Churchill Livingstone, Edinburgh

Grayson L 1997 Evidence-based medicine: an overview and guide to the literature. British Library, London

Greenhalgh T 1997 How to read a paper: the basics of evidence based medicine. London, BMJ Publishing

Hamer S, Collinson G (eds) 1999 Achieving evidence-based practice. Edinburgh, Baillière Tindall

Taylor M C 2000 Evidence-based practice for occupational therapists. Blackwell Science, Oxford

Trinder L, Reynolds S (eds) 2000 Evidence-based practice: a critical appraisal. Blackwell Science, Oxford

Journals and publications

Bandolier – http://www.ebandolier.com
Effective Health Care Bulletin -www.york.ac.uk/inst/crd/ehcb.htm
Best Evidence: A database on CD-Rom.
This provides abstracts and commentaries from ACP Journal Club and Evidence-based Medicine
Evidence-based Health Policy & Management
Evidence-based Mental Health
Evidence-based Nursing

Centres and web resources

Centre for Evidence-based Medicine	http://cebm.jr2.ox.ac.uk
Centre for Evidence-based Mental Health	www.cebmh.com/
Centre for Evidence-based Nursing	http://www.york.ac.uk/healthsciences www.york.ac.uk/depts/hstd/centres/evidence/cebn/htm
Centre for Evidence-Based Physiotherapy	www.cchs.usyd.edu.au/CEBP/index.htm
Critical Appraisal Skills Programme (CASP)	www.casp.org.uk/
Joanna Briggs Institute for Evidence-based Nursing and Midwifery	www.joannabriggs.edu.au
McMaster Occupational Therapy Evidence-based Practice Research Group	www-fhs.mcmaster.ca/rehab/ebp/

Netting the evidence	www.shef.ac.uk/uni/academic/R-Z/scharr/ir/netting.html
NeLH occupational therapy portal	www.nelh.nhs.uk/OT
NeLH physiotherapy portal	www.nelh.nhs.uk/physio
NHS Centre for Reviews and Dissemination	www.york.ac.uk/inst/crd/dissem.htm
OMNI	www.omni.ac.uk
PEDro	http://ptwww.cchs.usyd.edu.au/pedro
Unit for Evidence-based Practice and Policy	www.ucl.ac.uk/primcare-popsci/uepp/uepp.htm

5

Enhancing reflective abilities: interweaving reflection into practice

Gillian Brown and Susan E. Ryan

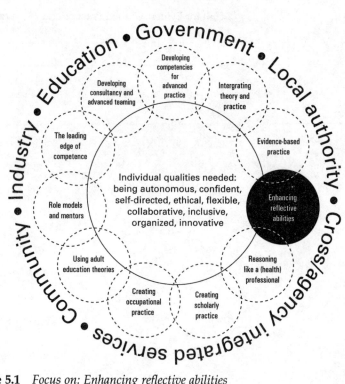

Figure 5.1 *Focus on: Enhancing reflective abilities*

Chapter outline

In this chapter Gill tells the story of Daniel who came to work in a department 9 months after he qualified as an occupational therapist. It illustrates, in a developmental way, how he was encouraged to become reflective in his practice. In this chapter the nature of reflection is explored while highlighting practical ways that the examples can be used in the practice setting. You can follow the exemplars to enhance your own reflective abilities as a practitioner. Further, you can use this chapter to advance your knowledge and skills to support and guide you in other roles such as team leader, supervisor, fieldwork educator or clinical supervisor, educator and researcher. The references and other contacts will enable you to develop your understanding of the concept and process of reflection.

Key words

Thinking, prospective reflection, retrospective reflection, experiential learning

Anticipated outcomes

As a result of reading this chapter we anticipate that you will be able to:

- appreciate the nature of reflection in relation to learning, particularly learning from experience
- recognize the range of overlapping constructs that constitutes reflection
- identify ways of enhancing reflective abilities for self and for others.

Introduction

Reflection is one of the most powerful growth factors for becoming an advanced practitioner (Martin et al 1992). There is a growing body of knowledge which suggests that reflective practice has the potential to transform who we are and what we do (Ghaye 2001). The concept has been around since 1910 when Dewey first described the process of reflection (Dewey 1910). Since the 1980s, however, a wide range of disciplines have adopted reflection as a concept. These include teaching, nursing, the therapies, and sports coaching.

Some professional education programs make reflection inclusive throughout the curriculum while others have designated parts of the program dedicated to it. Previously, educational programs of a more scientific nature tended to be objective and reflection was not integral to their practitioners' thinking. Also, some people are naturally reflective while others have great difficulty and are even unwilling to be reflective about their practice.

The clinical supervision is an area of Gill's expertise, so Daniel's story is told in the first person. The reflections about the supervision process and discussions about the theoretical frames of references and related research are in the first person plural, as these represent our shared work.

Gill's story: setting the scene

My beginnings in understanding about reflection and applying and using it in my work stem from the time I joined a post-graduate Master's-level program. In one module I studied clinical reasoning and reflection and subsequently became intrigued with the thinking that surrounds adult learning. This added to my knowledge and skills as reflection enabled me to see different ways of working in practice and other ways to facilitate the work of the members of the department where I work as Head Occupational Therapist and provided me with opportunities to enhance students' abilities on placement and in their educational settings.

Reflection became a subject of personal interest as I learnt to embed this new learning within my roles of clinician, team leader and educator. Adding an understanding of reflection to prior knowledge and experience has prompted me to ask how students, newly emerging therapists and working practitioners can develop their expertise by using reflection. In telling the story below I am going to make some assumptions about you, the reader. I am visualizing you as a working practitioner consolidating and practising your knowledge and skills. You probably want to develop your practice and to extend your thinking and understanding. Perhaps you have selected this text to help you on your way.

Figure 5.2 illustrates the different perspectives surrounding reflection and reflective practice that will be explored in this chapter.

I want to share some of my own experiences of using reflection by telling you a story that I have called 'A journey with Daniel'. This is a constructed story. I have used an amalgam of experiences that have resulted from many personal encounters with other therapists in supervision settings. Our team works closely with a number of other professions which contribute to the work of the centre and I have gained many insights into their ways of working and their thinking about their practice as a result. I believe that Daniel's experiences as told in this story are relevant and transferable across the range of health professionals.

A journey with Daniel: the beginning of the story

Daniel joined the department for a 9-month placement as part of a service-wide rotation to gain experience in different settings. The department is based at a Children's Centre. The 9-month placement

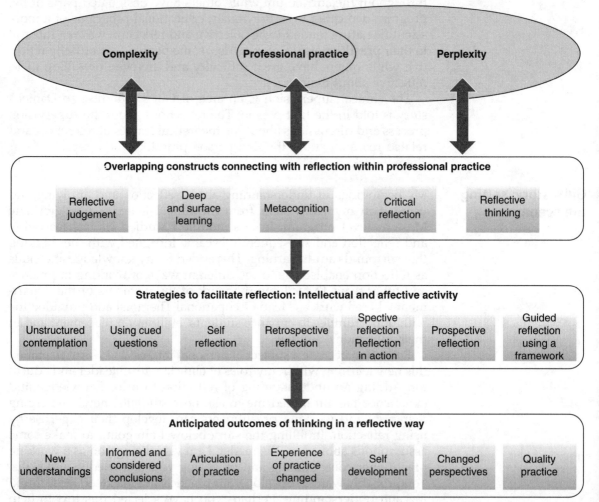

Figure 5.2 *Perspectives on reflective practice*

forms part of a selected series of work placements that move between different departments in the local area in the first years after qualifying. He had started his professional education as a mature-aged student at the age of 35 and had completed one other placement before this. This story will take you through the first months of Daniel's work and the experience of using reflection to support his learning and also to develop that of his supervision.

Point of embarkation: our first meeting

I invited Daniel for a planning meeting before the placement started. I wanted to negotiate and to map out with him his professional goals for this 9-month period. We shared information and explored our expectations of the roles he would be undertaking. I also wanted to get some understanding of his prior experiences and learning. We talked about his previous experiences of supervision. I wanted to understand how he viewed his developmental needs in terms of having supervision with me in the future. I believe it is important to establish a supervision framework and a provisional program at the beginning of a rotation but to make it clear that this is a starting point and that it can be modified at any time as learning progresses, and needs alter.

It was clear that Daniel had a variety of experiences about supervision to draw upon. These came from his days as an undergraduate, his time working in a junior practitioner post and his past experiences from his work in his previous career as a police officer. From hearing about Daniel's experiences and thinking about the way that he felt most at ease with reporting them, it became clear that he was rather 'scientific' in the way he spoke of facts and events. He struggled with expressing his own thoughts, feelings or reactions to the events he reported on. I asked Daniel to think about and tell me what he knew about reflection. He looked puzzled but made a brave attempt to give his own definition. He offered 'thinking about something that you have done'.

This seemed like Schön's (1983) 'reflection on action' or retrospective reflection where past events are examined. This type of reflection may occur in an unstructured mood of idle speculation or as a conscious effort to prepare for a future situation. Daniel was able to recall from his past learning that reflection had a place in learning from experience and he spoke of being introduced to Kolb's Learning Cycle (Kolb 1984). I encouraged Daniel by offering the comment that defining reflection was not easy. Many authors have provided definitions but it was clear that there were many different meanings of the term and much depends on which definitions you have come across, as you will see in Box 5.1.

The story continues

Daniel felt that learning from experience was important and that being able to use supervision effectively would help support his new learning. I asked him if there had been opportunities in his undergraduate program to challenge the knowledge and skills that he was developing at that time. He told me that he had been expected to produce a reflective diary at one stage in his second year but was given little guidance to begin with and no feedback afterwards. He felt that it had minimal value and may have contributed to feeling uncomfortable when he was expected to model 'being reflective'. He also talked about his experiences of thinking about his work in his previous placement. There, he had reported on the work he was doing and discussed his plans for the following week. Reflection had not been part of this way of working. After listening to him it was clear that Daniel had had few opportunities for using reflection in the past but it was very good that he had identified this as an area of skill that he wanted to develop. He felt that he had concentrated more on the procedural clinical aspects and departmental administration aspects of his work until now.

It was agreed with Daniel that we would aim to introduce 'thinking about what we have done' (i.e. retrospective reflection) into the supervision sessions, so that he could extend his understanding of this concept and become more comfortable in using this sort of reflection. A timetable for Daniel's first week in the placement was agreed and a time to meet for supervision each week was arranged.

Questions

1. Can you recall your first experiences of reflection in relation to learning?

   Record your responses in a way that you are comfortable with. Keep this work safely so that you can use it later as you read through this chapter to see how your understanding grows.

2. What does 'reflection' mean to you?

3. What everyday word(s) come to mind? Make a list to record your responses.

   Compare what you have written with the overview of other authors' work in Box 5.1. Does one of their definitions match something you have written?

   Kember et al (2000 p. 11) suggested that the last two definitions of reflection are 'moving towards the context of professional practice in that both view experience as the touchstone for reflection'. What kinds of settings are considered to be within the context of professional

---

Box 5.1   *Published definitions of reflection*

1. Reflective thinking is the 'active, persistent and careful consideration of any belief or supposed form of knowledge in the light of the grounds that support it and the further conclusion to which it tends' (Dewey 1933, p. 9).

2. Reflective learning is the process of internally examining and exploring an issue of concern, triggered by an experience, which creates and clarifies meaning in terms of self, and which results in a changed conceptual perspective (Boyd & Fayles 1993, p. 100).

3. Reflection in the context of learning is a generic term for those intellectual and affective activities in which individuals engage to explore their experiences in order to lead to new understandings

practice? Looking at all these ideas, when do you think reflective practice occurs?

Reflection as a component of professional practice

Being a reflective practitioner has become an essential component of being a healthcare practitioner. For example, the *Benchmark Statement: Health Care Programmes*, published by the Quality Assurance Agency (QAA) for Higher Education 2001 in the UK, includes the following statement: the award holder will be able to: 'reflect on and review practice' (p. 4). This is an expectation of the health professional who is providing patient and client services in health and social care services. The QAA document outlines expectations for reflective practitioners to be 'critical of what they do and to be able to be critical about why they do it in respect of the use of evidence in order to develop best practice' (p. 6).

What knowledge and skills are required to become reflective? A reflective practitioner needs to be proficient in using reflective thinking by being critical of existing published knowledge as well as experiential and newly gained knowledge.

The *Benchmark Statement* (QAA 2001, p. 12) states that professional competencies in reflection will include:

- self-reflection on the extent and limitations on the role of the healthcare practitioner in a variety of settings and the requirements for state registration and competence to practise
- the ability to reflect critically on their overall personal performance, and take responsibility under supervision for varying action in the light of this
- being reflexive in the formulation of the problems and identification of solutions.

Question

Can you list equivalent statements from your professional body's documentation?

'Busy messy day — can't make sense of it'

First supervision session

The story about Daniel continues.
I like to start supervision sessions with a 'thought for the day'. Daniel offered, 'it's been a busy messy day and I can't make sense of it'. His statement echoed the description of the nature of professional practice given by Schön (1987) when he talked about 'messy problems'. The situations, cases or problems tackled by professionals are often ill-defined and messy. When they present like this, the actual problem has to be defined. A judgement has to be made before embarking on any course of intervention or taking any action to bring about change.

The work of King and Kitchener (1994) introduced the concept of reflective judgement as the ability to deal with ill-structured problems or the messy problems of practice. They suggested a staged model of reflective judgement giving seven stages that take place over three phases that view a person's beliefs about knowledge. From starting beliefs about absolute answers students gradually learn to recognize that knowledge of ill-structured problems is constructed from inquiry. This ability leads to making reasonable solutions based on the evidence currently available. Perhaps understanding these stages will be helpful to those of you who are endeavouring to practise from a foundation of critical appreciation. These abilities will enhance your competence in this area.

Daniel began to report back on the events of the whole week. He gave detailed factual accounts of what actually happened but was still struggling to offer thoughts or comments about his reactions, feelings or questions that had arisen. To help him sort this out I asked him to select one of the events of the week that he would like to talk about in more detail. I then deliberately used a series of reflective questions and encouraged Daniel to gather his thoughts before answering. Through this support he gave well-considered responses. This showed me that he had indeed thought about what had happened and that his experience had prompted many reactions and questions. Constraints on our supervision time restricted our capacity to apply a similar approach to each of the experiences he had reported on. Therefore, I suggested that he come to the next supervision session having selected and thought about one of the situations he wanted to discuss. To do this, I thought he needed guidance and so I decided to select a simple process to guide his reflection and help him access his experience, describe his practice and explore his learning. I asked him to return to this experience and I suggested some headings to help him. I based these on the retrospective model of Boud et al (1985) entitled *Turning Experience into Learning*.

These headings were:

1. Return to the experience: what happened?
2. Attend to feelings: how did you feel?
3. Reevaluate the experience: how did it happen? What does it make you think about?

The story about this model is interesting. Meeting regularly, the authors reflected on their educational experiences when working with learners. The retrospective model above was the first part of the design of a larger model that was completed in 1991 (Boud and Walker 1991). While the first model highlighted aspects of returning to an experience, the later model included preparing for the experience (prospective reflection) as well as being in the experience (spective reflection).

I've been thinking!

Second supervision session

Daniel came to this session with a list of the issues and events he wanted to report back on. As agreed, he had chosen one to look at in more depth. It was about a visit to an orthotics clinic that was part of his induction program. Daniel had already spent some time trying to answer my reflective prompt questions so that he would be ready to talk about the visit in more depth. He told me that he had observed a session with the orthotist and the physiotherapist working with a family with a little boy. Using the prompt questions above as a frame Daniel told about this experience.

Using prompt questions

What happened?

They had been asked to see the boy because he seemed to walk unevenly. His mother added that he walked *'funny'*. As they started to go through their assessment, they first got him to walk up and down. They were obviously worried about the boy's back as he was leaning to one side when he was sitting. When they stood him up they were pointing out signs of a slight curve in his spine. The physiotherapist and the orthotist talked to the child's mother about their concerns and talked through the options for helping him. The child's mother was really upset and then the little boy started crying too. The boy's mother did not know whether to try and calm him down or whether to keep trying to ask questions.

Attending to feelings: how did you feel?

I thought she wanted to get out of there as quickly as she could! I felt really uncomfortable. The boy's mother did not know what to do for the best either. I felt really upset because it was so sad to see them so distressed.

Re-evaluating the experience: how did it happen?

Well, thinking back on it, I suppose it was just a routine appointment. Routine, but both the child's mother and the staff in the clinic had a bit of a shock when they started looking at the boy. They did a very careful assessment and I could see from their faces that they were unhappy about having to tell this mother something she was not expecting. After all, she went in to have his legs looked at because of his walking!

Daniel was still thinking about this and the experience had clearly made an impression upon him. Daniel then went on to the next question.

What does it make you think about?

So many things. My head was buzzing at the time and I did not really understand what was going on. But I've tried to think about it since then. For example, you get a referral, you send an appointment out and you don't really know what is going to happen when you meet. The physiotherapist and the orthotist really had to think on their feet about what they were doing and saying. What are you supposed to do if both the child and the child's mother get upset? There were many more children the practitioners had to see but they obviously wanted to be able to spend some time with the child's mother to try to help.

I went on to ask Daniel some more questions about his visit to the clinic. I have listed his ideas.

What questions did it raise for you?

What should I think about when I have to give information to a mother about her child which could be potentially difficult and distressing?
What does that mother do now? How will she cope?
What did the practitioners have to know about in order to do this assessment?

What was new?

Watching the collaborative orthotic/physiotherapy assessment of the child.

Understanding something about what they were looking for, like the structure of the body and how the boy moved.

Seeing how spinal problems can occur in children. I heard about this as they were explaining it to the mother. I'll need to get a book out and read about it too because I could only half-listen as I was so concerned for the child's mother.

The difference in the relationship with the child and the family and how it differed from the working relationships I had with people in my previous job.

How do you feel about it now?

Daniel sat quietly. I could see that he had thought a great deal about the session with the boy but it was not easy for him to put his thoughts into words. He said:

It was scary! . . . I was also feeling upset for the mother and realizing the effect of what we say on the people we work with. It really made me think about what and how I say things to people. I was very unhappy that we'd made the boy cry!

I was not expecting the child to cry and I was not expecting to react to his crying by getting upset myself.

To summarize this part of the story, Daniel had been provided a specific reflective framework to help think more deeply. A repertoire of prompt questions that would make him dig even further down into his thoughts and feelings was used. A sympathetic environment was created in the supervision session so that Daniel felt able to recount his true reactions.

Daniel found that by using this framework he was able to give a much more detailed account, including capturing his own thinking about what had happened. He was pleased with how the use of reflective questioning to prompt his thinking had helped. Daniel was becoming more aware of what other factors, like environmental factors, helped him to be more reflective. Box 5.2 gives further information about these environmental factors.

Box 5.2

Suggested environmental/organizational factors that support reflection

- Opportunities for open reflective discussion or comment
- Open working relationship with peers and seniors
- Appropriate supervision and performance monitoring
- Recognition of the value of reflective practice in delivering effective services
- Strategies adopted in delivering or accessing continuing professional development (CPD) and continual professional education (CPE)
- Service specifications and service-level agreements that accommodate beliefs about lifelong learning

Following this positive experience of using retrospective reflection, Daniel now wanted to know when it was appropriate to be reflective in practice. Was it possible to be reflective *all of the time*? I asked him to think about something in the week that had made him consciously stop and consider what he was observing or what he was doing. I wanted to find out when it happened. What had triggered his reflective thinking? We talked about the types of situations that are said to trigger reflection. Box 5.3 gives some examples.

Box 5.3	**Triggers for reflection**
	• Something that went really well
	• A crisis
	• An uncomfortable situation
	• A situation where what usually works was not working
	• An occasion when a usual explanation did not suffice prompting the need for a new explanation

Questions

1. Can you think about an event that has triggered reflection for you?
2. Can you identify one for each of the situations given above?

Reflection can take place privately on an individual basis and it can also be a social practice that takes place within groups or communities. It can also be seen in some qualitative research methodologies, such as in action research, as a way of structuring the reporting of findings and when exploring the researcher's own learning as the study progresses. You may recall a lecturer or practitioner using prompts to encourage you to reflect on your learning. It may also be about acquiring a self-disciplined approach to learning from experience by incorporating specific reflective techniques or frameworks into the way you choose to manage your life and work activities.

Our own practical experiences of using reflection and our appreciation of the literature indicate that *time* is an important factor in the development of reflection. This is about having the time to stop and consider what you are doing and why, and also to be able to look back at what you have done. Box 5.4 on page 128 gives a summary of the temporal nature of reflection.

The story continues

During our discussions about reflection, Daniel and I realized that affective influences and personal well-being can also be seen to have an effect on the quality of the detail recalled. When he had felt upset in the orthotics clinic he realized that his reflective abilities had not been as clear then compared to the other times he had tried to use it. But after these experiences Daniel was now convinced that reflection was deepening his learning. He told me that he was now keen to find out more about other frameworks that might help him access and widen his thinking.

Box 5.4

The temporal nature of reflection

- The activity of reflection requires opportunity, time and personal space (Ryan 1999)
- Thinking about Kolb's learning cycle and the action research cycle, there must be a time delay between the action and reflection (Kember 2000, p. 170)
- Categories of reflection differentiated by the depth of reflective thinking prompted or the extent to which perspectives are transformed (over years) also support the temporal dimension of reflection (Mezirow 1991, van Manen 1977)
- Deeper and more critical levels of reflection operate over an extended time frame (Kember 2000, p. 171)
- The time lapse between when the reflection takes place and the event being considered is important. Where reflection is retrospective, the impact of memory and other cognitive processes like recall will have an impact on the quality or depth or richness of the detail accessible and recalled

---

I directed him to another example that facilitates reflection, known as *strands of reflection* (Fish et al 1991). Box 5.5 gives the four named strands.

I thought that if Daniel could make time to look at this more complex example, we could begin to use it together. This framework was originally developed as a tool to support and facilitate reflection in supervision settings. We both agreed that this would be a further progression with the use of reflection in our supervision sessions and I promised that I would find the article for the next session so that he could examine it.

Cold analysis

During that week a different opportunity for reflection presented itself. At the team meeting a new document laying out a new framework for assessing children was introduced and I asked Daniel to make an appraisal of it and to analyse it to see what implications it might have for the service. To help him with this task the conversation about other frameworks was recalled. I gave him a different example of a framework that can be used to aid analysis and reflection for things like documents and Daniel went away with the headings from Atkins and Murphy's (1993) work. We agreed that this appraisal would be discussed in supervision the following week in preparation for presenting his findings at the next staff meeting. I wanted Daniel to use these headings: awareness of uncomfortable feelings and thoughts, critical appraisal, new perspectives.

Box 5.5

Strands of reflection (Fish et al 1991)
- The factual strand
- The retrospective strand
- The substratum strand
- The connective strand

Opportunistic—in the corridor: uncomfortable experience

Later that week we just happened to be passing each other in the corridor. Daniel had arrived back on site after being present during an interview with a family and he was feeling really unsettled by the experience. He asked me if he could talk about the experience in the next supervision as he was rushing off to do something else. I asked him to try to capture the event quickly in writing this time as a factual account and to try to add comments, as it was still fresh in his mind. This method would be like The *Factual Strand* from the model of Fish et al (1991). I was hoping that Daniel might feel ready to do this now so that he would not lose track of his thoughts. This was to be the start of him keeping a reflective diary.

The first strand, The *Factual Strand*, is outlined in Box 5.6. Chapter 9 also discusses the use of a reflective journal.

Questions:

1. Do you keep a reflective diary or use a diary to capture your thoughts?
2. Do you have a framework or a series of prompt questions that you use?

The factual strand

This draws on procedural knowledge and re-constructs and describes 'the practice' (i.e. the practical situation) in a loose narrative of the events and processes that are happening at the time. By constructing a narrative, the event is recalled but it is thought through and presented as if the narrator is still within the situation (Fish et al 1991). These authors refer to this strand as *debriefing*.

Daniel discovered that it takes several attempts to construct a narrative in sufficient detail. This is why it can be helpful to use this

---

Box 5.6

The factual strand: debriefing

1. **Recalling the practical situation**
Describe the context of the practical situation
Who was there?
Where did the practice take place?
Why was the situation created?

2. **Tell the story—in chronological order**
What was planned (procedural aspects)?
What actually happened? What was different from what had been planned?

3. **Can you pinpoint the critical incidents?**
What questions arose? What points seem to offer scope for learning?
What do you think you need to learn more about?
How did you feel and react at the time?
What have you learnt?

4. **Identifying views about future practice**
What should happen in the next piece of practice? This draws upon the views and intentions associated with the reconstruction. It is not yet at the stage for developing detailed plans for the next piece of practice

process in supervision or with a peer as discussing the story can help tease out the detail required. Helping learners reflect on uncomfortable experiences or engaging with uncomfortable feelings was one focus of an action research study in professional education (Kember 2000). In this study of undergraduate students across five healthcare disciplines the researchers explored the consequences for personal and professional development of the students in incorporating the affective dimension of reflection in the curriculum. The findings point to the reasons why people find reflection, and particularly writing reflectively, such a challenge. In summary, Wong et al (2000, pp. 139–151) found three themes with which people reported having difficulty. These were, firstly, the fear of new learning methods; secondly, specific aspects of the new learning method; and lastly, the workload that reflection presented. These findings echo our own experiences of trying to incorporate reflection into our own work but they also remind us of the responses we received from people with whom we have worked in both practice and academic settings. Reflection is not easy! Reflection is challenging!

I lose my thoughts—I freeze: the story continues

At the next supervision session Daniel explained that he had tried to work at recording his thoughts in a reflective diary but that his old anxieties about diaries had got in the way. I wanted to help him make progress with this way of reflecting so I suggested a way of working on his difficulty with writing so that he could capture his thoughts on paper. I knew that Daniel was able to find the words to express himself more easily now but that his main block was with actually writing down his thoughts. I asked him to make himself comfortable at a table and I gave him some paper and checked that he had a pen. I asked him to start writing and to keep writing for 20 minutes, trying to avoid stopping and to avoid taking his pen away from the paper. He had to do it on the spot and just keep writing. I told him not to bother about sentences or grammar but just to write down all his reflective thoughts. This is called *free-flow writing* and is one solution to writer's block.

Questions

- What helps or hinders you when trying to write down your thoughts?
- Have you discovered ways to capture reflection other than writing? (These methods might include recording your report of an event on a portable tape recorder or Dictaphone or using voice recognition software with a computer.)
- Do you think there will be a difference in the richness of the reflective thoughts or data captured if the activity is undertaken immediately after an experience, 1 hour later, the next morning or the next week?
- When do you reflect on your practice or on the events of the day?
- If the *essence* of your reflective thoughts is captured on audiotape or in writing, will the material be of a different nature? (How this detailed information is recorded will also have an impact on the richness of the description of the event.)

• If the incident or event invokes passion about a particular subject, will this affect the material accessed and captured? How will you address the impact of your 'passion' on your reactions and your reflections on these reactions?

Using writing in reflection and learning

There are many uses and applications of writing for these purposes. Nouns such as journal, log, diary and portfolio perhaps suggest different processes and anticipated outcomes. In Daniel's story we heard about the use of a reflective diary. The arenas in which these forms of writing may be used are also diverse, across the realms of both professional and personal development. (See additional resources section for further information.)

Being clear about how to work by using a defined process or framework and about the purpose of writing seems appropriate. The use of writing can help to monitor learning, and to capture affective and analytical thoughts in a deeper way. These can be freely captured but more practised *reflective* writers tend to adopt and to personalize some kind of framework. Reflective frameworks such as the prompt questions offered by Fish et al (1991) help to structure the writing process of producing a reflective journal or a portfolio. This kind of writing is more than an essay or a piece of descriptive writing. It does take practice, even for the prolific writer, and the techniques involved need careful development. Using the strands of reflection, strand by strand, can help to develop the capacity to capture your thoughts and to access deeper thinking in a developmental way. The differences between writing descriptively and writing reflectively have been teased out by one of our colleagues as she was marking reflective papers. The work shown in Table 5.1 is not published but is used with her permission.

Writing for a portfolio—formal reflection for professional development

By now, Daniel had been working with us in the service for 3 weeks and his Individual Performance Review (IPR) session was being arranged. He was asked to review his own professional portfolio in preparation for this session.

The local service uses the professional portfolio outline provided by the professional body, the College of Occupational Therapy (COT). This is used as a basic framework but individuals can elect to draw upon other frameworks if helpful. Most professional bodies have developed, or are in the process of developing, reflective portfolios. Further details can be found in Chapter 11, in the section on presenting the evidence of professional development.

Working with the material in Daniel's diary

Daniel was asked to think about whether the portfolio format worked for him or whether he might find it useful to draw from some of the other reflective frameworks he has recently tried.

Daniel had worked really well at capturing the event that had made him feel so uncomfortable and it was agreed that his experience would be explored further in supervision. Questions based on the other three Strands of Reflection—the *Retrospective Strand*, the *Substratum Strand*

Table 5.1   *The differences between writing reflectively and writing descriptively (concept developed by Sue Neville)*

Reflective	Descriptive
Descriptive account followed by some evaluation and ways of making sense of the information	Straight description given
Rich account, comes alive, brings own opinions, therefore the reader is aware of what matters to the person writing	No detail about what the writer thinks of the situation. It is written objectively and factually. Feelings, if mentioned, are not explained
Selects experiences and goes into depth	Tries to include too much detail and ends up with a chronological account
Is obviously asking 'why'?	No basis for the judgements made
Links to previous experiences	Little reference to previous experiences
Critically discusses extent to which the learning goals were met. Aware of personal learning	Tends not to refer to learning goals. Does not really articulate own learning

and the *Connective Strand*—were used to help him review and reflect on the event (see Boxes 5.7, 5.8, 5.9).

In the original text, the authors state that 'the details offered in the subsections are merely indications of the kind of issues occurring within that particular strand. They offer a flavour of an event but are not intended to be exhaustive, nor do they need to be considered on every occasion' (Fish et al 1991, p. 23). Each strand goes deeper and personal values and beliefs and future ideas are all captured. It is more effective if these strands are worked through separately to give time to this process. We advocate completing the first strand of the event during a specific period such as a placement or writing about a specific event before proceeding with the other strands (Alsop and Ryan 1996). The main purpose of using an approach such as the four strands is to develop insight into your practice over a period of time. It gives you a sense of the way you are, think and feel, and the way you work. Below are the prompt questions I used with Daniel for these three strands.

The Retrospective Strand

This strand focuses deliberately on the retrospective nature of reflection. It draws theory from practice and develops sensitivity and imagination by extending the appreciation of wider perspectives of practice. These were developed from the work of Fish et al (1991).

The Substratum Strand

This strand seeks to discover and explore the underlying assumptions and beliefs and value judgements about the events and ideas emerging from the *Factual Strand* and the *Retrospective Strand*. It focuses upon a critical exploration of personal theory and the links between personal theory and formal theory. It goes beyond the 'how' technicalities of the event and looks in detail at the intended goals. It extends the appreciation of personal theories emerging from the practice and expanded by an understanding of other people's perspectives by including challenges from formal theory. It encourages the practitioner to tolerate the idea that there is no right answer in many practice situations and that a range of views exist.

Box 5.7	**The Retrospective Strand**
	Looking back on the event, what patterns of behaviour and responses were evident?
	What did you think you expected to get out of it?
	What were the overall aims, intentions and goals?
	Were these achieved?
	Having thought initially about your own perspective about the practice, what viewpoints might the other people involved have to offer? How might they have felt about it?
	How does the context (background from the factual strand) relate to what actually happened?
	What existing knowledge did you draw upon?
	How and where did you apply that knowledge?
	What new things did you learn and from which part of the piece of practice?
	What can you say about the interactions occurring between the people involved?
	What could be said about human relationships as a whole?
	Think about the language used during the interaction. What might it tell you?
	What new discoveries did you make from the whole practice?
	What were the reasons, motives and emotions that might have been associated with actions?
	For you as the practitioner, what happened?
	What were the critical incidents? Were these connected?

Box 5.8	**The Substratum Strand**
	What customs, traditions and rituals were brought to the situation or were apparent?
	What beliefs, dogmas, prejudices or emotions were brought to the situation or were apparent?
	Where did they come from?
	Is an ideological pattern emerging?
	What basic beliefs and assumptions underlie the actions, emotions and decisions reported in the other strands?
	What beliefs are emerging about existing and new knowledge and how it is gained and used?
	What do you think about the theory and practice implicit in the practice and your reflection upon this?
	How can you explain the kinds of evaluation and justification used so far to guide the reflective process?
	What theories have you based your actions upon?
	What can you say about the ends or outcomes of the actions undertaken? On what grounds were they justified or were they defensible? Whose were the anticipated outcomes?
	What is your relationship with your work?

The Connective Strand

This strand pulls together new appreciation and insights about practice, of knowledge extended or newly gained from the previous strands. It does not examine detailed planning for future practice but seeks to focus attention to the wider world of other practical situations. It includes other professionals' experiences, views, reflections and expressions of theory as well as the practitioner's own personal theory. Through engaging with the professional literature it also combines formal theory. For Fish et al (1991) the information gained is fully contextualized.

Box 5.9

The Connective Strand

What have you learnt from this situation as a whole?

How has it related to past experiences? How might it relate to future ones?

What do you understand now about what drove your practice?

How do your thinking and your actions sit with the wider context of the action?

How might you modify your thinking and your actions specifically in this situation in the light of experience, further thought, and further reading?

Thinking about the ends of pieces of practice, what of the previous piece of practice? How were the ends considered in this one? How and when might they be considered in the next one?

What tentative further theories might be developed for future action?

What implications do your reflections have for future practice?

Using the Strands of Reflection

So how did these questions help Daniel? For him it was clear that using the framework of the four *Strands of Reflection* enabled him to access his thoughts and to talk about his practice. The first time the framework was used a selection of the questions were used to guide the conversation. Over time, Daniel felt more at ease and more confident in using the framework and the prompt questions to guide his own reflection. He began to use the guide questions to record his thinking and reflection in his reflective diary as well. For Gill, it offered a structure and direction within which to formulate and word questions, which could be geared to specific situations. Sometimes the factual and retrospective strands would be used in supervision. This gave Daniel an opportunity to work out his own thinking first so that he could bring his reflective thoughts, captured on paper, to the session ready to refer and discuss the issues. Where possible, the other strands would be used to explore significant situations in more depth within supervision so that we could work on them collaboratively. Daniel organized his diary so that he wrote on the left side only. The free page on the right-hand side was completed later. This allowed space to capture later reflections on his original entries.

Practitioners' group: the story continues

As a member of the staff team Daniel was encouraged to join the practitioners' group that met fortnightly. One of the activities that the group undertook each session was the presentation of a mini case story to look at practice. When Daniel's turn to present came round, he felt confident to use the Strands of Reflection (Fish et al 1991) to review and to present his case. He knew that he would have enough detail to share his thinking about practice, whereas before it had all seemed so messy and mixed up that he could not make sense of it. He was able to build on his own learning and on his gains in his self-confidence.

One of the group asked about reflection. She wanted to know when thinking was not considered to be reflection. Daniel was not sure and he offered to look into this with another group member. They agreed to report their findings at the next meeting. Through a search of the literature, Daniel discovered the work of Mezirow (1991), who distinguishes three types of *non-reflective action*. These are *habitual action*, *thoughtful action* and *introspection*. Further explanation of these terms is given in Box 5.10.

Box 5.10	**Mezirow's types of non-reflective action**

Habitual action

Habitual action is that which has been learnt previously, and through frequent use becomes an activity which is performed automatically or with little conscious thought, e.g. riding a bike, using a keyboard. These are examples of activities that would represent doing routine work in practice without much thinking.

This may also be likened to Schön's 'reflection in action' and proves to be an example of the inconsistencies in the use of terminology and definitions around reflection. For example, do you have time to think or to reflect when you are riding a bike? It may depend on your level of expertise and your success in staying on the bike and not falling off.

Thoughtful action

Thoughtful action is like making use of existing knowledge without any attempt to make an appraisal of that knowledge or to relate this knowledge to personal experiences. This is a cognitive process and is likened to Schön's 'knowing in practice' (Schön 1983, pp. 61–63). Reflection will only follow if there is a mismatch with the frameworks normally experienced.

Introspection

Introspection, from the affective domain, refers to thoughts or feelings about ourselves and also about others. It is that these thoughts occur, and not why they occur, that is considered to be introspection. If attempts are made to validate or reexamine this knowledge or to explore why these feelings occur then this can be considered to be reflective thinking.

So, from an understanding of what constitutes non-reflective action, Daniel and the practitioners' group were able to discuss their new understandings and use of reflection in more detail.

New technical skill—active learning

In a later supervision session Daniel highlighted a particular need to learn a practical task. He knew he would soon need to know how to use this knowledge with a family. Daniel would have to measure the depth of a seat for a child so that he could arrange a suitable chair for use by the child at home. Coincidentally, a similar situation was expected that week with another family being seen. I arranged that Daniel would join in and have the opportunity to work through the task. For a session like this a *coaching* approach, as offered by Schön (1987), was followed.

To explain this further I have chosen to use the example of measuring a child's chair, as it is a very practical task. It may help to identify a very specific task relevant in your own area of practice to which you can relate and compare.

Schön (1987) realized that much of the routine work that professionals do is tacit. That is, experienced professionals deal with familiar situations and judgements are made without thinking deeply about the reasons underlying why they choose to do something. Schön proposed that in *standard* cases professionals display an almost unconscious routine. He called this '*knowing in action*'. Because of this deep-seated knowledge expert professionals find it difficult to articulate their practice, to explain their reasoning and the processes undertaken as they do their work. In addition, Schön also realized that not all professional practice exists through this '*knowing in action*. He identified that both ordinary people and professional practitioners often think about what they are doing, sometimes while doing it. Schön viewed this more complicated procedure as *reflection in action*. He described an example of this reflection in action where the leader and learner in a learning situation work through a task together. They make their thinking explicit at strategic times during this process with the aim of developing the learner's thinking and appreciation of this practice. The practical task selected in the example in Figure 5.3 is chosen because it illustrates the kind of task and teaching and learning situation thought to be appropriate.

There are three stages within the coaching strategy. These are *Follow me*, *Joint experimentation* and *Hall of mirrors*.

We followed these cues shown in Figure 5.3 and as we cleared away after the session Daniel asked about the methods that he had been shown. I decided to respond with a question. I asked Daniel to think about what I was doing to guide his learning. After a while Daniel responded: 'You were showing me parts of the task and then gradually prompting me to question what you were doing. So the next time you do it I would know more about what I am looking at and the questions I should be asking myself when I actually do it!' This was a good start. In fact, Schön's *reflection-in-action* approach to teaching and

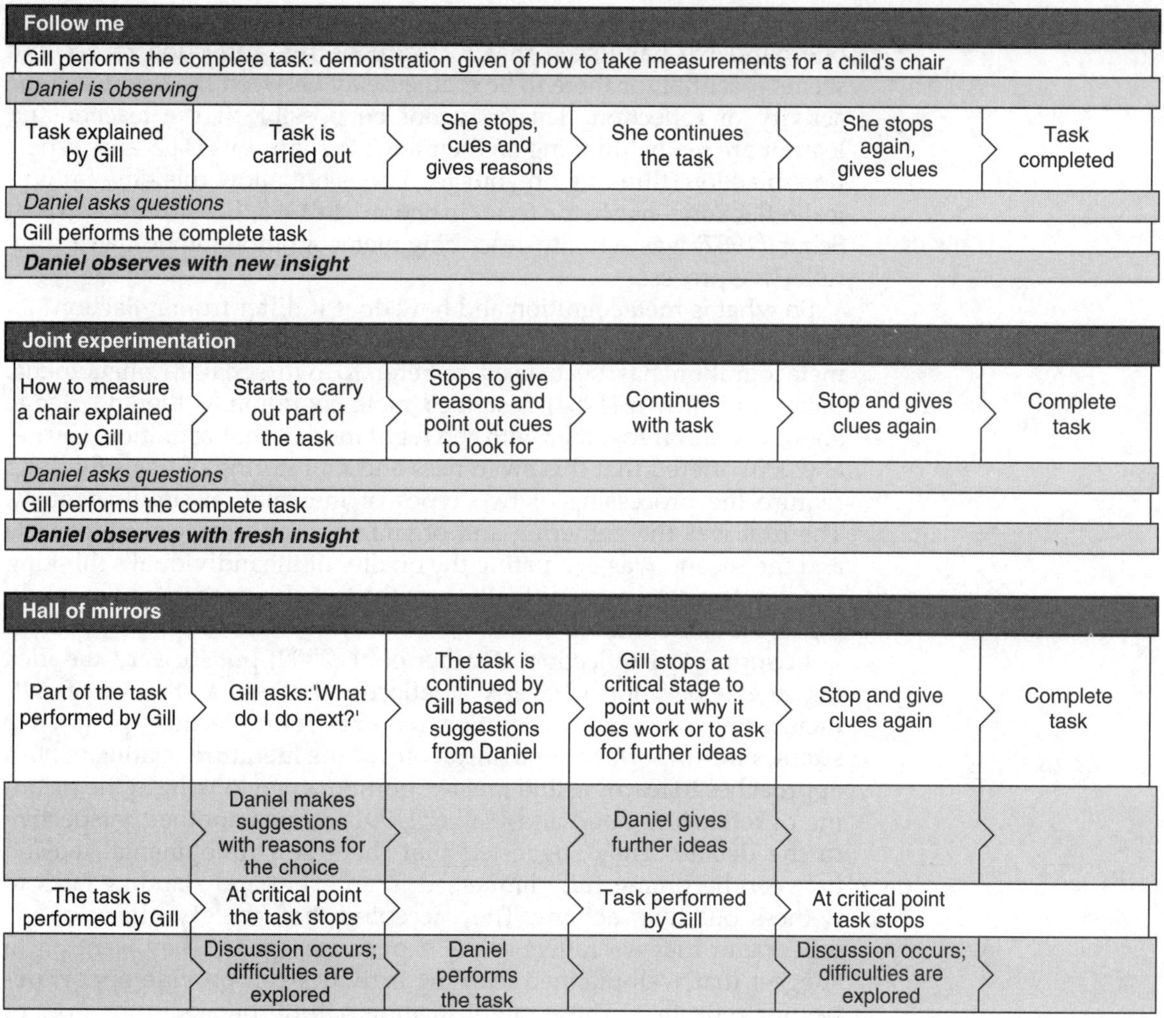

Follow me					
Gill performs the complete task: demonstration given of how to take measurements for a child's chair					
Daniel is observing					
Task explained by Gill	Task is carried out	She stops, cues and gives reasons	She continues the task	She stops again, gives clues	Task completed
Daniel asks questions					
Gill performs the complete task					
Daniel observes with new insight					

Joint experimentation					
How to measure a chair explained by Gill	Starts to carry out part of the task	Stops to give reasons and point out cues to look for	Continues with task	Stop and gives clues again	Complete task
Daniel asks questions					
Gill performs the complete task					
Daniel observes with fresh insight					

Hall of mirrors					
Part of the task performed by Gill	Gill asks:'What do I do next?'	The task is continued by Gill based on suggestions from Daniel	Gill stops at critical stage to point out why it does work or to ask for further ideas	Stop and give clues again	Complete task
	Daniel makes suggestions with reasons for the choice		Daniel gives further ideas		
The task is performed by Gill	At critical point the task stops		Task performed by Gill	At critical point task stops	
	Discussion occurs; difficulties are explored	Daniel performs the task		Discussion occurs; difficulties are explored	

Figure 5.3   *Using Schön's reflection in action*

learning can be considered to be like 'thinking on your feet' (Fish et al 1991). In this session with Daniel, I was taking the role of the teacher or coach and I was describing what was happening and what I was thinking about at the same time. As the task was repeated the teacher and learner, Daniel and I, explored the task collaboratively.

Question

Can you relate this approach to teaching and learning in practical tasks to similar situations you have experienced?

A debate about reflection

You may be puzzled and wonder whether this reflection in action does actually happen in such teaching and learning settings. There is a debate in the literature about whether this reflection in action is indeed reflection or whether it should be considered as meta-cognition. The question is whether this process is an example of cognitive and reasoning development. If it is, then it is not reflection.

Indeed, the concept of reflection-in-action has been challenged. On the one hand we have seen that for retrospective reflection to occur it seems essential for there to be a time delay between the event and the activity of reflection. This may not be possible if the teacher and learner are really 'thinking on their feet'. Perhaps this is because reflection in action (thinking on your feet) does not allow this time for critical reflection—hence the term 'in action'. In 1995, Eraut proposed that Schön (1987) was actually describing metacognition rather than a truly reflective process.

So what is metacognition and how does it differ from reflection? At another higher-level thinking process, in comparison to reflection, metacognition has been used to refer to two separate phenomena. Baker and Brown (1984) described meta-cognition as the knowledge about cognition together with the regulation of that cognition. Carr et al (2000) offered that this awareness and monitoring of one's thinking require the processing of two types of information simultaneously. The first was the gathering and organizing and synthesizing of facts and the second was evaluating the quality of the individual's thinking process. It is extremely difficult to do the two things that require thinking at the same time.

In support of reflection, Kember et al (2000) put forward the idea that meta-cognition is clearly a reflective process as the act of self-monitoring one's own cognition requires self-reflection (p. 15). He stresses the importance of being aware of the literature relating to both approaches to learning and meta-cognition when looking at the meaning of reflection. Boud and Walker (1991) offered another perspective to the debate. They suggested that there is a fundamental tension between becoming fully immersed in an event and standing back to witness our own actions. They accepted that 'we experience as we reflect and that we reflect as we experience' (p. 6). They went on to suggest that well-planned learning activities can provide opportunities for reflection. These might include natural breaks in the flow of events, time-out activities and selected exercises chosen for their reflective nature. Two other elements of the reflective process are also identified by Boud and Walker (1991). These are noticing and intervening. They are akin in some ways to the observing behaviour seen in Schön's (1987) 'Follow me' and the 'Joint experimentation' styles. Noticing is defined as 'the act of learners becoming aware of what is happening in and around themselves' (p. 7). 'Intervening is the action taken by learners within the event which can affect the learning milieu or learners themselves (including learners acting on themselves)' (p. 7). If we accept that by creating a structured learning situation by adapting Schön's coaching styles for use in specific practice settings, the structure and space and time provided can offer opportunity for reflection.

Deeper learning—a multidisciplinary team meeting: the story continues

One of the families with whom Daniel was working had an appointment with the multidisciplinary team to review their child's progress and to plan the next 6 months' intervention. Each team member would have the opportunity to share information and to hear viewpoints from other people too. Daniel found it useful to use Fish et al's (1991) *Strands of Reflection* to help him share his own thinking with the family through his contact with them and therefore he was happy to use this information and to contribute to the review session and meeting.

At the next supervision Daniel talked about his reactions to being part of that meeting, about the family's perspective of the event and what he might try to do differently the next time he would join such a meeting. He considered the information gained in the meeting in a structured way so that he could see where his new insights were developing. He recognized that his own new understanding of the family's situation had been shaped by learning from the different perspectives that had been shared about the family from the team. Daniel noticed that one professional may define the situation in one way and another may identify that quite different problems require attention.

Before decisions about problem-solving are made, issues of problem-framing have to be addressed. This latter concept encompasses an understanding of the uniqueness of each case. For each individual practitioner this problem-framing will go beyond applying professional theoretical knowledge and techniques involving procedural knowledge and technical problem-solving. Schön (1987) called this individualized practice 'Professional Artistry'. An ideal solution is rarely achievable. Some degree of agreement can be reached by recognizing the conflicts and ambiguities inherent in problem-solving within professional practice.

Daniel had demonstrated that he was able to use reflection to gain a deeper appreciation of his practice overall and also of the effect of his intervention and of other interventions, including the review session and meeting. His thinking had been logical and rational but he was also aware of the importance of care and compassion, as well as the passion of caring in professional practice.

Thinking about achieving deeper reflection leads us on to the question of whether there are different levels of reflection. Zeichner (1994), when writing about teacher education, summarized his analysis of the literature by highlighting three typologies or levels of reflection. Technical, practical and critical reflection can be seen as examples of these levels of reflection. Handal and Lauvas (1987) offered action, practical and theoretical reasons for action, and ethical justification for action. Additionally, Griffiths and Tann (1992) proposed the following levels:

- rapid reflection: instinctive and immediate
- repair: habitual, pause for thought, fast, on the spot
- review: time out to reassess over hours and days
- research: systematic, sharply focused, over weeks or months
- re-theorizing and re-formulating: abstract, rigorous, clearly formulated, over months or years.

These typologies show the types of reflection, the speed of reflection and the depth of reflection that it is possible to achieve, given time. However Zeichner (1994) argued against thinking about reflection in

Daniel: Using enhanced skills

During subsequent weeks Daniel needed little encouragement to continue developing his use and application of reflection in different ways in his work. He shared his interest in this extension to his skills with one or two of his colleagues and, when exploring ideas with them and the students who joined the department, Daniel was able to articulate practice. He showed an increasing self-confidence and demonstrated a sense of new understanding with a critical stance about his work. His experience of practice had changed. As he progressed to taking on more complex clinical cases his skills in using reflection enabled him to analyse his practice and to gain deeper understandings of the situations facing the families with whom he worked. His decision-making was clear and his conclusions and recommendations were informed and well considered. He was able to make sense of the complexity and perplexity of practice. These first few months provided a firm foundation from which Daniel was able to develop his reflective and practice skills still further. He began to take responsibility for elements of the practitioners' professional development program, building on his own expanding appreciation of the place of reflection in supporting learning from experience.

Strategies seen in use during Daniel's story

An overview of the range of techniques and frameworks that practitioners such as Daniel might discover and learn to integrate into their work is given in Table 5.2.

Synthesis and reflection – learning from writing this chapter

When we first embarked upon the task of writing this chapter it quickly became evident that we would need to revisit our own understandings and confusions about the topic of reflection. Each of us learns about reflection in different ways, but if we are being critical about our learning, we will continue to question our understanding as we arrive at each new situation. When we took on this task it prompted us to ask what it was about reflection that attracted us to become more interested in the subject. We discovered that it was important to find ways to capture our own thoughts more efficiently while studying at a higher level like a Master's program or doing doctoral research. We then wanted to find ways of helping our staff/faculty and students to do the same. We were able to incorporate some of our own learning into the way that we structure supervision sessions for staff/faculty and students and, indeed, this influenced the way that we approached and sought supervision ourselves.

We are still considering the questions of when, for example, it is appropriate to learn about *reflection* and *when* to learn more about *how* to apply this knowledge.

Table 5.2 *Key reflective techniques*

Technique	Example by author	Date	Scenario	Pros and cons
Reflective diary	Alsop and Ryan	1996	As a tool to capture thinking As a tool to support learning and develop critical thinking	Often difficult to sustain. Can seem unrelated to other developmental activities if not linked to supervision or peer support. Advantageous to use framework to guide structure
Reflective judgement	King and Kitchener	1994	To support critical appraisal of knowledge in *'messy problems'*, especially with peers	Most helpful to have other people around who can support or facilitate the process by offering challenges to the learner's beliefs and assumptions
Reflective questions/effective questioning	Fish	1995	Supervision Peer supervision	Offers a challenge to practitioners to seek to think more deeply about their practice
Preparing for an experience	Boud and Walker	1991	Before a visit to a new practice context, i.e. new ward, new clinic or new school	Finding space and time can be daunting but it can also assist time management and planning
Returning to the experience	Boud and Walker	1991	Personal debriefing, staff-room conversations and in supervision	Principles may not offer sufficient structure for the individual. Can be combined with strands of reflection
Strands of reflection	Fish et al Fish	1991 1995	As a guide to develop process and questions: supervision, reflective diary, research to support development of personal prompt questions or cues	Time involved initially will reap long-term gains. Helpful to be able to work with others as it is possible to become complacent about the quality of reflection if challenges are not available
Analysis and reflection	Atkins and Murphy	1993	Critical appraisal of a document	Records new perspectives. Also suitable for reflecting on other experiences besides responding to a document
Professional portfolio	Alsop Walker Professional body or equivalent	2000, Chs 2 and 3 1985	Provides structure to record professional activity and learning. Seen as a probable requirement for evidence of continuing professional development	Time involved can be a problem. Strategies need to be owned and developed by the practitioners and not implemented because they are dictated by rules. Requires a disciplined approach to recording and demonstrating learning
Group work with a facilitator	Alsop and Ryan	1996	Provides a structure to explore everyday challenges encountered in practice and to identify strategies and actions required	Facilitator acts as a resource. Responsibility for the process of running the group is shared between participants and facilitator
Coaching (reflection in action)	Schön	1987	Technical/practical skill in clinical setting	Learning context requires structure. Requires 'leader and learner' to have knowledge of process learning

There is some controversy about when reflection should be included. For example, should it be in the undergraduate curriculum? Alsop (1993) believed it should come later, while most other authors believe it should start from the beginning of professional education. As you have seen in this chapter, this debate may be on the fact that *'reflection'* is being interpreted in differing ways. This also prompts us to question how much *practice* has to be experienced before a *practitioner* can reflect on, and learn from, experience. We think that more use can be made of informal knowledge and life experience if this process starts early in professional education. Using reflection to discover the meaning of new experiences and the learning that has been derived from them is a skill that can be enhanced through reflecting at any stage of learning or career development.

Further questions

Terminology and language: global perspective

Reflection and reflective practice are established in the UK, in Australia, Scandinavia and in parts of North America, or other parts of the world in particular, where the language to communicate about the topic is English. It is not clear to what extent the concept of reflection or reflective practice exists outside the parts of the world, where English is read or spoken fluently. Think about your own beliefs and habits around reflection and how these influences may affect the way you interact with and apply any of the frameworks that have been discussed in this chapter. The above thoughts do not mean that reflection is culturally limited but it does manifest itself differently according to culture. Archetypal stories and myths and the use of metaphor are ways of enhancing reflection in many cultures. You may wish to pause here, and consider which countries in the world have cultures that use imagery and archetypal stories and how they contrast with written communication styles. How do you think this might affect communication at a global level?

Bridging the theory-and-practice divide

Intimately understanding the different perspectives on reflection enables the enhancement of reflective abilities. With increasing emphasis on the need for bridging the theory-and-practice divide in professional and continuing education, practitioners will be required to use strategies that bring about reflection across both contexts. Given that life-long learning is now recognized as part of professional practice, the ongoing extension of knowledge and skills around reflective thinking, reflective judgement and reflective practice is essential.

Question

Can you identify ways in which your department is working to incorporate strategies to support reflective thinking, reflective judgement and reflective practice? How do these strategies help you to blend practice and theory and bridge the divide?

Kember et al (2000) encouraged us to look at the relationship between the literature on educating the reflective practitioner with that of development of reflective judgement. These come from different disciplines and it would seem that authors have not acknowledged the work from these different disciplinary backgrounds, apart from a common acknowledgement of the original work of Dewey in the 1930s. Is this because the literature referring to reflective practice refers to the practice setting and the literature referring to reflective judgement sits within general education? Kember et al proposed that such compartmentalizing is limiting, as insights from those in other disciplines would often be relevant, particularly if adaptations were made.

Question

What action could you take to incorporate the work of King and Kitchener (1994) on reflective judgement? For example, how would you include these ideas into the educational programs in your clinical department?

This chapter has given you an overview of some of the different perspectives about the construct of reflection as a basis for extending your own appreciation of the nature of reflection. We hope it has stimulated some new insights for you.

References

Alsop A E 1993 The developmental model of skill acquisition in fieldwork. British Journal of Occupational Therapy 56:7–12

Alsop A 2000 Continual professional development: a guide for therapists. Blackwell Science, Oxford

Alsop A, Ryan S 1996 Making the most of fieldwork education: a practical approach. Nelson Thornes, Cheltenham

Atkins S, Murphy K 1993 Reflection; a review of the literature. Journal of Advanced Nursing 18:1188–1192

Baker L, Brown A L 1984 Metacognitive skills and reading. In: Pearson D, Kamil M L, Barr R et al (eds) Handbook of reading research. Longman, New York, p 353–394

Boud D, Walker D 1991 In the midst of experience: developing a model to aid learners and facilitators. Paper presented at the National Conference on Experiential Learning empowerment through experiential learning: explorations of good practice. University of Surrey, 16–18 July 1991.

Boud D, Keogh R, Walker D 1985 Reflection; turning experience into learning. Kogan Page, London

Boyd E M, Fayles A W 1993 Reflective learning: key to learning from experience. Journal of Humanistic Psychology 23:99–117

Carr J, Jones M, Higgs J 2000 Learning in physiotherapy programmes. In: Higgs J, Jones M (eds) Clinical reasoning in the health professions, 2nd edn. Butterworth-Heinemann, Oxford, p 198–204

Dewey J 1910 How we think. University of Chicago, Chicago

Dewey J 1933 How we think: a restatement of the relation of reflective thinking to the educative process. Heath, Boston.

Eraut M 1995 Knowledge creation and knowledge use in professional contexts. Studies in Higher Education 10:117–133

Fish D 1995 Quality mentoring for student teachers: a principled approach to practice. David Fulton, London

Fish D, Twinn S, Purr B 1991 Promoting reflection: the supervision of practice. In: Fish D, Twinn S, Purr B (eds) Health visiting and initial teacher training. West London Institute Press, London, pp. 23–70

Ghaye T 2001 FHS (faster, higher, stronger), issue 10. National Coaching Foundation, Leeds

Griffiths M, Tann S 1992 using reflective practice to link personal and public theories. Journal for Education for Teaching 18:69–84

Handal G, Lauvas P 1987 Promoting reflective teaching: supervision in action. Open University Press, Milton Keynes

Kember D 2000 Reflections on reflection. In: Kember D (ed) Reflective teaching and learning in the health professions. Blackwell Science, Oxford, pp. 167–175

Kember D, Wong F K Y, Yeung E 2000 In: Kember D et al (eds) Reflective teaching and learning in the health professions. Blackwell Science, Oxford

King P, Kitchener K 1994 Developing reflective judgement: understanding and promoting intellectual growth and critical in adolescents and adults. Jossey-Bass, San Francisco

Kolb D 1984 Experiential learning: experience as the source of learning and development. Prentice-Hall, Englewood Cliffs, NJ

Martin C, Thornberg K, Shepard K 1992 The professional development of expert clinicians in orthopedic and neurological practice. Physical Therapy 72:107–116

Mezirow J 1991 Transformative dimensions of adult learning. Jossey-Bass, San Francisco

Ryan S 1999 Layers of reflection: opportunity, time and personal space. College of Occupational Therapists' 23rd Annual Conference, Research, Reflect, Revise. Liverpool University, 20–23 July 1999

Schön D 1983 The reflective practitioner: how professionals think in action. Basic Books, New York

Schön D 1987 Educating the reflective practitioner. Jossey-Bass, San Francisco

The Quality Assurance Agency for Higher Education 2001 Benchmark statement: Health care programmes phase 1, occupational therapy subject bench marking group. Quality Assurance Agency for Higher Education, Gloucester UK

van Manen M 1977 Linking ways of knowing with ways of being practical. Curriculum Inquiry 6:205–227

Walker D 1985 Writing and reflection. In: Boud D, Keogh R, Walker D (eds) reflection: turning experience into learning. Kogan Page, London, p 52–68

Wong M W L, Kember D, Wong F K Y and Loke A Y 2000 The affective dimension of reflection. In: Kember D (ed.) Reflective teaching and learning in the health professions. Blackwell Science, Oxford, pp. 139–151

Zeichner K M 1994 Research on teacher thinking and different views of reflective practice. In: Calgren I, Handal G, Vaague S (eds) Teaching and teacher education in teachers, minds and actions; research on teachers, thinking and practice. Falmer Press, London, pp. 9–27

Further reading

Andrews J 2000 The value of reflective practice; a student case study. British Journal of Occupational Therapy 63:396–398.

Finlay L 1998 Reflexivity: an essential component for all research. British Journal of Occupational Therapy 61:453–456

Fortune T 1999 Student's fieldwork stories: reflecting on supervision. In: Ryan S E, McKay E A (eds) Thinking and reasoning in therapy. Stanley Thornes, Cheltenham, p 65–79

Mezirow J 1981 A critical theory of adult learning and education. Adult Education 32:3–24 (this paper discusses the role of critical reflectivity in adult learning)

Parham D 1987 Towards professionalism: the reflective therapist. American Journal of Occupational Therapy. 41:555–561 (this paper places reflection central to professional practice and offers a vision relevant across all elements of healthcare practice)

Progoff I 1975 At a journal workshop: the basic text and guide for using the intensive journal. Penguin Putnam, New York (this text provides a number of different frameworks applied within the field of counselling)

Additional resources

Institute of Reflective Practice
Twigworth Court Business Centre
Twigworth
Gloucestershire GL2 9PG
www.reflectivepractices.com
Journal of Reflective Practice

6

Do you reason like a (health) professional?

Joy Higgs

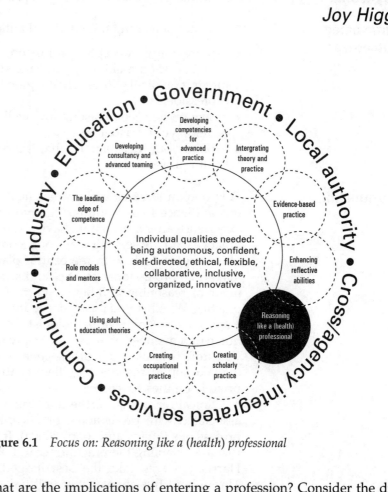

Figure 6.1 *Focus on: Reasoning like a (health) professional*

Chapter outline

What are the implications of entering a profession? Consider the differences between being a member of a profession and being a technician. Both can behave 'professionally' (with integrity and dedication), both can be well prepared for their role and both have a valuable part to play in work and society. However, professionals have the privilege and the obligation to work autonomously. This entails making quality, independent and accountable decisions and implementing them in a spirit of critical appraisal. Being a professional requires an ongoing commitment to education and to the generation of knowledge. All of these factors come together in the act of clinical reasoning or professional decision-making, which draws together a dynamic professional and personal knowledge base, the cognitive skills of reasoning, the heightened awareness of meta-cognitive and reflective practice, and a professional orientation to providing quality services for clients. This chapter asks you to consider the craft, science, artistry and human dimensions of professional reasoning and to examine ways of enhancing this reasoning as part of the journey to becoming an advanced practitioner (Figure 6.1).

Key words

Reasoning, professional, advanced practice

Anticipated outcomes

As a result of reading this chapter, I anticipate that you will be able to:

- explore these concepts: profession, professional, clinical/professional decision-making and advanced practitioner, and examine the integration of all of these challenging factors in the practice of health professionals
- reflect on how you reason, how well you reason and how you can develop your reasoning
- expand your ideas about what it means to reason like an *advanced* health professional.

Introduction

This book addresses early-career health professionals. In writing to this audience I am assuming that you have several years of practice experience after graduation, have acquired skills in reflecting on your practice, and are seeking ways of becoming an advanced practitioner. This chapter deals with the central place of reasoning and decision-making in professional practice and autonomy, and with the development of reasoning abilities as part of the move towards advanced practice. Whether you are an occupational therapist, a physiotherapist, a speech and language pathologist, an audiologist, a radiographer, a nurse or a member of one of the many other allied health professions, your role is to use your professional knowledge and reasoning skills to make sound, responsible, client-centred decisions and to act appropriately on these decisions.

Clinical reasoning, or the thinking and decision-making processes associated with professional practice, is a critical skill in the health professions (Higgs and Jones 2000a). It is a thinking process directed towards enabling the practitioner to take 'wise' action (Cervero 1988, Harris 1993); to take the best judged action in a specific context. Throughout this chapter you will have the opportunity to reflect on ideas and questions in order to explore how well you think you achieve the goals of competent reasoning and quality practice. Chapter 5 gives you further ideas about reflection.

Joining a healthcare profession

The health and nursing professions have expended a great deal of energy and angst, particularly in the last 50 years, to gain the title, position and respect associated with being a profession. While this endeavour has been led by professional associations and professional leaders, it is a responsibility shared by us all. Each individual in the profession contributes to the way the profession is regarded by our colleagues and the community.

Membership of a profession is permitted after recognized tertiary education which guarantees the quality and effectiveness of the practice of the profession's members (Cant and Higgs 1999). Because of this, professionals are accorded a privileged place in society, with their work being characterized by autonomy. This demands the capacity to make sound (credible and defensible) decisions to guide and evaluate practice.

Professionalism is portrayed by Eraut (1994) as an ideology, characterized by the traits and features of an 'ideal-type' profession. Professionals are expected to demonstrate social responsibility (Prosser 1995), accountability and a recognition of their limitations (Sultz et al 1984), to practise with integrity and personal tolerance and to communicate effectively across language, cultural and situational barriers (Josebury et al 1990). How well do you meet these expectations and criteria of being a member of a profession?

Being an autonomous professional in the changing world of healthcare

What does it mean to be an autonomous professional in the changing world of healthcare? We live in a society with changing views of health, where health is increasingly being viewed as wellness rather than the absence of illness, and where managers and governments consider health to be a commodity rather than a right (Higgs et al 1999). These changes have required a re-evaluation of the concept of healthcare. Health and other social service systems have become complex environments, with a global shift towards population and community health compared to curing individuals. Alongside the increasing costs of healthcare and social service systems there has been, in many countries, a trend towards reducing the scope of governmental services and the revenues derived through taxation, with a correspondingly decreased capacity of governments to fund healthcare and social services. This shortfall in funds is one of the driving forces behind such policies and strategies as economic rationalism, community-based services and transfer of costs to the consumer. Economic rationalism, discussed in Chapter 1, seeks to introduce corporate sector management philosophy and practices (e.g. market competition, privatization) into the public policy sector. At the same time the healthcare and social service systems are facing the increasing effects of globalization (see Table 6.1 on page 148).

Activity box 6.1

Reflective questions

What are the characteristics of your working environment in relation to changing health and social trends, concepts and management systems?

How does your work environment influence your professional autonomy, practice and decision-making?

Preparation for practice in tomorrow's workplace

What type of graduate does this changing, globalizing, market-driven workplace demand? What types of expectations face health professionals in the workplace? One way of considering these issues is to consider the type of graduate who was deemed satisfactory in the past and the type of graduate who will face the future with success and

---

Table 6.1   *Globalization effects on health and social services (derived from Neubauer 1998)*

Globalization means that:

- ideas and issues are quickly disseminated throughout the world; physical and national boundaries and time are no longer barriers to the dispersion of new medical products and procedures
- societies of the world are being restructured through the redistribution of employment and finance, generating health and social consequences (such as unemployment and illness associated with new regions of poverty) that are not immediately apparent or readily understood
- multinational corporations and finance capital are the primary players in the new system of globalization; maximization of return, rather than people concerns, is the new priority
- new social health problems and market style solutions are arising from national government and private sector restructuring
- reshaping of the job market is occurring, with changing levels of unemployment. Consequently, those typically requiring greater access to health and social services, i.e. people in lower socioeconomic groups, are less able to afford these services
- there is increased privatization and marketization of healthcare. Social services are being dehumanized and are increasingly viewed by governments and international agencies as a commodity and not a social responsibility

satisfaction (to self, clients and employers) (Higgs and Hunt 1999). Consider these different approaches:

- The traditional approach to the education of health professionals was the *apprenticeship model*. The focus of the apprenticeship system was on the practical knowledge, craft and art of the practice role of the healthcare worker.
- The move to the *health professional model* (built around the medical model) predominantly involved a shift towards professional–technical competence supported by a more scientific knowledge base.
- The *clinical problem-solver model* arose in conjunction with the knowledge and technology explosions and the threat of rapid knowledge obsolescence.
- The *competent clinician model* was the next major model. This had an emphasis on identifying and assuring professional competencies.
- The *reflective practitioner model* (Schön 1983) emerged from concerns about the growing gap between the research-based (propositional) knowledge taught in professional schools and the practical knowledge and actual competencies required of practitioners in the field. Reflection helped to bridge these gaps.
- The *scientist practitioner model* reflected the commitment of professional groups to scientific rigour (James 1994) and practice validation throughout the health disciplines.

Activity box 6.2	Reflective questions
	Did any of these models apply to your education?
	How has your education had an impact on your approach to practice, your competencies and your effectiveness in your practice role?

Clinical decision-making and professional practice

Clinical or professional reasoning and decision-making are the key processes whereby professional competence, knowledge growth and use, professional behaviour and client-centred practice are drawn together. A growing body of research and educational literature has examined clinical reasoning and the developments of clinical reasoning competencies (Higgs and Jones 2000b). A range of clinical reasoning strategies (Table 6.2 on page 150) has been identified, beginning with early research which recognized hypothetico-deductive reasoning (or hypothesis generation and testing) as a core process used in clinical reasoning and professional decision-making. This process is similar to the scientific method used in empirico-analytical research and to other applications of adult thinking. Recent interpretations and models of professional reasoning have been developed, particularly interpretive models such as that of narrative reasoning, which emphasize the social and human contexts of professional practice more than the biomedical nature of patients' illnesses (Higgs and Jones 2000a, Jones et al 2000). These models have particular relevance to non-clinical work contexts such as schools, industry and welfare settings. Table 6.3 illustrates the emerging pattern of professional distinctiveness in models and practices of professional decision-making.

Activity box 6.3	Reflective questions
	Where does reasoning fit in your practice priorities? Consider the nature of clinical/professional decision-making and the way it is practised in different professions (see Table 6.3). Is your reasoning characteristic of your profession?

Knowledge in reasoning

The importance of knowledge–reasoning integration as a basis for sound professional decision-making and practice is emphasized throughout the literature. In this section we examine the nature of professional knowledge.

Consider the different forms of knowledge (Higgs and Titchen 1995). The term 'propositional knowledge' refers to theoretical or research knowledge which has been ratified or supported by the field. Non-propositional knowledge is derived primarily through practice, without an attempt to generalize beyond practice experience. There are two forms of non-propositional knowledge—professional craft knowledge, which incorporates technical/process and tacit knowledge of the profession, and personal knowledge, which is tied to the individual's reality or experience.

A perceptible hierarchical value relationship has developed between propositional and non-propositional knowledge, with the former being accorded a higher status. This has limited the valuing and critical investigation of non-propositional knowledge. In a world where problems are not discrete nor solutions definite, we need knowledge beyond science (Higgs and Titchen 2000). Practitioners and researchers need to be aware of and to value the three forms of

Table 6.2   *Definitions of modes of reasoning (based on Edwards et al, 1998, Higgs and Jones 2000a)*

- *Hypotheticodeductive reasoning* involves the generation of hypotheses based on clinical data and knowledge, and testing these hypotheses through further inquiry in order to make clinical decisions as the basis for professional practice

- *Pattern recognition* or inductive reasoning has been identified in experts reasoning in non-problematic situations. It resembles pattern recognition or direct automatic retrieval of information from a well-structured knowledge base

- *Knowledge–reasoning integration* is a model of clinical reasoning which emphasizes the interdependence of knowledge and reasoning throughout the reasoning process

- *Diagnostic reasoning* is that reasoning which aims to reveal the client's impairment(s), disability(ies) and handicap(s) and the underlying pathobiological mechanisms. While diagnostic reasoning is the most familiar reasoning strategy, in clinical practice it is combined with other strategies to establish patient rapport and to educate and promote patient self-efficacy and responsibility

- *Interactive reasoning* occurs when dialogue in the form of social exchange is used deliberately to enhance or facilitate the assessment/management process. This reasoning provides an effective means of better understanding the context in which the patient's problem(s) exist while creating a relationship of interest and trust

- *Narrative reasoning* involves the use of stories regarding past or present patients to understand and manage a clinical situation. Such real-life scenarios bring credibility to the advice or explanation which they are used to support, and can be strategically employed by practitioners to strengthen their message

- *Collaborative reasoning* refers to the shared decision-making that ideally occurs between practitioner and patient. Here the patient's opinions as well as information about the problem are actively sought and utilized

- *Predictive* or *conditional reasoning* is part of the practitioner's thinking directed to estimating patient responses to treatment and likely outcomes of management, based on information obtained through the patient interview, physical examination and response to management

- *Ethical/pragmatic reasoning* refers to those less recognized but frequently made decisions regarding moral, political and economic dilemmas which clinicians regularly confront, such as deciding how long to continue treatment

- *Teaching as reasoning* occurs when practitioners consciously use advice, instruction and guidance for the purpose of promoting change in the patient's understanding, feelings and behaviour

Table 6.3   *Examples of clinical/professional reasoning approaches (derived from Higgs and Jones 2000b)*

- In *occupational therapy*, clinical/professional reasoning may be best described as the use of multiple reasoning strategies throughout the various phases of client management. Hypothetico-deductive modes of reasoning (including procedural reasoning, as presented by Fleming 1991a) are used when therapists think about client problems in terms of the disease and within the context of occupational performance. Interactive reasoning (Fleming 1991b) involves developing an understanding of the naming of existing problems from the client's perspective. It employs processes of narrative thinking (Mattingly 1991) and critical discourse with clients (Crepeau 1991). Conditional reasoning (Fleming 1991b) is a less definite process by which occupational therapists imagine the client in the future, and in so doing, imagine the therapy outcome and the therapeutic action required to achieve that outcome. Underpinning all these processes is a process of ethical reasoning and critical reflection (Chapparo and Ranka 1995, 2000)

- In *physiotherapy*, clinical reasoning refers to the thought processes associated with a clinician's examination and management of a client (Jones et al 1995). Modes of reasoning used in physiotherapy include hypothetico-deductive reasoning, pattern recognition, knowledge reasoning integration and integrated models of reasoning involving client-centred and collaborative decision-making (Edwards et al 1998, Jones et al 2000)

- In *nursing*, clinical reasoning can be defined as the cognitive processes and strategies that nurses use to understand the significance of client data, to identify and diagnose actual or potential client problems, to make clinical decisions to assist in problem resolution and to enhance the achievement of positive client outcomes (Fonteyn 1995)

- In the *speech and hearing sciences*, professional decision-making involves the application of relevant knowledge and skills to evaluation, diagnosis and rehabilitation, and is part of a larger practice decision-making system involving interaction between practitioner, client, task and environment. It is a dynamic system that acknowledges the natural complexity of the situation, and the interactive character of reasoning involving practitioner, client, task and environment (Doyle 1995) professional practice knowledge, because the focus of practice and research attention needs to be broadened from an active reliance on scientific and theoretical knowledge if professional craft and personal knowledge are to be articulated and made available for public scrutiny. All professionals are accountable for their practice and have a responsibility to review their professional knowledge base critically and to make it publicly available. Practitioners, therefore, need to understand the nature of this dynamic knowledge base, so that they can explore its complexity, apply it appropriately and participate in the never-ending process of critical appraisal, extension and review of the profession's knowledge base (Titchen and Higgs 2001).

Activity box 6.4

Reflective questions

What forms of knowledge do you use in your practice?

How do these different types of knowledge help in your clinical decision-making?

Seeking advanced practice — extending clinical/professional reasoning competence

Clinical reasoning or professional decision-making draws together the roles, acts and responsibilities of health professionals, the knowledge of the profession and the practitioner and the competencies of practice. That is, sound clinical reasoning is essential for the success of clinical practice. Clinical reasoning is, in addition, the key to advanced practice. Consider, for instance, the following propositions:

- Clinical reasoning can become the means of optimally melding together the art, craft and science of professional practice.
- Expert health professionals seamlessly integrate propositional knowledge, professional craft knowledge and personal knowledge in the practice of clinical reasoning, professional judgement and professional decision-making.
- Advanced practice goes beyond the technical 'epitome' of science to embrace the confusion and complexity of the situations in which people seek professional assistance to address their health and social needs.
- Expertise is a journey towards professional artistry, the essence of which is the ability to bring together technical competencies, the humanity of people-centred practice, the grounding of experience in the reality of practice and in the evidence from both practice and science, to support and give credibility to practice.
- Advanced professional practice can be thought of as metacognitive decision-making or reasoning which utilizes a raised level of awareness, self-critique, monitoring of thinking and knowledge use and reflections on both client's and practitioner's perceptions of practice aims, processes and effects.

• Clinical reasoning requires and contains a commitment to knowledge generation and ongoing learning. At the same time, professional reasoning, self-directed learning and research are parallel processes in which cognition/thinking, meta-cognition and knowledge refinement and use are integrated for purposes of self-development and professional service.

How can we facilitate or pursue advanced practice through the enhancement of clinical/professional reasoning? Here are some suggestions.

Re-frame the goals and outcomes of health professional education

Traditional health professional education curricula emphasized the acquisition of knowledge and technical skills and their application in clinical settings. Plans for treatment or patient care were often learned rather than created uniquely for each patient and situation. Curricula commonly taught problem-solving with an emphasis on the identification and solution of clinical or client problems. Clinical reasoning research has extended this vision, with increased attention to the process of reasoning and the complexity of practice contexts.

Learning professional decision-making was traditionally the responsibility of the individual on the job, particularly during the early years post-graduation. Educators have come to recognize the limitations of this approach, influenced by changes in educational theory and practices, and by the increasing body of research into the nature of clinical/professional reasoning and decision-making. As a result, health professional curricula have been challenged to introduce more explicit and self-evaluative strategies for teaching clinical reasoning (Cahill and Fonteyn 2000, Refshauge and Higgs 2000, Ryan 2000).

One way of addressing the challenge of enhancing the teaching of professional decision-making is to reframe the type of graduate our professional entry curricula are endeavouring to produce. The 'interactional professional' model (Higgs & Hunt 1999) focuses on this specific issue. In this model, the aim of curricula is to produce graduates who are capable of operating effectively within changing local and global contexts and who are effective situational leaders, competent to deal with changes, challenges and contingencies through the employment of creative, relevant, valid and effective strategies of reasoning, intervention, development and evaluation.

The interactional professional operates within an integrated, patient-centred approach to clinical/professional reasoning (Higgs and Jones 2000a) which includes the following components:

• cognition or reflective inquiry
• a strong discipline-specific knowledge base
• meta-cognition (thinking about your thinking), which links cognition and knowledge
• mutual decision-making, emphasizing the role of the client or patient in the decision-making process, within a humanistic framework
• contextual interaction between the decision-makers and the situation of the reasoning process

- consideration of task impact, or the influence of the nature of the client's problem(s) and the practitioner's tasks on the reasoning process.

Understand and pursue expertise as a deepening understanding of practice knowledge

In professional practice, health practitioners combine learned propositional knowledge with procedural knowledge to produce practice strategies which are unique to the specific health setting (Richardson 2001). Professional craft knowledge is important in the implementation of effective professional practice because it is composed of diverse, complex and dynamic knowledge derived from practice. Since professional craft knowledge is frequently tacit and embedded in practice, it is important for us to understand the nature of this knowledge if we are to access it, study it, further develop it and make it available for others to acquire expertise and improve their practice (Titchen and Ersser 2001). Professional craft knowledge arises from an awareness of cues from the physical, geographical and chronological location of a healthcare event which, together with expectations of the patient and others, define or situate action.

Most models of clinical/professional reasoning (e.g. hypothetico-deductive reasoning, pattern reasoning, knowledge–reasoning integration, narrative reasoning) emphasize the interdependence of knowledge and reasoning. This interdependence is emphasized by Boshuizen and Schmidt (1992, 2000) who contend that research has shown that clinical reasoning is not a separate skill acquired independently of medical knowledge and other diagnostic skills. Rather, the development of expertise can be interpreted through a stage theory in which knowledge acquisition and clinical reasoning go hand in hand (Table 6.4).

Table 6.4 *Knowledge restructuring and clinical reasoning at subsequent levels of expertise level (derived from Boshuizen and Schmidt 2000, p. 18)*

Expertise level	Knowledge representation	Knowledge acquisition and (re)structuring	Clinical reasoning
Novice	Networks	Knowledge is acquired and validated	Reasoning involves long chains of detailed reasoning steps through networks of biomedical knowledge
Intermediate	Networks	Through professional experience, the practitioner encapsulates prior learning in clinical knowledge	Reasoning becomes enriched and enhanced through the use of an encapsulated network
Expert	Illness scripts	With increasing experience the expert develops 'illness scripts' or narratives of medical conditions	Reasoning draws on the practitioner's rich knowledge base of generalized scripts or deep knowledge of illnesses, and also uses knowledge of specific cases to achieve expert reasoning

Learn to use meta-cognition and self-evaluation as essential components of reasoning

Meta-cognition is reflective self-awareness. It is thinking which occurs over and above normal conscious thinking (cognition). It refers to having knowledge of and examining one's cognitive processes. Research in this area identifies the value of meta-cognition in helping learners develop learning and problem-solving skills (Biggs and Telfer 1987). In developing a greater awareness of their mental processes, learners are better able to perform these mental processes. This is the basis for using learning strategies which involve articulation, critique and review of cognitive skills. Similarly, adoption of a higher level of meta-cognition allows practitioners to employ constant critical self-evaluation and to be more effective in sound reasoning, knowledge critique, and avoidance of reasoning errors.

Pursue professional artistry and professional practice judgement artistry

Recently the nature of expert professional practice has been re-examined against concepts such as artistry and connoisseurship. Professional artistry is defined as a concern for the invisible aspects of practice, the 'capabilities, assumptions, theories, beliefs, values and the moral dimensions of practice, including the practitioner's professional judgments' (Fish 1998, p. 2). Schön (1987, p. 13) describes professional artistry as 'an exercise of intelligence, a kind of knowing, though different in crucial respects from our standard model of professional knowledge'.

Related to these terms of artistry in knowing are the constructs of practice wisdom (Scott 1990) and professional practice judgement artistry. A practitioner who is using professional practice judgement artistry (Paterson and Higgs 2001) is using highly skilled practice judgements which are optimal for the given circumstances of the client and context. Such decisions are characterized by finesse and artistry, allowing advanced practitioners or professional artists to demonstrate advanced practice in the uncertain worlds of professional practice, as illustrated in Figure 6.2.

> There is an element of artistry at the heart or core of the kind of professional practice which is acknowledged to be outstanding and to which we all aspire. This artistry encompasses, but goes beyond, competence and what we might describe as technical expertise. It is owned by an individual who possesses a blend of qualities built up through extensive and reflective personal knowledge and experience (Beeston and Higgs 2001, p. 108).

Professional artistry, therefore, can be considered to be a broad term which includes technical, cognitive and attitudinal components (Figure 6.3). In the advanced practitioner, professional artistry is the meaningful expression of a uniquely individual view within a shared tradition (Higgs et al 2001) and it involves a blend of:

- practitioner qualities (e.g. attunement to self, others and events)
- practice skills (e.g. expert critical appreciation and meta-cognitive skills)
- creative imagination (imagining outcomes of personalized, unique care).

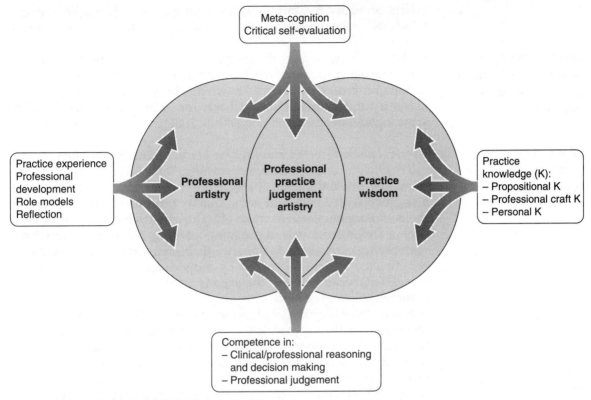

Figure 6.2 *Professional practice judgement artistry*

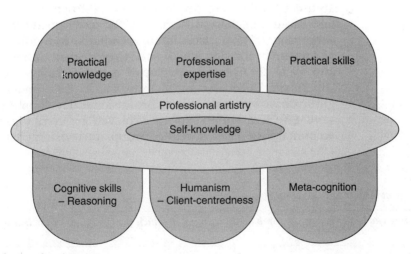

Figure 6.3 *Professional artistry*

These qualities, skills and processes and their blending are built up through extensive introspective and critical reflection upon and review of practice. According to Fish (1998), the development of artistry requires attention to dimensions of practice (such as values, beliefs, attitudes, assumptions, expectations, feelings and knowledge) which lie below the surface and behind the actions of the practitioner.

Develop strategies which deal effectively with ethical decision-making and practice

Without professional craft knowledge, ethically important matters about particular patients will be overlooked. The interaction between caring and professional craft knowledge in healthcare workers establishes a fundamentally sound basis for appropriate ethical understanding and decision-making (White 2001).

Take charge of your professional development

Are you a self-directed and lifelong learner in reality, not just rhetorically? Lifelong and self-directed learning (Table 6.5) is an essential prerequisite for enhancing professional competence. It is clearly associated with a commitment to quality professional practice and to the demonstration of accountability. The collective work of individual healthcare professionals in pursuing learning, continued competence and quality care serves to enhance their status and role. In addition, self-directed learning activities by individuals and groups of health professionals can result in the expansion and validation of their profession's knowledge base.

Since professional decision-making is a (largely) unobservable process, it is valuable to articulate your reasoning to your peers, to collaborate on decision-making, to gain support from your colleagues in difficult decision situations and to receive feedback. Knowledge and learning are facilitated when novice practitioners learn alongside their peers; this enhances professional competence and reasoning skills (Ladyshewsky et al 2000). Fostering peer discussion in the workplace setting is a way of promoting exposure of the learner's thoughts and arguments, allowing discussion and restructuring of knowledge to take place (Regehr and Norman 1996). For a successful peer learning experience to take place, interdependence, individual accountability and group processing ability need to be present (Johnson 1981). Amies and Weir (2001) have developed a model called 'reflective group supervision' utilizing such strategies. In this model, peer support groups assist in each other's professional development and supervision. Effective supervision is achieved by combining support and accountability. This process of group supervision enables workers to

Table 6.5 *Self-directed learning (based on Higgs 1993)*

Self-directed learning can be defined as an approach to learning in which the behaviour of the learner is characterized by:

- responsibility for and critical awareness of his or her own learning process and outcome
- a high level of self-direction in performing learning activities and solving problems which are associated with the learning task
- active input to decision-making regarding the learning task
- the use of the teacher as a resource person
- the effective interaction with other learners and the teacher in a collaborative learning manner

think past the limitations of their individual world view. It is a process of inquiry that provides an opportunity for people to extend themselves in relation to their work, and to think outside the parameters they would usually consider. Chapter 5 elaborates on these aspects of shared work.

Conclusion

To answer the question 'Do you reason like a (health) professional?' you need to understand what it means to be a health professional, what it means to be a member of your particular profession, which reasoning models are best suited to your profession and whether you adopt such approaches. Do you reason like an advanced health professional? What skills can you develop to extend your reasoning ability from a satisfactory to an advanced level of performance? This chapter provides you with information, arguments and stimulus questions to help you answer these questions, along with ideas for your further professional development.

References

Amies C, Weir S 2001 Using reflective group supervision to enhance practice knowledge. In: Higgs J, Titchen A (eds) Practice knowledge and expertise in the health professions. Butterworth-Heinemann, Oxford, p 135–141

Beeston S, Higgs J 2001 Professional practice: artistry and connoisseurship. In: Higgs J, Titchen A (eds) Practice knowledge and expertise in the health professions. Butterworth-Heinemann, Oxford, p 108–117

Biggs J B, Telfer R 1987 The process of learning 2nd edn. Sydney, Prentice Hall

Boshuizen H P A, Schmidt H G 1992 On the role of biomedical knowledge in clinical reasoning by experts, intermediates and novices. Cognitive Science 16:153–184

Boshuizen H P A, Schmidt H G 2000 The development of clinical reasoning expertise. In: Higgs J, Jones M (eds) Clinical reasoning in the health professions, 2nd edn. Butterworth- Heinemann, Oxford, p 15–22

Cahill M, Fonteyn M 2000 Using mind mapping to improve students' metacognition. In: Higgs J, Jones M (eds) Clinical reasoning in the health professions, 2nd edn. Butterworth-Heinemann, Oxford, p 214–221

Cant R, Higgs J 1999 Professional socialisation. In: Higgs J, Edwards H (eds) Educating beginning practitioners: challenges for health professional education. Butterworth-Heinemann, Oxford, p 46–51

Cervero R M 1988 Effective continuing education for professionals. Jossey-Bass, San Francisco

Chapparo C, Ranka J 1995 Clinical reasoning in occupational therapy. In: Higgs J, Jones M (eds) Clinical reasoning in the health professions. Butterworth-Heinemann, Oxford, p 88–102

Chapparo C, Ranka J 2000 Clinical reasoning in occupational therapy. In: Higgs J, Jones M (eds) Clinical reasoning in the health professions, 2nd edn. Butterworth-Heinemann, Oxford, p 128–137

Crepeau E B 1991 Achieving intersubjective understanding: examples from an occupational therapy treatment session. American Journal of Occupational Therapy 45:1016–1025

Doyle J 1995 Teaching clinical reasoning to speech and hearing students. In: Higgs J, Jones M (eds) Clinical reasoning in the health professions. Butterworth-Heinemann, Oxford, p 224–234

Edwards I C, Jones M A, Carr J, Jensen G M 1998 Clinical reasoning in three different fields of physiotherapy—a qualitative study. In: Proceedings of the Fifth International Congress. Australian Physiotherapy Association, Melbourne, p 298–300

Eraut M 1994 Developing professional knowledge and competence. Falmer Press, London

Fish D 1998 Appreciating practice in the caring professions: refocusing professional development and practitioner research. Butterworth-Heinemann, Oxford

Fleming M H 1991a Clinical reasoning in medicine compared with clinical reasoning in occupational therapy. American Journal of Occupational Therapy 45:988–996

Fleming M H 1991b The therapist with the three track mind. American Journal of Occupational Therapy 45:1007–1014

Fonteyn M 1995 Clinical reasoning in nursing. In: Higgs J, Jones M (eds) Clinical reasoning in the health professions. Butterworth-Heinemann, Oxford, p 60–71

Harris I B 1993 New expectations for professional competence. In: Curry L, Wergin J (eds) Educating professionals: responding to new expectations for competence and accountability. Jossey-Bass, San Francisco, p 17–52

Higgs J 1993 Physiotherapy, professionalism and self-directed learning. Journal of Singapore Physiotherapy Association 14:8–11

Higgs J, Hunt A 1999 Redefining the beginning practitioner. Focus on Health Professional Education: A Multi-Disciplinary Journal 1:34–48

Higgs J, Jones M 2000a Clinical reasoning in the health professions. In: Higgs J, Jones M (eds) Clinical reasoning in the health professions, 2nd edn. Butterworth-Heinemann, Oxford, p 3–14

Higgs J, Jones M (eds) 2000b Clinical reasoning in the health professions, 2nd edn. Butterworth-Heinemann, Oxford

Higgs J, Titchen A 1995 The nature, generation and verification of knowledge. Physiotherapy 81:521–530

Higgs J, Titchen A 2000 Knowledge and reasoning. In: Higgs J, Jones M (eds) Clinical reasoning in the health professions, 2nd edn. Butterworth-Heinemann, Oxford, p 23–32

Higgs C, Neubauer D, Higgs J 1999 The changing healthcare context: globalization and social ecology. In: Higgs J, Edwards H (eds) Educating Beginning Practitioners: Challenges for Health Professional Education. Butterworth-Heinemann, Oxford, p 30–37

Higgs J, Titchen A, Neville V 2001 Professional practice and knowledge. In: Higgs J, Titchen A (eds) Practice knowledge and expertise in the health professions. Butterworth-Heinemann, Oxford, p 3–9

James J E 1994 Health care, psychology, and the scientist–practitioner model. Australian Psychologist 29:5–11

Johnson D 1981 Student–student interaction: the neglected variable in education. Educational Researcher 1:5–10

Jones M, Jensen G, Rothstein J 1995 Clinical reasoning in physiotherapy. In: Higgs J, Jones M (eds) Clinical reasoning in the health professions. Butterworth-Heinemann, Oxford, p 72–87

Jones M, Jensen G, Edwards I 2000 Clinical reasoning in physiotherapy. In: Higgs J, Jones M (eds) Clinical reasoning in the health professions, 2nd edn. Butterworth-Heinemann, Oxford, p 117–127

Josebury H E, Bax N D S, Hannay D R 1990 Communication skills and clinical methods: a new introductory course. Medical Education 24:433–437

Ladyshewsky R, Baker R, Jones M 2000 Peer coaching to generate clinical-reasoning skills. In: Higgs J, Jones M (eds) Clinical reasoning in the health professions, 2nd edn. Butterworth-Heinemann, Oxford, p 283–289

Mattingly C 1991 The narrative nature of clinical reasoning. American Journal of Occupational Therapy 45:998–1005

Neubauer D 1998 Some impacts of globalization on health and healthcare policy. Occasional paper. Centre for Professional Education Advancement, Faculty of Health Sciences, University of Sydney, Sydney, Australia

Paterson M, Higgs J 2001 Professional practice judgement artistry. Occasional paper 3. Centre for Professional Education Advancement, University of Sydney, Sydney, Australia

Prosser A 1995 Teaching and learning social responsibility. Higher Education Research and Development Society of Australasia, Canberra, Australia

Refshauge K, Higgs J 2000 Teaching clinical reasoning. In: Higgs J, Jones M (eds) Clinical reasoning in the health professions, 2nd edn. Butterworth-Heinemann, Oxford, p 141–147

Regehr G, Norman G 1996 Issues in cognitive psychology: implications for professional education. Academic Medicine 71:988–1000

Richardson B 2001 Professionalisation and professional craft knowledge. In: Higgs J, Titchen A (eds) Practice knowledge and expertise in the health professions. Butterworth-Heinemann, Oxford, p 42–47

Ryan S 2000 Facilitating the clinical reasoning of occupational therapy students on fieldwork placement. In: Higgs J, Jones M (eds) Clinical reasoning in the health professions, 2nd edn. Butterworth-Heinemann, Oxford, p 242–248

Schön D 1983 The reflective practitioner: how professionals think in action. Basic Books, New York

Schön D A 1987 Educating the reflective practitioner: towards a new design for teaching and learning in professions. Jossey-Bass, San Francisco

Scott D 1990 Practice wisdom: the neglected source of practice research. Social Work 35:564–568

Sultz H A, Sawner K A, Sherwin F S 1984 Determining and maintaining competence: an obligation of allied health education. Journal of Allied Health 13:272–279

Titchen A, Ersser S J 2001 The nature of professional craft knowledge. In: Higgs J, Titchen A (eds) Practice knowledge and expertise in the health professions. Butterworth-Heinemann, Oxford, p 35–41

Titchen A, Higgs J 2001 A dynamic framework for the enhancement of health professional practice in an uncertain world: the practice–knowledge interface. In: Higgs J, Titchen A (eds) Practice knowledge and expertise in the health professions. Butterworth-Heinemann, Oxford, p 215–225

White K 2001 Professional craft knowledge and ethical decision making. In: Higgs J, Titchen A (eds) Practice knowledge and expertise in the health professions. Butterworth-Heinemann, Oxford, p 142–148

Additional reading and resources

Alsop A, Ryan S 1996 Making the most of fieldwork education: a practical approach. Chapman and Hall, London

Fish D, Coles C 1998 Developing professional judgement in healthcare: learning through the critical appreciation of practice. Butterworth-Heinemann, Oxford

Fleming M, Mattingly C 2000 Action and narrative: two dynamics of clinical reasoning. In: Higgs J, Jones M (eds) Clinical reasoning in the health professions, 2nd edn. Butterworth-Heinemann, Oxford, p 54–61

Fonteyn M 1998 Thinking strategies for nursing practice. Lippincott, Philadelphia

Fonteyn M E, Ritter B J 2000 Clinical reasoning in nursing. In: Higgs J, Jones M (eds) Clinical reasoning in the health professions, 2nd edn. Butterworth-Heinemann, Oxford, p 107–116

Hart G, Ryan Y 2000 Teaching clinical reasoning to nurses during clinical education. In: Higgs J, Jones M (eds) Clinical reasoning in the health professions, 2nd edn. Butterworth-Heinemann, Oxford, p 276–282

Higgs J 1997 Learning to make clinical decisions. In: McAllister L, Lincoln M, McLeod S, et al (eds) Facilitating learning in clinical settings. Stanley Thornes, Cheltenham, p 130–153

Higgs J, Bithell C 2001 Professional expertise. In: Higgs J, Titchen A (eds) Practice knowledge and expertise in the health professions. Butterworth-Heinemann, Oxford, p 59–68

Higgs J, Edwards H (eds) 1999 Educating beginning practitioners: challenges for health professional education. Butterworth-Heinemann, Oxford

Jensen G M, Gwyer J, Hack L M, Shepard K F 1999 Expertise in physical therapy practice. Butterworth-Heinemann, Oxford

Jones M, Higgs J 2000 Will evidence-based practice take the reasoning out of practice? In: Higgs J, Jones M (eds) Clinical reasoning in the health professions, 2nd edn. Butterworth-Heinemann, Oxford, p 307–315

Mattingly C, Fleming M H 1994 Clinical reasoning: forms of inquiry in a therapeutic practice. F A Davis, Philadelphia

McAllister L, Rose M 2000 Speech-language pathology students: learning clinical reasoning. In: Higgs J, Jones M (eds) Clinical reasoning in the health professions, 2nd edn. Butterworth-Heinemann, Oxford, p 205–213

McKenzie L 2000 Teaching clinical reasoning in clinical education: orthoptics. In: Higgs J, Jones M (eds) Clinical reasoning in the health professions, 2nd edn. Butterworth-Heinemann, Oxford, p 270–275

Perry A (ed) 1997 Nursing: a knowledge base for practice. Arnold, London

7

Creating scholarly practice: integrating and applying scholarship to practice

Susan A. Esdaile and Linda M. Roth

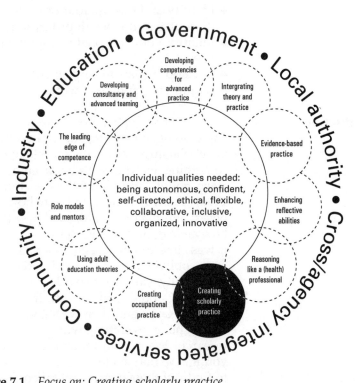

Figure 7.1 *Focus on: Creating scholarly practice*

Chapter outline

In this chapter we present the scholarship of practice in terms of an integrated model in which basic research from both the physical and social sciences informs practice, and practice generates further questions for research. We focus on four areas of scholarship: *discovery* that includes, but is not limited to, research; *integration*, or the process of using information; *application* of the information to practice; and *teaching*, which includes both formal education and learning through practice. We discuss professional issues in healthcare practice, including how professional knowledge is generated, the characteristics of a profession, the dissemination of its knowledge, intellectual debate, and education. We provide illustrations of concepts, and issues are provided through interviews with four early-career practitioners: a medical technologist, an occupational therapist, a physical therapist, and a radiation therapist. To assist readers to plan for their future scholarly development, we have included a variety of techniques, exercises, discussion questions, and references.

Key words   Scholarship of discovery, integration, application, teaching

Anticipated outcomes   As an outcome of reading this chapter, we anticipate that you will be able to:

- describe four factors that comprise the scholarship of practice
- identify and discuss four or more issues that comprise professional discourse in the health professions
- identify your personal strengths in relation to scholarship in practice
- develop a plan to implement scholarly practice for yourself, and within your sphere of work.

Introduction   Let us think about scholarship as a way of organizing the work we enjoy doing, believe in, and want others to know about. In the process of scholarship, we create knowledge and pass it on to others. This is something we did with great enthusiasm when we were young. A story about Jane Goodall as a child illustrates this point (Goodall 1999). She was curious to know how chickens laid eggs, and being an observant, realistic child, she knew that the chicken would not like to be watched. So, she hid in the coop waiting for the chicken to decide it was time to lay an egg. Goodall waited for hours, crouched in the coop, oblivious to time or the discomfort of her cramped situation. But, finally, she was rewarded; the chicken did come to lay her egg. Politely, Goodall waited until the chicken had performed the task in her own time, and then with great enthusiasm, she rushed to tell her family, her eyes shining with joy at the discovery. Eureka! Discovery is research! We can all remember the fun of discovery when we were young. We may have collected shells at the beach, gone to the library to find out their names and taken them to school to show our friends and our teacher. We even listened attentively when the teacher gave us more information about shells. We may have had similar experiences watching the sky and learning about the stars, going fishing, learning the basics of cooking and baking our first batch of cup cakes, or planting seeds and being impatient to see them grow.

Memories like these can make us smile. But, what has this got to do with scholarship? Well, a lot actually, as the elements and process of scholarship are the same. First there is discovery, driven by curiosity. We call this *research*. The newly discovered information becomes part of our life. We have new knowledge, our understanding has expanded; this is *integration*. We then put our new knowledge to a useful, practical purpose. We may raise chickens and sell the eggs, build a shell collection, bake different cakes. This is *application*. Often we prefer to do these activities with others, perfecting our skills together, sharing our knowledge and enthusiasm for the discoveries that have enriched our lives. Thus, we take our friends to the beach to collect shells, we garden and cook with others, and we point out the stars to our younger siblings. This is *teaching*.

Scholarship starts with ordinary curiosity and is a regular part of our life and work. In our everyday life, we can be curious about things that interest us and become quite scholarly in our knowledge about our interests without needing to document and organize too much. For example, you may enjoy walking in the woods and identifying the plants without needing to structure your knowledge or scholarship beyond your personal need. In the scholarship of our practice, we need to extend the organization and documentation beyond our personal need, to document and evaluate our scholarship objectively. Professional accountability requires us to be able to identify our knowledge and modify it through new discovery, our own and that of others; to integrate new knowledge; to apply our integrated knowledge in practice; and, through these scholarly endeavors, to teach others. So, let us take a closer look at the scholarship of practice.

Four elements of the scholarship of practice

The scholarship of practice is important in any profession. Donald Schön's (1983) book *The Reflective Practitioner: How Professionals Think in Action* has been influential in bringing the notion of scholarship in practice to the attention of many. He used the practice example of architecture. However, other professions, in health and social sciences, such as anthropology and occupational therapy, have embraced his ideas (Mattingly and Fleming 1994). You were introduced to Schön's work in earlier chapters about clinical reasoning and enhancing reflective abilities. We believe that the model of scholarly practice described in the discipline of academic medicine is particularly useful for health professionals, so we have used it as a framework for examining scholarship in practice in this chapter (Boyer 1990, Glassick et al 1997). The focus is on four areas of scholarship in practice:

- Discovery
- Integration
- Application
- Teaching

Discovery

Discovery includes not only research, but also observation of practice and its context in the immediate and broader environment, staying well-informed and curious. Increasingly, the scholarship of practice involves collaborations of individuals engaged in basic and clinical sciences. These interactions are important. Basic research, for example, investigations in biological sciences, may identify underlying causes of disease. A continued cycle of interaction between basic and clinical research is emphasized in current literature in the field of medical education (Beattie 2000). The recorded and debated clinical observations of all health professionals contribute to clinical research. This interaction between basic research and its clinical application is an important aspect of advancing scholarship in all the health professions. Basic research in physics and inorganic chemistry has led to the development of effective new techniques to treat cancer through radiation therapy. In another example, current studies that examine aspects of motor neuron function in bilateral and unilateral grasp have relevant implications for clinical practice in occupational and physical therapy (Conti 1998, Hurvitz, et al 2000).

Integration

Integration includes using evidence-based practice information from all the sciences, keeping up to date with the socio-political contexts of practice, and not losing sight of a good clinician's common sense. Integration often involves stepping back from a more narrow, problem-based focus in order to make connections between different approaches. The process of integration will cause the scholarly clinician to reflect on the meaning of new findings in the differing contexts of practice. The explosion of communication technologies has accelerated our ability to share and integrate new information. Using e-mail to facilitate scholarship is an example (Ribbons and Vance 2001).

Successful integration involves moving beyond discipline-specific boundaries. Considering this point in a historical context can provide us with some pertinent examples of the application of basic knowledge to practical purpose. Compact disks (CDs) are used extensively in the processing and integration of knowledge. However, making CDs that could play accurately involved using a coding system derived from set theory, an invention by Gaulois, an 18th-century French mathematician. As a more recent example, scholarship that led to the discovery of nuclear magnetic resonance in 1938 was integrated decades later to enable the development of diagnostic tools that improve the early detection of diseases (Dauphinée and Martin 2000).

The scholarship of integration is greatly enhanced through collaboration among professionals from different disciplines and education that encourages interdisciplinary, creative problem-solving within a broader societal context. Current government publications in both the UK and the USA address the importance of innovation and collaboration in healthcare practice (National Health Service 2000, US Department of Health and Human Services Public Health Service 1999). They underscore the importance of the scholarship of integration in healthcare practice of the future. One of the most important aspects of the scholarship of integration is linking academic institutions that educate health professionals with the communities that they serve.

Application

Through the scholarship of application we can assess how an intervention works when it is applied in practice. The many different ways that basic and clinical research are used in the treatment of individuals are illustrations of the scholarship of application, as is the day-to-day work of most health professionals (Shapiro and Coleman 2000). Examples range from the prescription and dispensing of drugs found to be effective through clinical trials, to the application of neuroscience research in treatment techniques used by a physiotherapist. Application includes evidence-based techniques as well as using insights from colleagues, clients, their families, and others. It also includes consideration of the ethics of the techniques, protocols, and other factors determining the application of the outcomes of scholarship to individuals and communities.

The development of treatment models is an example of the scholarship of application that is predicated on the scholarship of discovery and the scholarship of integration. For example, basic research in bio-psycho-neuroscience can be integrated into clinical practice by an interdisciplinary healthcare team that is working to create an optimal recovery and rehabilitation model for the treatment of persons with a closed-head injury. Similarly, committees that review policies and establish guidelines and protocols for practice are using the scholarship of application (Shapiro and Coleman 2000, p. 896). The service-learning model used in the clinical education of health professionals is an excellent example of the scholarship of application that is directly relevant to the community. Supervised by their academic preceptors, senior nursing, occupational therapy, and social work students may apply this model to assist in the development of a community-based center for people with chronic mental health problems. In another setting, pharmacy, physical therapy, and occupational therapy students may work together doing clinical fieldwork to set up a volunteer service to enhance opportunities for meaningful, active occupations, or to monitor use of prescription medications for older adults attending a church-sponsored community center.

Teaching

Teaching, in terms of scholarship, includes teaching oneself as well as students and colleagues, translating information for clients and their families, and teaching by example. The education of health professionals is an aspect of the scholarship of teaching that has been highlighted in many recent publications in academic medicine and health sciences. Wales et al (1993) advocate that academics charged with educating future professionals must teach students how to use effectively what they learn. During the education process students learn what *has been* discovered and *has been* done, but they cannot know what *will be* discovered and what *should* be done (their emphasis). Thus, the newly minted practitioner leaves the educational setting with well-ingrained 'habits of mind' and is able to think the way a professional thinks (Dewey 1933).

To educate students, rather than train them, academic staff themselves must be educated. Academic leaders in health professions are frequently charged with assisting the transition of clinicians who wish to become educators in universities and colleges (Esdaile and Roth 2000). Given the importance of the contribution of clinical teachers, who are practicing their professions as well as educating their future colleagues, increasing attention is given to the enhancement of clinical education. Roth et al (2001) conceptualize the academic educator in a clinically based profession (in their example, medicine) as a professional who performs at one of three levels. Firstly, academics need to be competent professionals, according to established criteria (such as certification and registration) set by their profession. Secondly, in addition to the professional base outlined above, they need to have exceptional competence in an area of knowledge. Thirdly, academics whose interest and curiosity about their area of expertise extend to research may be termed investigators.

In order to achieve excellence in the scholarship of education, maintaining and enhancing professional autonomy is important across healthcare professions. Autonomy allows professionals to make unique contributions, to be self-governing, self-regulating, and self-directed. Thus, a profession is able to respond more readily to societal needs. However, if autonomy is not based on altruism and governed by high ethical standards, an autonomous profession may become self-seeking and focus its regulations and control on the promotion of its own interests, rather than on the needs of society. The medical profession has been criticized for such self-interested professionalism. However, it is also taking a scholarly lead in educating professionals who are in the service of healing, and who understand and accept the obligations of being a professional (Cruess and Cruess 1997). Other issues related to professional autonomy have been discussed in Chapter 1, in the context of the power discourse that impinges on health professionals.

Interviews with early-career practitioners

Reading the professional literature of your own and related disciplines is an essential part of professional practice. It helps to add some human interest. How do others view this topic? How have they used this information to enhance their learning and practice? It is more fun to read if you can discuss the readings with colleagues; this is why journal clubs are a useful adjunct to becoming an advanced practitioner. Journal clubs were discussed in Chapter 4; we shall discuss them from our perspective later in this chapter (see Table 7.2). Firstly, we want to share with you the views of four early-career health professionals whom we interviewed about scholarship in practice.

For early-career professional, we are using the definitions provided in a study of 392 early-career medical technologists (MTs) that can generalize to other professions (Summers et al, 2000). The authors were motivated by their belief that professional development activities can strengthen professional commitment. We share this belief. In their study, the authors tracked MTs for the first 5 years after their graduation and described an early-career stage as having two distinct periods–*establishment* and *achievement*. The focus of the *establishment period* is learning the technical aspects of a job, and the norms, rules and values of the employing organization. The *achievement period* involves an increase in professional activities and organizational contributions. Early career development is supported when organizations sponsor continuing education, create opportunities for sharing of ideas in teams, and create work opportunities that provide growth in responsibility. The specific goals of this study were to determine whether there are distinct types of professional development for MTs (that may also apply to other health professions). The variables included were gender, continuing education, task complexity, work satisfaction, shift (to different work), team participation, and organizational commitment. Two key factors that described career progress emerged in the data analysis. These were scholarly professional development that focused on activities designed to advance the knowledge base of the profession, and administrative professional development that focused on advancing the process of organizing and supporting professional needs. Both are valid areas of professional development, and the choice of direction is dependent on individual skills and inclinations. Ideally, institutions employing health professionals invest in their continued professional development and support individual choice based on skills and performance. In reality, employees need to be proactive to ensure that this happens. One of the main reasons that we wrote this book is to assist early-career practitioners to be proactive in planning their careers. Given the cuts in the resources allocated to professional development in many places, we believe that many early-career practitioners have to find support and resources outside their work situation in order to develop themselves professionally.

We hope that the views and experiences of the early-career professionals we interviewed will assist readers at similar stages of their careers. In order to protect their privacy, we have changed their names and other details which would identify them. *Alex*, aged 25, had graduated with a Bachelor of Science degree in medical technology a year and a half before our interview. He worked in the blood bank of a large university teaching hospital. *Lisa*, aged 23, had graduated with a Bachelor of Science degree in occupational therapy 4 months prior to our interview. She was working part-time in home-care and about to start working part-time in a special school as well. *Mary*, aged 25, had graduated with a Master of Science degree in physical therapy a year prior to our interview. She worked in the rehabilitation department of a large urban hospital. *Don*, aged 28, had graduated with a Bachelor of Science degree in radiation therapy/technology 2 years before our interview. He worked in the oncology unit of a university teaching hospital.

After obtaining approval from our employing university's human subject investigation committee, we interviewed each of these young healthcare professionals separately, asking them the questions listed in Table 7.1 on page 168. We audiotaped the interviews so we could analyse and synthesize their comments. We started by describing our concept of scholarship in practice.

Each of these early-career healthcare practitioners readily gave us different examples in response to question 1. *Alex* discussed problem-solving in relation to cross-matching of blood samples. He described a recent experience when he thought that he had found a rare antibody, as his tests were showing a cold agglutinin reaction. As this can be a critical factor when a person's temperature is lowered below 15°C, as is done in some surgical procedures, it was important to make sure that the test results were correct. Re-testing confirmed his original test results. He remarked that 'part of the job is troubleshooting' and described another recent experience when he came to work to find that the irradiator was not working. He was able to test the equipment, identify the problems and do what was needed to have it functioning again.

Table 7.1   *Questions asked in the interviews*

Our questions relate to scholarship in practice. By scholarship in practice, we mean discovery through observation, being well informed and staying curious, using information from many sources to stay up-to-date, including published evidence, and people that can add insights such as patients, their families and our colleagues. Scholarship in practice also includes sharing knowledge with others through formal and informal teaching.

Question 1
We all learn from experience as we practice our profession. Can you describe a recent work situation where you learned from experience?

Question 2
As you reflected on this learning experience, did you read any articles or books related to this experience, or go to a website for more information?

Question 3
How did you integrate this new learning experience with what you had learned about this subject previously?

Question 4
How did you apply this new learning experience and your further investigations/study in your practice?

Question 5
Did you share this new information with any of your colleagues or students?

Question 6
Overall, what have you learned from this experience of scholarship in practice?

Lisa's examples of learning from experience hinged around having to resolve communication problems with patients. In her first example, the patient was aphasic, and *Lisa* quickly had to find ways to communicate with him. In the second example, she had to communicate with a patient who could not speak English. Again she had to find alternative techniques. With the aphasic patient, she found that drawing pictures was helpful, and the non-English-speaker responded to non-verbal gestures and touching. She showed professional insight in quickly ascertaining that the same technique may not work with both patients. 'I learned a lot from the experience, because I had to approach the situation (differently for each person) to make the experience positive for the patient and myself.'

Mary said that she was trying to learn as much as possible through taking advantage of the rotations offered to new graduates in the rehabilitation unit where she works. These rotations include orthopedics, neurological disorders and surgery; she had just completed an orthopedic rotation. Whenever she was unsure of her clinical decision-making, she was able to ask one of the more senior therapists with advanced qualifications. *Mary* described her work as an ongoing process of new learning experiences that she welcomed. 'I feel there is so much to learn. [I] need to continue to progress and learn more.' The next learning challenge she was setting herself was to become confident to work in an intensive care unit. Part of this experience would require her to learn more about wound care and to acquire the competencies needed to handle the complex equipment used in treating critically ill patients.

The hospital where *Don* works uses very advanced radiation equipment for both photon and neutron radiation treatment for cancer. Only a few centers use both neutron and photon radiation in cancer treatment. This is a source of pride to those working in the unit, but also a challenge. *Don* said that he frequently has to learn to use new equipment. The treatment of each patient is also a new challenge, as the radiation therapist is responsible for making sure that all the equipment is correctly positioned for treatment. This requires special skill, as the positions of organs and individual body proportion have to be considered each time. 'The goal is to get it as accurate as possible and as quick as possible.'

The learning experiences of all four early-career practitioners involved mastering new techniques and, in the case of *Alex*, *Don* and *Mary*, the ongoing learning experience of using new equipment. We would anticipate that as *Lisa* has more working experiences she would also have to learn about new equipment. However, this is probably the greatest, most continuous challenge in *Don*'s occupation. All four mentioned discussing new experiences with more accomplished colleagues as well as peers, in order to help reinforce the learning. Workplace seminars were also mentioned as an effective way of learning more about a new experience. *Alex* said that following the experience of learning to confirm the cold agglutinin reaction, he went to a seminar by the Red Cross that 'hit the nail on the head'. It was exactly what he needed to extend his knowledge in this particular area. *Don* also found that seminars on use of new equipment, held regularly in his workplace, were very useful. *Lisa* said she re-read relevant sections from her text books and also read additional references related to her new learning. *Mary* also said that she frequently went back to her text books and looked for articles on special topics. She actively sought new learning experiences through her membership in the state and national branches of her professional association, and she had recently joined the acute care special interest section of the American Physical Therapy Association. During the past year she had also attended several workshops offered at her hospital, and two conferences, one state and one national.

All four mentioned integrating new learning by discussion, by sharing with colleagues, and by application to patient care. *Alex*, although not in direct contact with patients, was aware of the implications of his work to patient care, and took advantage of opportunities to discuss the progress of patients whose blood he was testing with medical and nursing staff. He also talked about integrating learning through documentation. In his unit, staff keep a procedure manual where new techniques are carefully written down step by step, so any person facing the problem for the first time is able to follow clear instructions. *Lisa* described integration as a good experience in which she was first able to brainstorm, and later read and reflect in more depth. *Mary* described integration in terms of the on-going clinical decision-making process, as she learned what to look for, what to do and when to ask a more expert colleague for assistance or advice. All four mentioned honing observation skills and then applying the skills to new learning opportunities.

Alex, Mary and *Don* had been able to share their own experiences with students and peers as a regular part of their jobs. It seemed to be a particularly critical part of *Don*'s job. In his workplace, therapists constantly had to learn to use new equipment and this was largely done through on-site training. Radiation therapy students start by working 20 hours a week in clinical settings, and instructing them was part of *Don*'s work. Because *Lisa* had started working so recently, and was moving to combine two part-time positions in home care and in a school for children and young adults with developmental disability, she was eager to practice what she had learned in college. She stressed the importance of observational skills, and was aware that she would need to adapt treatment to meet individual patient's needs, and to work collaboratively with others. *Mary* was planning to develop advanced clinical skills leading to specialist credentials. For the present, she was focused on becoming competent in acute care. *Alex* was especially enthusiastic about hands-on learning experiences: 'I have to physically do it myself and work it out and then I know'. For the future, he was thinking about doing graduate studies, but was not sure whether to focus on research in his own field, education or business management, as he was aware of the importance of running a laboratory well. He said that management appealed to the people-oriented side of his personality. *Don* saw his future work as a continuation of the process of adapting to new equipment and learning new skills.

All four early-career practitioners saw their work in terms of the patients whom they could assist. Best practice in terms of patient care was a primary motivation for them to be observant, collaborate with others, and continually improve their skills. *Mary* was the most fortunate in terms of having many opportunities to attend workshops and also getting some financial support and time off to attend conferences. Apart from the on-site seminars to orient staff to new equipment, *Don* had no support for continuing education. If he wanted to attend a conference, he had to use his own funds and vacation time.

How can we best use the information from these interviews to inform our own scholarly practice? At this point it would be useful to pause, and reflect on how your own experience compares with what *Alex, Mary, Lisa* and *Don* have said. How would you compare and contrast what they said with what you read in other chapters? For example, did reading *Alex*'s thoughts on deciding a future career-path and choice of a higher degree make you think back to what you read in Chapter 2? Were you able to identify anyone's preferred learning style? Did *Lisa*'s, *Mary*'s or *Don*'s comments mean more to you because you read about reflection in Chapter 5, and clinical reasoning in Chapter 6?

Scholarship and health sciences

In this section we present a general overview of issues that *Alex, Don, Lisa* and *Mary* will be considering as they progress towards becoming advanced healthcare practitioners. We have used examples of current scholarly discussion in a sample of health professions that include behavioural science, dental hygiene, medical technology, nursing, occupational therapy, physical therapy, and radiation therapy. The number of professions identified as health professions is very large. We prefer to leave out the frequently used adjective 'allied', as this is not congruent with the concept of autonomy that we believe is needed for scholarly development. If a profession is considered to be 'allied' to another profession, the implication is that the 'allied' profession is dependent, and the profession to which it is 'allied' can exert a strong influence in determining and limiting its scope of education and practice. The exact number identified as (allied) health professionals varies from 50 to 200 in some publications (Karni et al 1995). The list may include credentialled, registered professions that require practitioners to have higher degrees as well as technicians with certificate qualifications earned through participation in a brief course of 6–12 weeks. In documents that describe allied health practitioners collectively, there is a tendency to describe them in terms of work setting rather than expertise. Some of the problems inherent in this clustering of health professions have been discussed in Chapter 1.

First, some general comments will serve as a useful guide for more in-depth reading. Scholarship is a product of knowledge (Van Doren 1991). The accumulated philosophical perspective of a discipline is often referred to as a paradigm. In practical terms, when we debate our scope of practice and how to articulate this to others we are considering aspects of our professional paradigm. Kuhn (1996) described four stages in the professional evolution paradigm:

1. the *preparadigm* period, which precedes the formalization of a profession
2. the *paradigm* period, during which the discipline accepts and consolidates a dominant ideology
3. the *crisis* period, in which members of the discipline become aware that the paradigm fails by leaving some major problems unsolved
4. the final stage is the *acceptance* of a new paradigm that redefines the discipline.

(See Chapter 3 for additional information about paradigm development.)

Professional scholarship has been viewed from a number of different perspectives that include discussion of:

- the way the profession's body of knowledge is generated (discovery)
- the characteristics of the profession (integration)
- how scholarship is disseminated and used in practice (application)
- the level of intellectual debate within a profession (integration and application)
- how the members of the professions are educated (teaching).

An integrated profession in which practice is both the source and conduit for ideas (Figure 7.2) is the overarching concept in the discussion of these perspectives (Yerxa 1994). Practice creates the critical incidents and frustrations that raise questions for the profession. Professionals seek to understand and create new approaches for

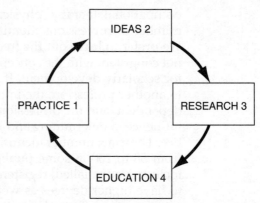

Figure 7.2   *Model of an integrated profession. Reproduced with permission from Yerxa EJ (1994) In search of good ideas for occupational therapy. Scandinavian Journal of Occupational Therapy 1:7–15*

practice. 'It is also where we make ethical decisions about which ideas may serve practice appropriately because they reflect our value system' (p. 7). These ideas, tested through research, are made available to the profession and are incorporated into the education of the profession. The new graduates bring new energy and new ideas to vitalize the profession. In turn, they will have new ideas that lead to further research. Each of the early-career professionals we interviewed talked about situations in which needed to solve a clinical problem. For example, *Mary*'s interest in acute care could lead her to advanced work, including research in this area of practice.

A profession's body of knowledge (discovery)

The way a profession's body of knowledge is generated involves the scholarship of discovery. Professional differentiation based on discussion about a profession's body of knowledge can lead to elitist views that some professionals may find exclusive. An academic discipline may not be synonymous with the profession that it informs; for example, microbiology informs medicine, nursing, pharmacy, and other professions, but is still separate from these professional disciplines. In discussing the scholarship of practice, we used examples from scientific disciplines such as physics and neuroscience to highlight the integration of knowledge with professional practice. In order to promote scholarly development within an academic profession, we need to consider the academic discipline and the academic profession separately as well as together. An academic discipline can inform practice, but may not provide any immediate practice-related answers (Ottenbacher 1996). The practice of a health profession is informed by a number of disciplines. These include basic sciences such as mathematics, social sciences such as anthropology, and physical sciences such as kinesiology. We have accepted this in terms of more established discipline/professional collaborations, e.g. physics and radiation therapy, kinesiology and physical therapy, or psychology and all the health professions.

We need to pause here to add that we are aware that most health professionals are motivated by human concerns and want to be involved 'hands-on' in practical work and client-centred discussion. As health professionals, we like to get to the point where we intersect with the real issues affecting our clients, and feel less motivated to become involved with more abstract concerns. However, it is important to remember that knowledge is an important base for power. Therefore, we do need to consider how knowledge-related issues impinge on our professions. This notion of how disciplines inform our practice is more challenging in respect to emerging disciplines that grow out of, but are not part of professional practice, and aim to inform practice, not develop treatment techniques for it. Microbiology grew out of medical practice, but the struggle for the establishment of this discipline occurred before our time. The emerging discipline of occupational science is a current example of a developing discipline (Yerxa et al 1989, Zemke and Clark 1996). It is a bio-psycho-social science with roots in occupational therapy as well as social and biological science. As an academic discipline, it has the potential to enhance practice by providing a conduit for basic as well as applied research and scholarly debate. An understanding of the contribution of occupation to health in general is an example (Hocking 2000). The application of concepts of occupation to healthcare professions more generally is outlined in Chapter 8. The relationship between knowledge and power has been described in Chapter 1. It enhances the status of a profession if it can claim specific disciplines as its knowledge base.

Characteristics of a profession (integration)

The characteristics of a profession relate to the scholarship of integration, and include the integration of individual type and skills with practice, as well as integration of knowledge within the profession as a whole. Professional characteristics may also impinge on the scholarship of teaching in making decisions about the parameters of education.

The identification of individual differences that characterize professional groups, for example in work values and role salience, of physiotherapists and occupational therapists, has been discussed in detail in Chapter 2, with particular reference to the International Work Importance Study (Super and Sverko 1995). A recent study in the state of Michigan, USA, compared the job choice and personality profiles of 294 occupational therapists and physical therapists (Lysack et al 2001). This study confirmed previous findings that personality exerts an influence on career choice. However, along with the mainstream of literature on career counseling, the authors caution against using personality type to influence selection into professional programs. However, they endorsed its relevance to matching teaching and learning styles to enhance professional education. *Lisa, Mary, Don* and *Alex* gave many examples of their preferences, firstly, for learning by doing, extra learning through discussion with mentors, and colleagues, as well as reading related literature. As *Alex* said: 'Personally I have to do it. I have to physically do it myself and work it out and then I know'. The others made similar comments, and also acknowledged the importance of professional literature. *Mary* said: 'I receive journals on all those areas, which are applicable to what I do'. *Lisa* added: 'I integrated the learning experience by going home, reading my text and getting a better base of knowledge in that specific area'.

The valuing of a broader skill base and educational experience through a science or liberal arts degree, prior to embarking on profession-specific education is reflected in the move to entry-level Master's degrees in health professions such as speech and language therapy, physical therapy and occupational therapy. Physical therapy education has moved from the Bachelor to the entry-level Master's degree in the USA, and differences between students at the Bachelor's and Master's levels of education have been examined. Significant differences have been found between the two groups. For example, Warren and Pierson (1994, p. 342) found that:

> Master's degree respondents anticipated greater involvement in research and teaching and felt better prepared to practice across a broad spectrum of clinical practice and to perform activities related to research, teaching, management, and direct access practice than did Bachelor's degree respondents.

Thus they concluded that the move to post-baccalaureate entry-level education was a positive outcome for education, practice and research in physical therapy. The occupational therapy profession in the USA has also endorsed the development of post-baccalaureate entry-level education. Bachelor-level programs are being phased out, as entry-level Master's becomes the educational requirement by 2007. The arguments supporting this change are similar to the ones identified in respect to the physical therapy example cited above. These arguments center on the benefits of professional autonomy that can facilitate growth and enhance scholarship (Gourley 2000, Kornblau 1999). In the USA, both the occupational therapy and physical therapy professions campaigned hard and long to achieve this advanced entry-level for their educational programs. Other health professions in the USA, such as speech and language pathology, audiology, and clinical psychology, have required entry-level Master's education for some time. Entry-level Master's professional education in the health professions has also been introduced in some Australian and British institutions of higher education. There is no doubt that the altruistic aim of this upward trend in education is evident in other countries beside the USA. It is motivated by ideals that enhance scholarship in practice and professional autonomy. However, there are those who disagree and have many concerns that escalating costs of health care will be exacerbated if health professionals demand higher salaries commensurate with their higher level of education. There are also concerns that a fast upward trend in basic educational requirements could create a shortage of health professionals and suitably qualified educators of health professionals, particularly in countries where a shortage of both is already evident (Waters 2000). It is outside the scope of this chapter to engage in this debate. However, we do not share this concern, as we believe that the complex, culturally diverse, and rapidly changing societies in which healthcare practitioners work demand the expertise of highly educated, autonomous individuals. Among our interviewees, *Mary* has an entry-level Master's degree in physical therapy and *Alex* talked about the possibility of doing a higher degree in the near future, in either education or business administration. *Don* and *Lisa* have Bachelor of Science degrees and were focused on developing their clinical skills. How to make the right choice about further education to match your own needs was discussed in detail in Chapter 2.

Dissemination and use of scholarship in practice (application)

The dissemination of scholarship within a profession addresses the scholarship of application. Understanding the interplay between health-related law and professional ethics is an important aspect of professional development in clinical, educational, and research settings. For example, the blending of law and ethics that is pertinent to physical therapy practice (Scott 2000) is also relevant to other health professions, as the level of individual accountability increases with an emphasis on evidence-based practice and the high cost of healthcare. Quality assurance in many different contexts is an important aspect of ensuring best practice in the health professions and among other professional groups (Fogarty et al 2001). This topic is discussed more fully in Chapter 1. However, we agree with Jensen and Paschal (2000) that the motivation for ethical practice and professional excellence needs to be internal. Writing eloquently from a perspective predicated on extensive work with physiotherapists, from students to expert clinicians, they stress the importance of concepts that are discussed in this and other chapters of this text, namely, multidimensional knowledge, collaboration, patient-centred focus, clinical reasoning, and reflection. These are the elements that can facilitate a practitioner to develop 'skills and habits of mind that will contribute to virtuous practice'. The merging of moral virtue and professional excellence is congruent with all aspects of scholarship in practice discussed so far. Jensen and Paschal (2000 p. 42) present a concept of virtuous practice that is enduring because it resonates with the basic tenets of a civilized society. They noted:

> The original Aristotelian concept of virtue was that virtue was a mark of excellence in function and that one *becomes* virtuous. The act of becoming is not through practiced drills, but by developing habits that require self-awareness and the freedom to choose to act.

Alex, Don, Lisa and *Mary* voiced their concern about implementing best practice, focused on their clients' needs, as they progress towards becoming advanced practitioners. *Mary* demonstrated this self-awareness when she said: 'I have been working with a supervisor and we have been going there [intensive care unit] every opportunity we have, which has been good for me. We can treat patients together until I am ready for her to observe me, and give feedback. Eventually I will be confident to treat more critically ill patients'.

Ethical dilemmas in healthcare reform are of particular concern to health professionals (Fisher 1997, Yerxa 1991). A growing body of literature in the health professions, for example in behavioural science, medicine, and occupational therapy, has highlighted and explored the spiritual dimensions of practice. Discourse about spirituality and health is not limited to prayer and formal religious orientation, but includes a holistic approach that enhances the individual's ability to develop hope and engage in meaningful occupations that are uplifting and affirming to the human spirit. These may include prayer meetings, training in relaxation techniques and poetry reading (Antonovsky 1993, Collins 1998, Horsburgh 1997, Peloquin 1997, Propst 1996, Rosenfeld 2000).

Intellectual debate within a profession (integration and application)

Intellectual debate relates to the scholarship of integration, as well as to the scholarship of application, in deliberating about what is appropriate to integrate and how it may be applied to practice. Vigorous intellectual debate in the health professions is in a developmental stage in comparison with disciplines that have been autonomous for a longer time. Engaging in intellectual debate in writing through published letters to a journal may be the preferred, albeit not frequent, method of intellectual debate for many. A major advantage over discussion at a seminar or conference is that those engaged in the discussion have had time to think and consider. Also, their views are exposed to a wider professional group who may choose to get involved in the discussion, in public, or among their peers. An article written by a group of doctoral students in occupational therapy is an excellent example of constructive scholarly debate (Dunn et al 1999). The topic of their debate centred on two published papers: the first by a well-respected clinician and educator whose article described a conceptual model of life style performance (Fidler 1996), and a second article that was critical of this model, written by two more junior, but reflective and scholarly clinical academicians (Hocking and Whiteford 1997a). The debate continued in the form of letters to the editor of the *American Journal of Occupational Therapy* (Hocking and Whiteford 1997b). The students overcame some initial discomfort and undertook a scholarly analysis of the two articles and related correspondence by examining the issues from several perspectives. They concluded by saying that they were excited about their newfound ability to engage in debate and thereby contribute to development in their profession. They encouraged further critical discourse as a mechanism for facilitating professional growth and for educating students. Many journals, for example, the *British Journal of Occupational Therapy*, welcome letters from readers that debate current issues such as the research priorities of the profession (Creek 2001, Forsyth 2001).

We realize that given all you have to do at work and the need to plan for your continuing professional development, writing letters to the editor of a professional journal may be a low priority. So, we suggest that you wait until some issue really stirs you, and you feel that you want to voice your opinion, because you have something important to say. Getting involved in professional organizations can give you the taste for discussing issues that are important to you. *Lisa* was very positive about her experience as a student representative at a national meeting: 'That was a phenomenal experience because it allowed me to first look at the organization, and look at how occupational therapists can really promote their profession'.

Professional education (teaching)

Here we address the scholarship of teaching. The education of professionals is best sustained through close collaboration between education, research, and practice (Yerxa 1994). Leadership in education is critical to the development and continued growth of scholarly practice. In an invited comment that prefaced a special issue on leadership in physical therapy education, Rothstein (1998) first outlined a crisis in education due to a shortage of suitably qualified university educators who meet academic criteria set by universities as well as clinical criteria required by a practice profession. She emphasized the importance of professionals contributing to the knowledge base of their profession. The challenge is for academic leaders to excel in the broad contexts of higher education, not just in physical therapy education. At the same time, she urged academic leaders to retain their ties to clinical practice. These multiple–even conflicting–challenges are faced by other practice-based health professions that juggle the dual demands of academe and the clinic. In a study conducted by academic educators whose professional discipline is medical technology, the investigators sought to explore the extent to which the health professions' deans and directors were actively involved in scholarship and research (Waller et al 1999). They found that, although two-thirds of their informants' time was spent in administration, they remained active in scholarship in all the areas outlined earlier in this chapter. They integrated their research, publication, and teaching with clinical involvement within their profession, thus acting as appropriate role models for their academic staff members and students. In Chapter 10 you can read the positive comments of our early-career interviewees about their clinical and academic role models and mentors.

Schmoll's (1998) holistic conceptualization of leadership in physical therapy education provides a model for supporting sustained scholarly professional development. She includes the socio-political organizational culture on the one side, and socio political organizational needs on the other. A skilled leader is at the center interacting with patients, to address their needs and interests and to implement educational programs to meet the needs of both patients and students. The attributes of the leader she describes include vision to move forward, skills in communication, process skills that can facilitate change and resolve conflict, empowering skills to build community, entrepreneurial skills that tolerate ambiguity and risk-taking, and personal qualities that include a sense of humour and self-knowledge. Schmoll also distinguishes between leadership and management. Health professionals educated by leaders who practice within this model would have had the benefit of excellent role models and mentors and would be well prepared for the scholarship of practice. *Alex* described these qualities about one of his instructors, who even made him consider a career educating clinical laboratory scientists: 'She taught it in a way that I just understood it. I also started thinking towards the end of the course whether I wanted to pursue teaching and if I wanted to teach in a university'.

It is great to be curious and enthusiastic about being better at our job. We also need to organize our professional development, evaluate the success of our scholarly endeavors and articulate the outcomes for our future plans. So, to assist with this process we shall share with you some ways of scholarly organizing that we have found to be useful (Table 7.2).

Table 7.2   *Techniques and exercises that can be used to develop scholarly practice*

- Fawcett Hill's (1969) learning through discussion (LTD) to ensure that written information is understood before it is integrated with other knowledge and applied in practice

- Action research to establish a system of identifying issues, implementing related action, reflection and evaluation of the outcomes

- Writing a memoir of all our pre- and professional work experiences to increase our self-knowledge about our strengths and preferences

Techniques to assist in developing a scholarly practice

Fawcett Hill's learning through discussion

Fawcett Hill's learning through discussion (LTD) (Fawcett Hill 1969, Rabow et al 1994) is a process that can be used to ensure that we understand what we read, and have a clear concept of the author's message. It is important to note that one can understand a written piece on a personal level of understanding that may not be the same as understanding the author's message. LTD aims to teach the reader to do the latter. It can be used in respect to an article, book, chapter, or report. The LTD process comprises eight steps that ideally take 60 minutes to complete (Rabow et al 1994, p. 8; Table 7.3). Although it was designed to be used as a group learning exercise, part of it can be used to enhance individual understanding of any written text. If you are using LTD process for individual study, follow steps 2–7, take notes, then review and edit your notes. Your previous reading about the use of reflection in Chapter 5 will assist you in this editing. These edited notes can then become part of your annotated bibliography of useful references.

1. The group meets at a previously determined time to discuss a paper that each member has read prior to the meeting. It is a good idea to select a timekeeper who will ensure that the discussion does not go beyond time for each section of the discussion. This role can be rotated.

2. Group participants agree on definitions of key terms. This stage requires individual preparation before the group meets. The article or chapter is read, and each person notes words or concepts that are new, or unclear, and, using a dictionary or other sources, writes a definition or explanation. When the group meets, these definitions and explanations are shared and briefly discussed. Another person can be responsible for taking the lead in this section of the discussion.

Table 7.3 *The stages of learning through discussion (LTD)*

1. Checking in, when group members greet each other	2–4 minutes
2. Vocabulary, when difficult words and concepts are defined	3–4 minutes
3. General statement of the author's message	5–6 minutes
4. Identification of major themes and subtopics	10–12 minutes
5. Application of material to other works	15–16 minutes
6. Application of material to self	10–12 minutes
7. Evaluation of the author's presentation	3–4 minutes
8. Evaluation of the group and individual performance	7–8 minutes
Total time	60 minutes

Adapted from Table 2.1, p. 8., in Rabow J, Charness MA, Kipperman J et al 1994 William Fawcett Hill's Learning Through Discussion, 3rd ed. Reprinted with permission of the publisher. Waveland Press Inc, Prospect Heights, IL. All rights reserved.

3. The purpose of identifying the author's message is to obtain an overall understanding of the paper being read. This can be easy if the author has stated the overall purpose of the article, or chapter, but in some cases, for example, where the writing is related to complex theoretical material, it may be more difficult.

4. The major themes are identified and discussed. This may be easier when the author has provided clear headings, but breaking down the themes and making logical connections between them enhances understanding of the reading. If there are many themes, it is a good idea to select only three or a maximum of four for discussion; otherwise, it is easy to lose the thread and end up with a discussion that is confusing or superficial.

   Time management is an important part of this process. Setting time limits helps to keep the discussion focused. At this stage it takes discipline not to relate the reading to other works or start discussing the application of the material. However, once you get into using the LTD method to read and review professional literature, we are sure that you will agree that it is helpful to understand the author's message and identify the major themes before doing anything else with the information.

5. Now, the group is ready to apply this reading to other works with which they are familiar. This ensures that the new learning does not stay fragmented. This is where the group can think laterally and make links between discipline areas. This is part of the scholarship of integration that we discussed earlier in this chapter.

6. It is really satisfying to get to this stage of personal application after working through the earlier part of the exercise. Many readers have a tendency to jump to this stage almost immediately. Therefore, they may never have a clear understanding of the material they have read, and they could be making incorrect assumptions in its application. We all have a natural tendency to focus on the application of the new information to our own, sometimes immediate,

needs. The connection between analytical concepts, research evidence, and one's own life experience as a professional and individual makes new information more exciting.

7. Personal reactions are an important part of the process of evaluating the author's presentation. Sometimes an article or chapter may be very complex because it is theoretical, full of statistical data, and written in a dry, dense style. This can be frustrating, and some complaining is legitimate, but it is also important to remain objective and constructive, so difficult material with potentially useful information is not dismissed.

8. This final step is a very important part of the discussion. This is when the group evaluates its own performance. Some checkpoints to consider include how well the subject was covered; what agreements were reached; whether there were questions that needed further clarification; was anything not answered; who contributed to the discussion and to what extent.

Many professional groups find that having a journal club is a useful way to keep up-to-date. You will also find references to journal clubs elsewhere in this text. We certainly recommend this as an adjunct to scholarship in practice. Some people choose to meet at lunchtime, at designated intervals such as the first Friday of the month. Lunchtime meetings will ensure that more people will attend, but the time is limited, and the discussion will be as well. If the group finds this frustrating, or not very useful, meeting more frequently, e.g. once a week, will make it possible to carry over discussion of the same article in greater depth over 2 or 3 weeks. Other groups may prefer to meet for a longer period after work. Whatever your preferred choice, we recommend that you use the LTD method to structure the discussion. We also think that it is important to rotate roles, so that everyone gets a chance to choose the article, prepare the first stage by bringing the definitions and explanations, and do the summary. The social role is also important. Whether it is a lunchtime or evening meeting, discussion flows better with good food. Taking turns to organize the food, or prepare part of the text gives a nice balance to this whole scholarly, social process.

Action research

Action research (Kemmis and McTaggart 1988, Lewin 1946, 1952) is a continuous method of incorporating planning, action, observation, reflection, and evaluation. It is noted for going beyond theory building or interpretation to effect relevant change in practice (Conway et al 1994). The research model is thus a continuous approach to improving a process, as new research questions replace those that have been resolved. Gummesson (1991) points out that the understanding developed during an action research project is holistic, as opposed to studying in detail one or a few isolated factors. Such an approach requires cooperation between all the participants involved in a project and requires continuous adjustment to new information and events. Oja and Smulyan (1989, p. 12) note that action research is a collaborative method: 'collaboration allows for mutual understanding and consensus, democratic decision making, and common action'. Frequent and open communication between participants that may include senior management staff and junior employees is essential throughout the process to avoid possible conflicting perceptions and assumptions that result from their different positions in an organization.

Action research addresses the process and the outcomes of an investigation simultaneously (Figure 7.3). There is an expectation that involvement in the process itself will affect change, and that outcomes are not only reported, but also used to generate further documented action and evaluation (Stringer 1996). Thus action research is well suited to working with diverse communities engaged in shared goals

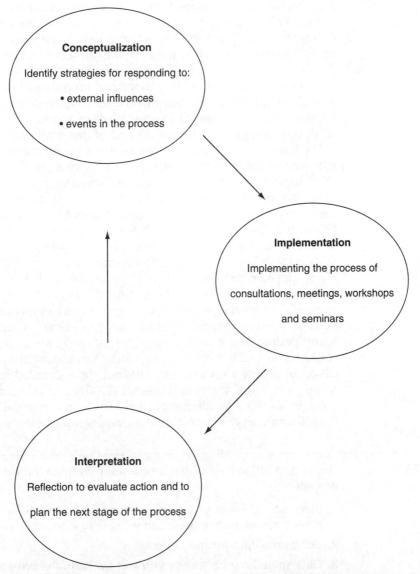

Figure 7.3   *The action research model. Reproduced with permission from Roth LM and Esdaile SA (1999) Action research: A dynamic discipline for advancing professional goals. British Journal of Occupational Therapy 62:498–506*

and objectives, for example hospitals, community organizations, and university departments. Both organization development and action research are variants of applied behavioural science. They are problem-solving, social interventions that are action-oriented, databased, and require collaboration between insider and outsider. French and Bell (1995, p. 151) further state that 'a sound organization development program rests on an action research model'. Wilcock (1998) advocates using an action research model for an occupational approach to public health. She advocates using this model because action research, in line with critical social science, 'aims at facilitating social change through self-reflecting inquiry and consciousness raising which enlightens participants' (p. 225). Self-reflection is essential to increase awareness of our actions and provide support for collaborative reflection and informed action, which has the potential to change our natural and social environments. Thus, participatory action research can provide the support needed to change environments and health services. However, Wilcock (1998) warns that if we are not aware of why we do what we do, and do not take time to reflect on the actions and outcomes of the results of our work, we can become disorganized and self-defeating. In order to implement action research in your place of work, we refer you to the additional resources section at the end of this chapter.

We have found that action research is a useful method for ensuring that work, required as part of professional practice, is done in a scholarly manner. We used this method effectively in a 2-year project designed to enhance individual and organizational development in a university-based department within a faculty of health professions (Roth and Esdaile 1999). Examples of situations where the action research process may be used effectively include evaluating the objectives and outcomes of regular departmental meetings and the planning, implementation and evaluation of skill-based continuing education offered over a period of time (Hyrkäs 1997). You do not need to develop a special project. The on-going work of any department can become more scholarly through the application of action research. Many people find that departmental meetings are unproductive. You could try to make these meetings more productive through the application of action research. You will find clear, detailed instructions for focus groups in Krueger and Casey's (2000) practical guide to the topic. Stringer's (1996) handbook on action research also includes instructions that are easy to implement as the example below indicates.

Activity box 7.1   Goals and objectives of departmental meetings: an action research project

1. Start with a focus group of all those who attend the meetings to determine what they think and what they want to achieve.
2. Set a time limit for the project.
3. Determine how frequently you will evaluate the project. For example, if you set the time limit to 6 months, you may want to evaluate the process every 2 months.

Activity box 7.1 *cont'd*

4. Decide on who is going to do what: set the agenda, allocate action statements and time limits to issues identified as needing action, take detailed minutes of meetings, evaluate the process, write the interim evaluation and final evaluation reports.

5. Decide whether all these tasks will be allocated to people within your department, or whether you will use an outside consultant to assist with part of it, e.g. the focus group and/or the final evaluation.

6. Remember that action research is a cyclical process. When you have completed the evaluation and decided on what is to be implemented, you can continue the action research process to determine how the new system is working, and finetune it.

7. Because the work and needs of your department are dynamic, you will find that even systems that work well for a time, will have to be revised in the future.

Writing a memoir of pre- and professional work experiences

Becoming an advanced healthcare practitioner will take time and effort, and this also involves emotional investment. So, it is important that you take time to decide what you really like to do. What type of work is most meaningful and satisfying for you? Everyone who has completed a course of studies and obtained a professional qualification will have learned how to prepare a succinct résumé as well as a more comprehensive, curriculum vitae (CV). But these professional exercises may not help an individual to identify his or her real work preferences at a deeper level. The reasons we choose to do certain jobs may be pragmatic, related to availability rather than preference. The importance of knowing more about our personality type and work values was discussed in some detail in Chapter 2. Knowing more about our individual preferences and personality is very useful. But it isn't as useful if we try to take short cuts and make do with a superficial understanding. The Myers-Briggs Type Indicator^R (Briggs Myers et al 1998), and Super's Work Importance and Role Salience Inventories (Super & Sverko 1995) are predicated on complex theories that can't be well understood quickly. This is a good example of material that could be used for an LTD exercise.

Writing an autobiography requires the writer to use correct dates and facts. A memoir is more subjective and allows the individual to write about impressions and feelings that would not be included in a résumé or CV. Writing a memoir is not just for old people; it can be useful at any stage in one's life, and can be used to address specific aspects of life, such as work. The process of writing will add richness and texture to all that you have learned from using the standardized tests referred to above and described in Chapter 2. Even a short memoir of a working life will help to identify not just how you think and what you value, but what you really enjoy doing and what you don't, even if you may be quite good at it. Using a format to guide you may be helpful. For example, *The Autobiography Box*, by Brian Bouldrey (Bouldrey 2000) is designed to provide a structure for constructing a memoir. The title is a little misleading. The key words Bouldrey uses are *remember, discover, structure* and *dramatize*.

Your first step will be to set aside a morning or afternoon to write the first draft of your memoir. You can then add to it whenever you wish. Start by *remembering* your very first job. It may have been baby-sitting, delivering the local newspaper or an after-school or weekend job working in a store or a restaurant. Start by jotting down what you recall. This will help you to *discover* recurring words or themes in what you remember. Are the memories pleasant? Are you happy thinking about them? Or was some of this tough to write, as you recall the frustration of having to work for weeks to save so little, or cold winter mornings when all you wanted to do was sleep? Did you skip anything because you may have thought it was too obvious or dull? Now, *structure* your memoir according to the themes you identified. It may be your experiences in dealing with the people in charge, or the things you bought with your earnings. You may want to arrange events in chronological order, or juggle inner and outer stories, what happened and what you did (outer) and how you felt about it (inner). Next, try to *dramatize* the memory by imagining that you are reliving the experience, and telling one of your friends about it at the time. One way to do this is to pretend you are writing a letter to a friend from that period of your life. Or you could try writing in the present tense. You could even try writing it as a movie script, adding lots of extra detail for 'visual effect'.

Telling your story, discovering more about it, structuring it, then dramatizing it can build up interconnected vignettes of each of your jobs, through your school, college or university days to the present time. Thus, you may find that you enjoy the hands-on learning type of problem-solving experiences. This can emerge as a theme in your work memoir, because you have discovered that you really liked working in a bicycle repair shop after school when you were 15 years old. Later, the laboratory classes were what you looked forward to when you were in college or university. Now, in your current job, you like getting new equipment and doing the testing to make sure it functions effectively.

Someone else doing this exercise may discover that she has always enjoyed organizing and reorganizing things. Back in grade 5, she got the other children on the block to make lemonade to sell to the neighbors on hot summer days. She volunteered to help the teacher, became class captain, then student union representative. Now, she makes it her business to know the organizational structure of the hospital where she works and is chair or secretary of several committees. These are very different examples that provide knowledge that can help an individual to decide where to focus his or her scholarly efforts. Organizations thrive on the scholarly input of diverse skills from all members. Most of us don't mind doing extra work if we enjoy what we do and others value it. But we need the confidence to know what we are naturally good at doing and where we want to put our long-term efforts, so we are not drifting into work about which we are ambivalent. It is important to feel empowered to enhance your scholarship in practice in areas of your profession where you are most comfortable and motivated.

Conclusion

Jensen and Paschal's (2000, p. 44) comment about the outcomes of qualitative studies of expert practice in physical therapy may be applied to all healthcare professionals. They state:

> the experts draw their knowledge from multiple sources, including formal education, literature, people (mentors, patients, colleagues), and interpretation and reflection on data gathered through the senses. Most notable is their focus on continued learning and transforming their knowledge over time as they engage in practice.

Along your own journey of scholarly practice, you will be using all the reflections, skills and competencies described in the chapters of this text. You will also continue to add to your knowledge, and rethink and reshape ideas that inform your practice as you respond to the clinical irritations, or problems for which you need to find new solutions (Yerxa 1994). The early-career practitioners we interviewed–*Mary*, the physical therapist, *Lisa*, the occupational therapist, *Alex*, the medical technologist and *Don*, the radiation therapist–highlighted the concepts and issues discussed in this chapter. They are in the process of becoming advanced healthcare practitioners. Along their journey, they are discovering new knowledge through practice and observation and through reading professional literature; they are also becoming more familiar with the ways that their professional knowledge is generated. In the process of integrating their own discoveries and those of others, they are developing clearer professional identities and better skills for applying their knowledge, working within interdisciplinary teams and engaging in professional debate. They are also continually engaged in the process of teaching through sharing their skills with, and learning from, others.

Activity box 7.2

Questions for further discussion

Do you think that your profession is also a discipline?

If you responded in the affirmative, what arguments would you use to support that it is a discipline?

Identify the positive and negative aspects of your own professional education. Now, identify your views about formal professional education, including clinical education, and list the five factors that you consider most important.

How can you put these into practice to assist students or less experienced colleagues?

How is your profession regulated? What aspects of the regulations enhance and what aspects limit your own professional practice?

Did you identify with any of the people interviewed for this chapter? What could you add from your own unique experience and insights that could help others?

References

Antonovsky A 1993 The structure and properties of the sense of coherence scale. Social Science and Medicine 36:725–733

Beattie D S 2000 Expanding the view of scholarship: introduction. Academic Medicine 75:871–876

Bouldrey B 2000 The autobiography box. A step-by-step kit for examining the life worth living. Chronicle Books, San Francisco, CA

Boyer E L 1990 Scholarship reconsidered: priorities of the professoriate. Carnegie Foundation for the Advancement of Teaching, Princeton, NJ

Briggs Myers I, McCaulley M H, Quenk N L, Hammer AL 1998 MBTI: a guide to the development and use of the Myers-Briggs type indicator, 3rd edn. Consulting Psychologists Press, Australia

Collins M 1998 Spirituality and occupational therapy. British Journal of Occupational Therapy 61:280–284

Conti G E 1998 Clinical interpretation of 'grip strengths and required forces in accessing everyday containers in a normal population'. American Journal of Occupational Therapy 52:627–628

Conway R, Kember D, Sivan A, Wu M 1994 Making departmental changes through action research, based on adult learning principles. Higher Education 28:265–282

Creek J 2001 Letters to the editor. Response. British Journal of Occupational Therapy 64:421

Cruess R, Cruess S 1997 Teaching medicine as a profession in the service of healing. Academic Medicine 72:941–952

Dauphinée D, Martin J B 2000 Breaking down the walls: thoughts on the scholarship of integration. Academic Medicine 75:881–886

Dewey J 1933 How we think. Heath, Lexington, MA (originally published 1910)

Dunn E, Schulz E K, Schulz C H, Honaker DeL, Wiley A M 1999 The importance of scholarly debate in occupational therapy. American Journal of Occupational Therapy 53:398–400

Esdaile S A, Roth L M 2000 Viewpoint. Education not training: the challenge of developing professional autonomy. Occupational Therapy International 7:147–152

Fawcett Hill W 1969 Learning through discussion. Sage, Newbury Park, Beverly Hills

Fidler G S 1996 Life-style performance: from profile to conceptual model. American Journal of Occupational Therapy 50:139–147

Fisher G S 1997 Ethical dilemmas in healthcare reform. Occupational Therapy in Health Care 11:1–27

Fogarty G B, Hornby C, Ferguson H M, Peters I J 2001 Quality assurance in a radiation oncology unit: the chart round experience. Australasian Radiology 45:189–194

Forsyth K 2001 Letters to the editor. Occupational science as a selected research priority. British Journal of Occupational Therapy 64:420

French W L, Bell C H 1995 Organization development, 5th edn. Prentice Hall, Englewood Cliffs, NJ

Glassick C E, Huber M T, Maeroff G I 1997 Scholarship assessed: evaluation of the professoriate. Jossey-Bass, San Francisco, CA

Goodall J 1999 Reason for hope. A spiritual journey. Warner Books, New York, NY

Gourley M 2000 Postbaccalaureate requirement facilitates OT growth. OT Practice 5:9

Gummesson E 1991 Qualitative methods in management research. Sage, Newbury Park, CA

Hocking C 2000 Occupational science: a stock take of accumulated insights. Journal of Occupational Science 7:58–67

Hocking C, Whiteford G 1997a The issue is—what are the criteria for development of occupational therapy theory? A response to Fidler's life-style performance model. American Journal of Occupational Therapy 51:154–157

Hocking C, Whiteford G 1997b Letters to the editor. Authors' response. American Journal of Occupational Therapy 51:710

Horsburgh M 1997 Towards an inclusive spirituality: wholeness, interdependence and waiting. Disability and Rehabilitation 19:398–406

Hurvitz E A, Conti G E, Flansburg E L, Brown S H 2000 Motor control of upper limb function after botulinum toxin injection: a case study. Archives of Physical Medicine Rehabilitation 81:1408–1414

Hyrkäs K 1997 Can action research be applied in developing clinical teaching? Journal of Advanced Nursing 25:801–808

Jensen G M, Paschal K A 2000 Habits of mind: student transition toward virtuous practice. Journal of Physical Therapy Education 3:42–47

Karni K R, Lang A, Beck J B 1995 Why a school of allied health? Journal of Allied Health 24:187–202

Kemmis S, McTaggart R (eds) 1988 The action research reader, 3rd edn. Deakin University Press, Geelong, Victoria

Kornblau B 1999 Say 'yes' to resolution, Journal of Advance for Occupational Therapy, April 5, 7

Krueger R A, Casey M A 2000 Focus groups. A practical guide for applied research, 3rd edn. Sage, Thousand Oaks, CA

Kuhn T S 1996 The structure of scientific revolutions, 3rd edn. University of Chicago Press, Chicago

Lewin K 1946 Action research and minority problems. Journal of Social Issues 2:34–46

Lewin K 1952 Group decision and social change. In: Swanson G E, Newcomb T M, Hartley F E (eds) Readings in social psychology. Holt, New York, p 459–473

Lysack C, McNevin N, Dunleavy K 2001 Job choice and personality: a profile of Michigan occupational and physical therapists. Journal of Allied Health 30:75–82

Mattingly C, Fleming M H 1994 Clinical reasoning. Forms of inquiry in therapeutic practice. F A Davis, Philadelphia, PA

National Health Service 2000 Meeting the challenge: a strategy for allied health professions. Department of Health, London

Oja S, Smulyan L 1989 Collaborative action research: a developmental approach. Falmer, London

Ottenbacher K 1996 Academic disciplines: maps for professional development. In: Zemke R, Clark F (eds) Occupational science. The evolving profession. F A Davis, Philadelphia

Peloquin S 1997 Nationally speaking—the spiritual depth of occupation. Making worlds and making lives. American Journal of Occupational Therapy 51:167–168

Propst L 1996 Cognitive behavior therapy and the religious person. In: Shafrenske E (ed). Religion and the clinical practice of psychology. American Psychological Association, Washington, DC, p 391–407

Rabow J, Charness M A, Kipperman J, Radcliff-Vasile S 1994 William Fawcett Hill's learning through discussion, 3rd edn. Waveland Press, Prospect Hill, IL

Ribbons R, Vance S 2001 Using e-mail to facilitate nursing scholarship. Computers in Nursing 19:105–110

Rosenfeld M S 2000 Spiritual agent modalities for occupational therapy practice. OT Practice 5:17–21

Roth L M, Esdaile S A 1999 Action research: a dynamic discipline for advancing professional goals. British Journal of Occupational Therapy 62:498–506

Roth L M, Schenk M, Bogdewic S P 2001 Developing clinical teachers and their organizations for the future of medical education. Medical Education 35:248–249

Rothstein J M 1998 Invited comment. Will our leadership inspire? . . . Or just wield power? Journal of Physical Therapy Education 12:3–5

Schmoll B J 1998 Educational leadership from a holistic perspective. Journal of Physical Therapy Education 3:6–10

Schön D 1983 The reflective practitioner: how professionals think in action. Temple Smith: London

Scott R 2000 Supporting professional development: understanding the interplay between health law and professional ethics. Journal of Physical Therapy Education 14:17–19

Shapiro E D, Coleman D L 2000 The scholarship of application. Academic Medicine 75:895–898

Stringer E T 1996 Action research. A handbook for practitioners. Sage Publications, Thousand Oaks, CA

Summers S H, Blau G, Ward-Cook K 2000 Professional development activities of medical technologists: management implications for allied health. Journal of Allied Health 29:214–219

Super D E, Sverko B (eds) 1995 Life roles, values and careers. Jossey-Bass, San Francisco, CA

US Department of Health and Human Services Public Health Service 1999 Building the future of allied health. Report of the implementation task force of the National Commission on Allied Health. Health Resources and Services Administration, Rockville, MD

Van Doren C 1991 A history of knowledge: past, present and future. Ballantine Books, New York

Wales C E, Nardi A H, Stager R A 1993 Emphasizing critical thinking and problem solving. In: Curry L, Wergin, J F (eds), Educating professionals. Responding to new expectations for competence and accountability. Jossey-Bass, San Francisco, CA

Waller K V, Karni K R, Wilson S L 1999 Scholarship and research of allied health deans and directors. Journal of Allied Health 28:1–7

Warren S C, Pierson F M 1994 Comparison of characteristics and attitudes of entry-level bachelor's and master's degree students in physical therapy. Physical Therapy 74:333–347

Waters B 2000 Master's degree as a pre-registration qualification: a need for caution. Opinion. British Journal of Occupational Therapy 63:500–502

Wilcock A A 1998 An occupational perspective of health. Slack, Thorofare, NJ

Yerxa EJ 1991 Nationally speaking–seeking a relevant, ethical and realistic way of knowing of Occupational Therapy. American Journal of Occupational Therapy 45:199–204

Yerxa E J 1994 In search of good ideas for occupational therapy. Scandinavian Journal of Occupational Therapy 1:7–15

Yerxa E J, Clark F, Frank G, Jackson J, Parham D, Pierce D, Stein C, Zemke R 1989 An introduction to occupational science. A foundation for occupational therapy in the 21st century. Occupational Therapy in Health Care 6:1–17

Zemke R, Clark F (eds) 1996 Occupational science. The evolving discipline. F A Davis, Philadelphia, PA

Additional resources   Morton-Cooper A 2000 Action research in healthcare. Blackwell Science, Oxford

8 Creating occupational practice: a multidisciplinary health focus

Clare Hocking

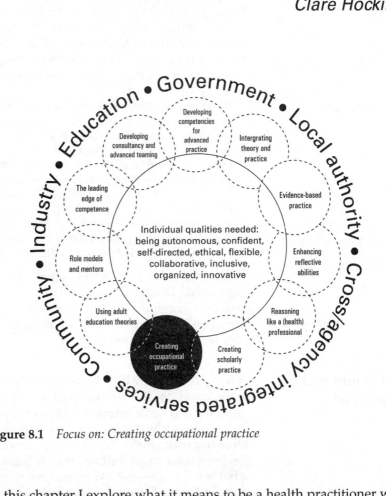

Figure 8.1 *Focus on: Creating occupational practice*

Chapter outline

In this chapter I explore what it means to be a health practitioner who is concerned about the things people with health problems are able to do in their day-to-day lives. It focuses on all the things people usually do that occupy them and it looks at the ways disease and disorder affect those occupations. The chapter is also concerned with the ways our occupations sustain and improve health. Consistent with the World Health Organization's (WHO) *International Classification of Functioning, Disability and Health* (ICF: WHO 2001), it proposes that a key purpose of health services is to help people to participate in the everyday occupations that give life meaning. I believe that this requires health practitioners who look beyond the injury, disease or disorder to focus intervention towards occupations that are important to their clients. My hope is that thinking in more occupational ways will also result in questioning established practice where it does not best support clients' return to occupation.

Key words

Occupation, participation, health, outcome measurement

Anticipated outcomes

As a result of reading this chapter, I anticipate that you will be able to:

- explain the importance of occupation in people's lives
- explain how helping people to do the things they want and need to do is the ultimate goal of all health interventions
- give examples of health issues that affect occupation
- reflect on personal and professional experiences to develop occupation-oriented interventions and health services.

Introduction

What was petrifying me was the thought of returning home, not as the skinny, long-legged Millie who used to run so fast and jump so high that people used to joke 'You'd think she was training for the Olympics'; not as Millie who used to swim like a fish and who, on a good day, could hold her breath under water for longer than all but one or two of the gang; not as the Millie who used to walk or cycle for miles along the beach and the track; not as the Millie who used to dance like Michael Jackson and Bobbie Brown (well, as James Brown, then). No, it wasn't the thought of returning home that was frightening me. It was the thought of arriving home, not as the runner, the dancer, the cyclist, but as Millie the wheel-chair user! (Hill 1994, p.143)

Millie was a different person when she returned home, and she was frightened. Disabled by a spinal cord injury, Millie knew that she could no longer do the things she used to do, the things that defined her as an individual in her community. She was worried about how people would react to her.

The importance of occupation

When people like Millie leave the health services, they return to lives made up of day-to-day occupations. By occupations I mean all of the ordinary and extraordinary things people do at home, at work and in their community that occupy their time. Occupation, here, refers to more than our work roles. As Millie's story illustrates, our occupations are important to us. In part, that is because we know who we are by what we can do—our skills, successes and failures, the things we've done in the past as well as those we expect or hope to do in the future. It is through occupation that we learn about ourselves. The things we do are also important because that is how we support our families and ourselves, and because our daily round of occupations provides structure and meaning to our days. Further, our social identity hinges on our occupations—Millie was known as a runner, a dancer and a cyclist. Her occupations provided a context for interacting with others. They made her not just a person, but a particular person (Christiansen 1999). Look at Figure 8.2 on page 191.

But what has occupation got to do with being a health practitioner? Why should nurses, speech and language therapists, physical therapists podiatrists and audiologists be concerned with clients' occupations? Surely that is the role of occupational therapists and vocational counsellors? In the first section of this chapter, I will put the case that, as a health practitioner functioning at an advanced level,

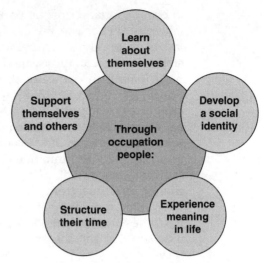

Figure 8.2   *The role of occupation in everyday life*

you will increasingly be concerned with occupation. The discussion will identify three primary reasons for this.

The first reason to be concerned with occupation is that there is a strong relationship between occupation (the things people do) and health. People's occupations can keep them healthy or make them unhealthy. During recovery from disease or injury, health practitioners are concerned with what their clients need to do or not do to promote recovery. People who have had a hip replacement need to start mobilizing—they will be encouraged to walk to the bathroom. People who have had a skin graft may need to stay on bed rest, accepting assistance with all self-care occupations. As an advanced health practitioner who is aware of the relationship between occupation and health, you will be concerned with:

- how your clients' everyday occupations are affected by their health status
- how those occupations support or undermine their ongoing physical and mental health.

The second reason why occupation is an important concern of all health professionals is that people's occupations give meaning to their lives. When we do things that are fun, feel good, challenge and excite us, or express our love for and care of others, life is worth living. Health professionals understand that people who believe that life is worth living, despite hearing loss, immobility, pain, dysphasia, poor mental health or an array of other health problems, will be motivated to work hard at the business of getting well and will generally achieve a better outcome. Working at an advanced level will involve finding out what makes your clients' life worth living and what occupations they are motivated to work hard for.

The third reason for being concerned about occupation is that health and the outcomes of health services are increasingly described in occupational terms. Of particular note is the work recently undertaken by WHO. The WHO's ICF describes health in terms of impairments of bodily structures or functions, limitations in performing activities or occupations, and restrictions individuals experience when participating in educational, self-care, communication, social, vocational and civic occupations. (See Table 8.1 for a summary of the ICF categories of activity and participation.) Over time, the WHO envisages that health services and health professionals will begin to measure and report the effectiveness of health interventions in terms of reducing activity limitations and restrictions to participation. To do this demands an advanced level of practice, because it will require a change in focus from the biological consequences of disease and observable reductions in symptoms (Peters 1995) to the longer-term outcomes of intervention. Adopting the ICF will challenge you to provide services and measure health outcomes in highly individualized ways.

Having explored why it is important to focus on occupation, I would like to move on to a discussion of the advanced practice skills required to deliver a health service that addresses clients' occupational

Table 8.1 *Summary of activity and participation categories identified in the International Classification of Functioning, Disability and Health (World Health Organization 2001)*

Categories of activity and participation

Learning and applying knowledge

- Purposeful sensory experiences
- Basic learning
- Applying knowledge

General tasks and demands
Communication
- Receiving messages
- Producing messages
- Conversation and using communication devices and techniques

Movement
- Maintaining and changing body position
- Moving and handling objects
- Walking and related activities
- Moving around using transportation

Self-care
Domestic life areas
- Acquisition of necessities
- Household tasks
- Caring for household objects and assisting others

Interpersonal interactions
- Interpersonal interactions
- Particular interpersonal interactions

Major life areas
- Education
- Work and employment
- Economic life
Community, social and civic life

needs. This section of the chapter will be framed around four key questions:

1. *What occupations?* People who experience the same impairment may be affected in different ways. Some find ways to do things that others struggle with. In addition, different people do different things. Even the things that most people do, such as getting dressed and having a conversation, are important for some and mundane for others. How will you know which occupations are important to clients? And how might that knowledge influence your practice?

2. *What kind of occupation is your intervention?* Most healthcare services require the recipient at least to cooperate with what is being done to them. Many interventions require clients' active participation. But what is it like to do the things you ask your clients to do? Could it be a more pleasant or health-enhancing occupation?

3. *Are your clients ready for occupation?* When people present to a health service, they often need to be cared for. At some stage, however, most will need to resume doing things for themselves or having their usual care givers do things for them. How will you know when they are ready?

4. *What occupations does your practice setting enable?* Acute healthcare is often provided in hospital settings. Many of these health services, at least in the western world, employ people to make the beds, maintain the buildings, provide meals and beverages, and assist with personal care if required. Employees answer the phone, keep the records, and manage the finances. With so many occupations done for them, what opportunities exist for clients to exercise and maintain their capacity for occupation?

Dispersed throughout these discussions, I have provided activity worksheets to help you to apply the discussions to your own practice. As you complete the worksheets you will generate new insights into your own practice and build up an individualized plan for becoming an advanced, occupationally focused practitioner. To begin the process, please complete Activity worksheet 1, which focuses on the kinds of occupational challenges your clients may experience.

Being concerned about occupation

As previously mentioned, there are three primary reasons for health professionals to be concerned about their clients' occupations. These are now discussed in more detail.

Occupation and health

The first reason is that there is an implicit relationship between health and occupation. Wilcock (1998) in particular has argued that occupation is a biological necessity for human kind, stating that it is through occupation that humans meet basic needs, exercise their capacities, and experience meaning, purpose and satisfaction. These, Wilcock argues, are the foundations of health. The notion that engaging in occupation underpins health is presented pictorially in Figure 8.3.

Activity worksheet 1

Identify someone that you know reasonably well who fits the profile of the clients or some of the clients with whom you typically work, or have worked in the past. That is, someone who is the same gender and in the same age range as your client group. If you work with people of all ages, select anyone of the people you know reasonably well. This may be yourself, a member of your family, a friend or someone you work with.

Write the person's name here: _____

Now list two or three of the impairments your current or previous clients typically exhibit(ed) that might affect their ability to do the things they want and need to do.

1. _____
2. _____
3. _____

If the person you identified above developed these impairments, what occupations that are important to them would be affected? Try to name three or four occupations that would really make a difference to the person you identified. Make sure you identify specific occupations — not just eating, but eating evening meals with the family; not just working, but walking from their desk to the meeting room or understanding customers' requests in order to place their orders accurately.

1. _____
2. _____
3. _____
4. _____

Now write a brief paragraph about what it would be like for the person you are thinking of to have this experience. How do you think it would affect him/her to have difficulty doing these important occupations? Would he/she think about him/herself differently? Would other people react to them differently? Are there people he/she might try to hide his/her problems from? If this went on for a long time, might the experience change him/her as a person? In what ways?

_____
_____
_____
_____
_____
_____

Activity worksheet 2 will ask you to build on the thinking you have started in Activity worksheet 1.

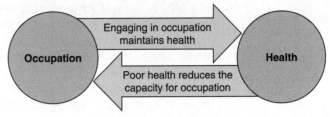

Figure 8.3 *The two-directional relationship between occupation and health*

Health itself can be defined in a variety of ways. It can be viewed as a goal, something people should aspire to and strive to achieve. However, each individual will aspire to different aspects of health. As Dubos (1970) suggested, top executives, lumberjacks, jockeys, pilots and newspaper deliverers have different requirements for health, depending on the different physical and mental requirements of their chosen occupations. This is a perspective of health that emphasizes having the capacity to meet occupational demands (Sim 1990).

Illness, disease and injury, however, often compromise an individual's capacity to meet the demands of familiar and valued occupations. Looking at Figure 8.3, for example, people who survive having a stroke typically experience residual impairments that may disrupt perceptual and cognitive function, expressive and receptive communication, and their ability to walk and manipulate objects. Stroke survivors commonly report limitations in their ability to perform the everyday activities involved in caring for themselves and managing their home, especially those activities that are strenuous or involve working outside. Those unable to participate in their pre-morbid life style have been found to have the greatest difficulty adjusting to their losses and accepting residual physical limitations (Huijbregts et al 2000).

In addition, stroke survivors often report a reduction in activity levels, spending more time being inactive because of their mobility problems or reduced ability to stand for any length of time (Trigg et al 1999, p. 345). This can and does lead to further health problems. At a physical level, this may involve loss of fitness and unwanted weight gain. For example, one participant in the study undertaken by Trigg and his colleagues had previously maintained a high level of fitness. After his stroke he reported sitting on the sofa 'since January' and gaining 30–40 lb (13–18 kg) in weight 'not for the food that I'm eating. I've kept a strict check on it, it's just through lack of exercise'.

Stroke survivors typically also experience decreased participation in social and leisure activities (Drummond 1990). This reduction is frequently attributed to decreased access to valued occupations, for example an inability to drive, or to have impaired performance due to motor, communication or cognitive impairments. In addition, previously meaningful occupations may be less satisfying when stroke survivors are unable to perform to the same level of competence or with the same ease as prior to their stroke. Three further factors reported as contributing to the decline in social and leisure participation are feeling that others do not understand the difficulties they are experiencing, embarrassment about changed physical appearance, and that social and leisure occupations are not seen as essential. As Trigg et al (1999) report, many stroke survivors direct their energy elsewhere. It has been suggested, however, that this reduction in leisure occupations is directly related to the high levels of depression following stroke. Alternatively, the high incidence of depression and anxiety following stroke may be associated with problems with physical functioning, as it is for people diagnosed with human immunodeficiency virus or HIV (Nixon and Cott 2000). Whatever the causative factor, stroke survivors who receive leisure rehabilitation have been found to have significantly higher psychological well-being (Drummond and Walker 1996). Furthermore, perhaps because engaging in leisure occupations involves walking, recipients of the leisure rehabilitation intervention Drummond and Walker studied also had significantly better mobility.

While this example has focused on stroke survivors, the same change processes can be expected to apply to people with other health conditions. Just as is the case for stroke survivors, individuals who acquire impairments are likely to experience difficulty with some aspects of occupational performance and are likely to derive less satisfaction from social and leisure occupations. Like other people from affluent industrial countries, they will be subject to social expectations that people should work to be independent in their self-care activities, and many will share the cultural perspective that work takes precedence over leisure. As an advanced health professional tuned to the health-giving properties of occupation, however, you will appreciate that, as Mulley (1994) has asserted, 'maintaining optimum levels of activity and life satisfaction is of supreme importance' (pp. 61–62). Perhaps, like Drummond Walker, you will question whether leisure rehabilitation might be most effective if integrated into all aspects of healthcare, and all stages of rehabilitation. Certainly, you will support your clients in continuing with previous social and leisure occupations, or finding new, satisfying things to do. Perhaps you will guide them towards accepting help with self-care or household tasks, or work with them to access support services, to ensure they have enough energy to be involved in those occupations that will be satisfying and maintain their psychological well-being.

Occupation and motivation for rehabilitation

As well as having long-term health implications, occupation relates to clients' motivation for rehabilitation and the outcomes they achieve. In particular, Guthrie and Harvey (1994) suggest, the way individuals think about themselves and the things they will do in the future is central to their success in rehabilitation. Those who believe that a positive future is possible despite their health issues rate their abilities highly and set demanding goals for themselves. These optimists are highly motivated and make the best progress. However, the goals they set are frequently perceived as unrealistic by health professionals, who have failed to understand the relationship between specific, challenging goals and motivation.

To enable clients to set challenging goals about what they will do in the future, and to support their commitment to achieving them, requires an understanding of their 'previous achievements, occupations, hobbies and enthusiasms' (Mulley 1994, p. 62). It means understanding how people think about themselves in terms of what they can do, what is difficult or enjoyable to do, and what is worth doing. It also means understanding that it is not just the frequency of engagement in occupation, but the quality of performance and enjoyment derived through occupation that are important (Trigg et al 1999). Understanding healthcare clients in this way is a foundation for understanding their intentions for participation in home, work and community life (Thoren-Jonsson and Moller 1999). Clients of a community-based pulmonary rehabilitation program, for example, reported goals such as being able to laugh without coughing, walk two holes of golf, visit relatives, look after themselves and being able to 'do what I want to do when I want to do it' (Folden 1993, pp. 31–33). Although encompassed in the overall goal of the program—to return clients 'to the highest level of health'—these goals are characterized by being both challenging for the people in this rehabilitation program and specific to their interests and life style. As Guthrie and Harvey (1994) emphasize, it is only by developing an occupationally focused understanding of clients as unique individuals that healthcare professionals can work with them to set individualized goals about what they will do in the future. Furthermore, Folden (1993) warns us that not tuning into the occupational goals of recipients of healthcare causes dissatisfaction because they perceive that their individual goals are not being met.

Occupation as a health outcome

The third reason why advanced health practitioners are concerned with occupation is that WHO initiatives will, over time, influence how the outcomes of health interventions are described. As outlined in the introduction, the revised ICF focuses on individuals' ability to engage in activities and the extent to which they participate in a normal range of occupations within their home, work place and community. This signals a major change from the predominant pathology or impairment focus of most health professions to focusing on the consequences of diseases and disorders (Enderby 1992, Dekker 1995). Furthermore, it is not just the WHO that is supporting this shift. Since the mid-1970s, the rehabilitation literature has increasingly identified that goals targeting change in activity and participation rather than impairment are the most important (Bussmann and Stam 1998), or indeed the ultimate goal of rehabilitation (Cardol et al 1999). Some professional associations, such as the American Speech Language Hearing Association, also now emphasize the ways in which disability affects people in their day-to-day life (Yaruss 1998).

Occupational goals

For some professions, refocusing practice towards activity and participation will be more challenging than for others. Podiatrists, for example, have been found to focus all treatment goals towards alleviating impairments, while physical therapists focus 68% of goals towards impairment and the remainder towards disabilities. Client goals reported by both occupational therapists and SLTs are primarily directed towards reducing disability and to a lesser extent handicap (Dekker 1995). SLTs, however, identify treatment goals aimed at impairments for virtually all clients (Raaijmakers et al 1998), while only 23% of occupational therapists' goals address impairments (Dekker 1995).

Refocusing practice does not, however, mean that all of the separate health professions will slowly merge into one profession. Rather, each will make its unique contribution towards shared goals that address returning the client to occupations they value. What the WHO initiative highlights is the need for all health professionals to be mindful of what they contribute to overcoming the disadvantage experienced by people living with the consequences of disease or disorder. Thus, physical therapists need to understand how spasticity, paresis, pain, neuropathy, decreased respiratory function and so on relate to handicap (Nixon & Cott 2000). Podiatrists who have become advanced practitioners will continue to evaluate the extent to which their clients' feet deviate from normal and to address the pain and fatigue this causes (impairment level). But they will also tailor intervention to take account of the occupations their clients engage in that exacerbate or relieve those problems, and the choices the client makes about

Activity worksheet 2

Think back to the person you identified in Worksheet 1 and the occupations that would be affected if he or she acquired an impairment.

1. Write down one occupational goal the person might have. (An example might be to resume cooking for the family before Christmas.)

2. Identify the contribution your profession might make towards achieving that goal.

3. Identify the contribution another profession might make towards achieving the goal.

N.B.: Activity worksheet 3 will continue the same case study.

continuing to participate in occupations which contribute to pain and fatigue. Thus, an attribute of advanced practitioners will be that their intervention is highly individualized because it is directed towards the occupations important to each individual client. Refer to Activity worksheet 2 before moving on.

Occupational language and occupational outcomes

Making the shift towards practice that addresses activity limitations and restrictions to participation, however, will not be easy because of the change in thinking that it involves. One change relates to the language used to describe the health issues with which you typically work. As Raaijmakers et al (1998) point out, health professionals have traditionally followed a medical model and categorized health concerns in terms of impairments. We have talked about limited range of movement, perceptual dysfunction, dysarthria and hearing thresholds. At least, some professions have talked of disorders of movement, others of disorders of speech, still others of disorders of hearing, and so on. Rethinking clients' concerns in terms of the consequences of disease and disorders for activity and participation, and identifying the environmental factors which contribute to or compound health consequences will lead health professionals to identify concerns not previously considered within their domain. Nixon and Cott (2000, p. 195), for example, recommend that physical therapists work with people diagnosed with HIV to address issues of social integration and economic self-sufficiency, as well as their ability to occupy time through participation in 'family roles, schooling, volunteering and recreation'. In essence, these are the health consequences highlighted by the WHO. Faced with such challenges, practitioners working towards creating practice that encompasses occupational concerns will be well advised to adopt the standard terminology of the ICF. In this way and over time, led by advanced practitioners, all health professions may come to speak the same language and be able to communicate with each other more effectively (Yaruss 1998).

A second change in the way that you think, as you advance towards occupational practice, may be in the assumptions you make about the outcomes of your intervention. Just as medicine has assumed that curing disease makes people well, other health professionals involved in rehabilitation services have tended to assume that decreasing impairment would automatically help people achieve the things they want to do within their normal living situation. We thought that improving people's balance, increasing the intelligibility of their speech, teaching them essential skills such as managing their medication, and so on, would restore people's ability to return to normal life. However, there is now mounting evidence that changing the level of impairment does not necessarily improve the functional outcome. Sometimes, this will be because even the increased level of function is insufficient to accomplish the occupational performance. For example, increasing an older woman's standing tolerance from a few seconds to a minute may not enable her to bake cookies for her grandchildren because measuring and mixing the ingredients takes a few minutes.

Some authorities in the field of rehabilitation have pointed to a growing awareness that 'the mechanical approach—repairing and restoring the human machine—has not always served our patients well' (Mulley 1994, p. 62). Others have concluded that, although there is some association between impairments and function, at times 'this relationship appeared to be or is assumed to be absent or complex' (Bussmann and Stam 1998, p. 458). Given such evidence, practitioners advancing towards occupational practice will accept that people with improved balance may not be able to walk more confidently. People whose speech is more intelligible may continue to avoid social situations. People capable of accurately managing daily medications may not do so. This finding implies that, if the purpose of your intervention was to change function, you will need to check that this is in fact the outcome.

Activity worksheet 3

Consider the occupational goals you identified on Worksheet 2.

1. What might you observe that would indicate that the person was making progress towards his or her goal?

_____

_____

2. What might the person concerned report that would indicate progress?

_____

_____

Now review what you wrote for questions 1 and 2. Have you identified a reduction in impairment or a change in performance? If you framed progress in terms of a reduction in impairment, please go back and try again.

This is the end of the case study you have been developing. The remaining activity worksheets that follow address broad professional issues.

Occupational practice

One strategy to help develop advanced skills in thinking about your practice and its outcomes for clients in an occupational way may be to examine the theories, models or frames of reference that inform your practice. (See Mitcham's discussion of the relationship between theory and practice in Chapter 3.) Do the theories that guide you address the consequences of impairments? Are interactions between impairment, activity and participation identified? For example, Bartlett and Palisano (2000, p. 599) have proposed a model of the determinants of motor change for children with cerebral palsy. Their model is intended to help physical therapists establish 'realistic and attainable goals', and the authors claim that it is based on the ICF. However, it does not fully incorporate activity and participation, and fails to account for impairments that might arise from lack of opportunity to participate in the normal range of activities. For example, a child that was excluded from playground activities in case he or she was injured may feel less valued as a person in that setting. The loss of esteem (impairment) may trigger further withdrawal from physical activity (decreased participation), and result in lost opportunities to develop or practise motor skills. Yet this dynamic is not represented in the model. Thus, although the model addresses 'change in basic motor abilities' (p. 600) it fails to account for external factors which may influence such a change. (For more on being a critical consumer of the professional literature, see Esdaile and Roth's discussion of published critiques of the lifestyle performance model, the section on intellectual debate within a profession in Chapter 7.)

A further strategy, on the way to becoming occupationally aware, is to re-examine the assessments traditionally used by your profession. The challenge, in a nutshell, is knowing what to measure and how to measure it. As an illustration of this challenge, SLTs have well-developed assessment tools to evaluate impairments, including voice and articulation disorders, developmental language disorders, disorders of speech flow, and so on. If the SLT needs to diagnose the cause of the communication problem, in order to determine how to intervene, the existing tools will suit the purpose. However, since we know that reducing the level of impairment may not improve function, these same tools may not be suited to measuring the outcome or effectiveness of intervention.

Furthermore, at the disability level, deciding what to measure means determining what aspect of performance is important—level of dependence or independence of performance, quality of performance or competence of performance (Keith 1995). To return to the example of the SLT, reducing dependence might mean reducing individuals' reliance on having with them someone familiar with their speech to interpret their meaning to others. Improving the quality of performance might mean being reasonably successful in conveying meaning on one's own or having sufficient confidence in one's ability to speak intelligibly to risk initiating a conversation with a new acquaintance. Improving the competence of performance might mean improving how close one's speech is to normal speech patterns. Existing evaluations of impairment may or may not be suitable for these purposes.

Attempting to measure outcomes at the level of handicap would reveal a further problem—within any discipline a profound lack of well-developed evaluation tools that address participation or participation restrictions (Keith 1995, Wilkerson 2000). The SLT in the example above faces the problem that there are no suitable formal assessments with which to evaluate the participation restriction experienced by a teacher who has developed a voice impairment (Raaijmakers et al 1998). Even the few handicap questionnaires currently available have been criticized for not capturing the perspective of the person experiencing the handicap (Cardol et al 1999). Neither is there a recognized, cross-disciplinary evaluation tool to determine the occupations in which a client is most likely to participate, so that intervention can be tailored to meet the demands of those occupations. This implies that practitioners with advanced skills in creating occupational practice will develop personal strategies to find out about occupations that may be affected by their clients' changed or changing health status. The skill will lie in working with clients to identify occupations they expect to perform in the future and the aspects of participation that are important to them. As Burton (2000) reminds us, however, short-term rehabilitation approaches are unlikely to achieve participation goals or deliver the quality of life increasingly demanded by disability groups.

Activity worksheet 4

Write the names of four or five evaluation tools commonly used by members of your profession. Beside each tool, record whether it primarily addresses impairment, activity/participation or environmental barriers to participation. Use the summary of activity and participation categories in Table 8.1 as a guide.

1. _____
2. _____
3. _____
4. _____
5. _____

Have you managed to identify any evaluation tools that address participation?
The next worksheet considers the outcomes of occupation.

Consequences of occupation

Creating occupational practice also involves envisaging the long- and short-term consequences of participating in valued occupations despite impairments. The skill here will lie in tailoring interventions in ways to allow for and support ongoing activity, and supporting clients to modify domestic, work-place and community environments to enable participation, and to predict and manage threats to their health or quality of life.

An example of advanced skill in identifying and addressing the long-term occupational impact of functioning despite permanent impairment is provided by two physical therapists. Sinnott and Mercer (2000) were concerned about the prevalence of rotator cuff disorders which typically occur 12–15 years post injury in people with paraplegia who mobilize in a manual wheelchair. According to Sinnott and Mercer, cumulative strain on the shoulder musculature of individuals with poor trunk stability results in difficulty with activities of daily living, wheelchair propulsion, and participation in sporting activities. Contemporary restorative rehabilitation practices, they claim, do not adequately address the long-term effects of transferring into and out of the wheelchair for individuals with a high-level paraplegia. They recommend individualization of rehabilitation, taking into account the level of the spinal cord injury, along with educating clients about how to prevent and manage shoulder problems.

While this example involves the predictable problems of a specific population, practitioners who create occupational practice will also work at an individual level, helping clients to predict and manage the longer-term effects of participating in valued occupations. Here the detailed breakdown of activities of learning, communication, movement and moving around, and self-care, domestic, interpersonal activities and tasks provided within the ICF will prove a valuable resource. Firstly, it may serve as a checklist to guide your thinking about occupations which are particularly likely to be impacted by the impairments of concern to your profession. If this is so, you will be better prepared to assist clients to predict difficulties they may encounter in everyday life.

Activity worksheet 5

Think of the clients with whom you typically work. Given the nature of their health condition, can you think of an occupation in which a client might wish to engage on a regular basis that would exacerbate his or her impairment? Use Table 8.1 as a reference if needed.
What might the long-term health consequences be?

_____

_____

Suggest one thing people might do, or do differently to manage those consequences.

_____

_____

This activity sheet has asked you to think about working with clients to support their occupational performance. The next moves on to look at how we might measure the outcomes of occupationally focused interventions.

The ICF supporting occupational practice

As well as using the ICF as a checklist, its widespread adoption may address concerns that a majority of rehabilitation goals, at least in some fields of practice, are only moderately specific or non-specific and thus fail to individualize treatment to meet specific client needs (Arns & Linney 1995). Armed with the ICF, you will be equipped to develop precise, holistic treatment goals at the level of both disability and handicap and adjusted to the specific needs of your clients (Raaijmakers et al 1998). In addition, you'll be working in a way that will enhance collaboration between team members, as we are increasingly able to communicate our unique contribution to shared goals of enabling the occupations valued by our clients.

Having said all that, I need to acknowledge that, although comprehensive, the ICF cannot identify every nuance of every occupation, nor every activity limitation and participation restriction your clients might experience. The activities of producing spoken messages, for example, specify simple and complex messages, humor, sarcasm and so on, but do not capture the different skill requirements of talking face-to-face versus leaving a message on an answer phone. Meeting these challenges may require the development and adoption of new evaluation and intervention strategies.

In the same way that the ICF cannot be all-inclusive, no assessment tool can provide all the information you might need about the consequences of impairment for your client. Becoming an advanced practitioner means recruiting the available tools to help you think critically about your practice. The ICF, for example, can be used to guide your decisions about which evaluation tools to use to capture information about activities and participation. For example, a comparison of four evaluation tools commonly used in physical rehabilitation settings revealed, amongst other things, that only one included using transportation, and none incorporated activities of caring for possessions and assisting others (Haley and Langmuir 2000). Comparing evaluations against the ICF will help you create occupational practice by helping you identify aspects of function that you will need to assess directly, if they are particularly relevant to a client.

Consequences of occupational practice

Creating occupational practice may increasingly take you out of the hospital or clinic and into the community. For instance, there is a growing consensus that it is more valid to evaluate function in its natural, everyday setting rather than in clinical settings (Bussmann & Stam 1998, Keith 1995). Measuring the symmetry of walking, for example, may be better conducted in a shopping mall than on a treadmill (Bussmann and Stam 1998), or on a forest track if that is where the person intends to walk. Treatment may also increasingly follow clients into the community. For example, it has been suggested that physical therapists working with stroke survivors need to expand their role, which would involve 'moving beyond the physiotherapy gym' to determine what help their patients require from care givers 'to be mobile at home and in the community' (Huijbregts et al 2000, p. 303). It was envisaged that this would necessitate intervention continuing beyond discharge from hospital to ensure a smooth transition, and that it may require physical therapists to 'become advocates for their patients to ensure community mobility' (Huijbregts et al 2000 p. 303).

As well as using formal assessment tools to monitor the progress of individual clients, many of these tools can be used to measure outcomes, which have increasingly come to mean 'the results for the person served' (Wilkerson 2000, p. 43). By aggregating the outcomes for different individuals, information can be generated about the effectiveness of health interventions or the adequacy of services. This information is useful to health funders and to individuals wishing to make informed choices about their treatment options (John and Enderby 2000). If assessments are to serve these purposes, they need to be valid, reliable and sensitive. As well as having these psychometric properties, there is a growing awareness that outcome measures need to be relevant. This is generally taken to mean that they address the ultimate goal of rehabilitation—'the patient's ability to reintegrate into normal patterns of life' (Trigg et al 1999, p. 342).

Recognition of the need to measure more than resolution or reduction of impairment has contributed, for example, to physical therapists being advised of the need to measure activity, as defined by the WHO, as well as impairments (Huijbregts et al 2000). Other calls to action, such as that from Mulley (1994), identify resumption of normal activities after hospitalization as the only measure of effectiveness of rehabilitation after hip fracture. In order to achieve this, Mulley urges health practitioners to begin collecting information about clients' occupational goals from the first contact. Similarly, Wilkerson (2000) has suggested that, even though there are few well-developed evaluation tools to measure participation, practitioners can achieve the same end by collecting information relating to participation in work, leisure and other roles.

Ensuring the reliability of outcome measures that address aspects of activity and participation, such as resumption of normal occupations, may however be problematic. Research undertaken on an outcome measure developed for SLTs, for example, suggests that in general assessments are likely to be less reliable in the measurement of participation than impairment and disability (John and Enderby 2000). The researchers attributed this to the fact that fewer established assessment tools address handicap and so health professionals are less experienced in evaluating the consequences of health in this way. Moreover, they found that therapists lacked knowledge of the disadvantages their clients experienced that would have been necessary to make an accurate judgment about participation restrictions.

Summing up

To summarize the discussion to this point, I have argued that there is a strong, two-directional relationship between occupation and health (Figure 8.3). In one direction, it is through engaging in occupation that people maintain and hone their health status and meet their health needs. In the other direction, poor health often compromises individuals' ability and opportunities to engage in occupation. This can and does lead to further health problems, such as further decrease in physical fitness, as well as psychosocial problems such as depression, anxiety and withdrawal from social activities.

In rehabilitation settings, it has been found that occupation is a powerful motivator and a strong predictor of outcomes. Indeed, optimistic clients who identify challenging occupations to work towards achieve the best outcomes, despite being perceived as unrealistic or lacking insight by healthcare professionals. In addition, there is some evidence that supporting individuals with significant health problems such as stroke to resume previous leisure occupations or develop new ones has benefits for both physical and mental health.

Because the relationship between health and occupation is so fundamental, I have argued that all health practitioners need to be concerned with their clients' occupations. This includes being concerned with the limitations to activity that clients experience as a result of impairment to body structure or function, as well as restrictions to participation arising from the physical environment and from attitudinal and legislative barriers. I have identified that some health professions will intervene primarily at the level of activity and participation. Others may focus on the reduction or management of impairment, whilst considering the ways in which their clients' impairments limit activity and how participating in occupation may exacerbate, maintain or alleviate impairments. In all cases, health professionals need to individualize their interventions in order to support and enable clients' engagement in valued occupations and to demonstrate the effectiveness of their services by measuring clients' participation in domestic, self-care, work and community activities.

Activity worksheet 6

The focus of this section of the discussion has been occupation as a health outcome. Each health profession focuses on a different aspect of returning people to health. This Worksheet challenges you to think about the contribution your profession makes to achieving occupational outcomes.

If you can, identify three occupations that your clients typically want to do but, because of their health condition, may not have the same opportunity to participate in as other people of their age and gender:

1. _____
2. _____
3. _____

If participation in these occupations became the outcome measure for your service, how might you gather information about your clients' involvement in it?

_____
_____
_____

This activity is the last to consider general professional concerns. The next provides an opportunity to hone your skills in implementing occupational practice.

Because of the relative lack of valid and reliable assessments of activity and participation, this may require the development of skill in gathering information about activities clients engage in and the barriers to participation they experience on an individual basis. It may also mean following clients into the community to evaluate the status and impact of their impairments on occupation in natural settings. What contribution does your profession make to achieving occupational outcomes (see Activity worksheet 6).

Skills for occupational practice

The next section of the discussion addresses specific practice skills and perspectives that will enable health practitioners to deliver services that effectively meet clients' occupational needs. The discussion is organized around four questions that focus on key issues for clients.

What occupations are important to your clients?

While rehabilitation services have tended to focus on self-care and vocational activities, 'involvement in the wider social world, including family roles and responsibilities, social activities, [and] life style' has also been found to be crucial to maintaining quality of life (Burton 2000, p. 597). But how will you know which occupations are crucial to a particular client? Creating practice that addresses occupations important to your clients may require you to develop a new set of skills. This means, firstly, acknowledging that general rehabilitation goals such as returning clients to the highest level of health are unlikely to mirror clients' goals. The discrepancy between clients' and practitioners' goals, according to Folden (1993), is due to differences in how health is perceived. While relatively healthy people generally cite notions of physical, mental, social and spiritual well-being, people with a diagnosed illness that affects their functional ability are more likely to define health in terms of the symptoms that impede participation in valued occupations. To understand what health means to individual clients, occupational practitioners will ask them what they want and need to do and what occupations are most important to maintain their quality of life.

Creating occupational practice will also require that you develop skill in working with clients to identify occupations limited by the illness itself, or by environmental barriers. People with hearing loss, for example, may cope well in everyday conversations but find it impossible to hear enough of what is said in a lecture theatre to be able to function as a student. People with visual deficits may be passed over for a promotion at work because of managerial assumptions about their potential to perform, despite the availability of enabling technology (Roulstone 1998). Implicit to recognizing environmental barriers and their impact on social participation and functioning is a further set of skills to elicit relevant environmental information (Badley 1987). Although no satisfactory assessment tools have been developed to date, the Impact on Participation and Autonomy which is being developed in the Netherlands looks promising (Cardol et al 1999). Designed to measure handicap from the perspective of the person concerned, it is based on the ICF. Occupational practitioners are likely to find the test items and questioning format informative, even in advance of the assessment being finalized. A final skill is communicating this information to the rest of the health team, so that each member is working towards achieving the same goal (Folden 1993). As previously acknowledged, the detailed listing of activities within the ICF offers an invaluable guide to assist in the precise definition of activity limitations and restrictions to participation.

What kind of occupation is your intervention?

Creating occupational practice for your clients means thinking about what kind of occupation your intervention is. That is, what is it like to experience the things we do to clients, such as giving them a bed-bath or fitting them with a hearing aid? What is it like to do the things that you ask your clients to do, such as learning to use a communication board, or the things you do together, such as helping them get dressed? Are your interventions painful, arduous, embarrassing or impersonal? How does having to do something like that affect people's hopes for the future or their relationship with you? Thinking about your intervention as an occupation includes thinking about the ways you evaluate clients, and what it is like for them to be involved in those evaluations (Hocking 2001).

Some insight into the experience of being a client in a health service comes from an investigation into what made an occupational therapy group therapeutic. The group was for people with long-term mental illness who attended a day-care program (Eklund 1997). One factor to emerge as therapeutic was occupational—participants reported positive benefit from being occupied, from the specific activities each enjoyed, and from opportunities to develop new skills. One factor that was particularly revealing was that, although the program included routine household tasks such as cooking and doing the dishes, only occupations that were self-initiated were identified as therapeutic.

Further insights into the ways occupations that are intended to be therapeutic may be perceived come from an analysis of the outcomes of a transitional residential program for homeless people with severe and persistent mental illness (Baier et al 1996). People on the program were involved in two kinds of occupations. They were required to take turns doing household chores and to attend programmed group activities designed to develop skills thought to be essential to maintaining independent housing. Programmed activities included vocational rehabilitation, living-skills classes and self-help groups such as Alcoholics Anonymous. Analysis of the outcomes of the program revealed that those who successfully completed it attended significantly more activities than those who did not. What made the scheduled occupations effective for some but not others was not determined. However, there is some suggestion that, at least for some of the unsuccessful participants, the program may have been too structured. Having learned to cope with the dangers and anonymity of living on the street, the authors speculate, these people may have felt incompetent within the rules and daily timetable of activities.

Although both of these examples are drawn from a review of outcomes for people with severe mental illness, the findings confirm that the nature of occupations intended to be therapeutic affects the outcome. Furthermore, the same occupation may be therapeutic for some and not for others. As you work towards creating occupational practice, you will need to be aware of how your clients experience the occupations of care. In particular, health professionals need to remember that occupations familiar and comfortable to us may be unfamiliar, unpleasant or meaningless to our clients.

Are your clients ready for occupation?

In your own life, or from your observations of others, you will know that at times people are reluctant to do things for themselves. How will you know if your clients are ready to do the things for which your intervention prepares them, or whether they need ongoing assistance and encouragement? Here the notion of 'occupational self' is informative. 'Occupational self' refers to the way individuals think about themselves in terms of what they can do, what is difficult or frightening to do, what is enjoyable to do and so on. Our understanding of ourselves as occupational beings develops over the life course and has three components—body image, sense of competence, and values and goals (Thoren-Jonsson and Moller 1999), which suggests that events that strengthen or threaten any of these components are likely to influence occupational identity. Accordingly, for example, dyspnea may threaten body image, particularly in individuals who have prided themselves on their physical prowess, and consequently undermined their occupational self. On the other hand, learning new skills or strategies to manage impairment or remove a barrier to participation may give a new sense of competence and strengthen occupational self. For example, when people experiencing the long-term sequelae of poliomyelitis have a positive experience of using an assistive device, they may subsequently feel more competent and be more willing to take part in physically demanding activities such as going shopping or to an amusement park, or travelling abroad for a holiday (Thoren-Jonsson and Moller 1999).

One implication of the notion of occupational self for practitioners striving to create occupational practice is the need to think about the health issues our clients face in terms of possible impact on body image, sense of competence and valued goals. A second implication is that, even for routine interventions, it is important to talk to our clients about how they perceive themselves as occupational beings, what they imagine they might do in the future and how the health issues they face might change that. In particular, we need to provide opportunities for clients to develop competence despite their impairments. An example might be allowing a child time to fit a hearing aid or new prosthesis for him- or herself, rather than doing it for him or her.

At times, however, clients or their care givers may be unable to take action on their own behalf. At times this is recognized and responded to by health professionals. For example, older people admitted to hospital because of an acute medical event may experience immense relief when nursing staff take responsibility for looking after them (Gooder 2001). Here, the need to provide care is made evident by the person's physical state. In other circumstances, health professionals may be unaware that the recipients of their advice are unable to carry it out.

For example, while parents of children with cerebral palsy are struggling to come to terms with their children's diagnosis, they are unlikely to carry out the home exercise programs prescribed by physical or occupational therapists (Piggot 2000). Perhaps because they feel guilty about not carrying out the program, or do not like to admit they have not understood what to do, they are also unlikely to admit their lack of action to therapists. This example illustrates that health professionals need to consider more than physical health in determining readiness to carry out health-giving occupations.

What occupation does your practice setting enable?

A final consideration in creating occupational practice is the occupations in which healthcare recipients are able to participate within healthcare settings. Sim (1990, p. 426), for example, espouses an ethically based vision of healthcare for physical therapists which entails 'the removal of obstacles to the achievement of human potential' by supporting the capacity to act. The first venue of concern in enabling clients to act is the healthcare setting itself. Yet, as Mulley (1994) points out, hospitals typically support activities that may diminish patients, such as replacing clothes with pyjamas. He also points to failure to provide, or perhaps request patients or their families to bring to the hospital, belongings that would support occupational performance—braces to hold up loose trousers and footwear to enable safe ambulation. Further, he charges hospitals with neglecting to provide privacy for occupations that most people prefer to complete alone, such as cleaning their dentures. Clients are not enabled to engage in occupation in comfort.

Even more concerning are instances of health settings unnecessarily removing the potential for occupation. An example is Gooder's (2001) finding that patients in one rehabilitation ward were expected to go to bed after dinner, whereupon their walking frames were removed until the next morning. This resulted in patients in hospital for rehabilitation being dependent on nursing assistance to go to the toilet, or move from their beds to do anything else, from 6.30 p.m. each evening. Whatever the reason for this practice, it results in lost opportunities to restore positive body image through exercising returning capacities, experience competence in the hospital setting and work towards goals of building physical strength, and to action values of self-reliance.

Health practitioners who take an occupational perspective would challenge this practice as removing rather than creating opportunities for occupation. They may actively look for ways to provide opportunities for occupation. Examples might be as straightforward as notifying people booked for non-essential surgery to bring clothing and shoes suitable to wear in hospital corridors with them. It might also be ensuring that patients able to mobilize independently can get in and out of their bed, and on and off their bed side chair on their own (Gooder 2001). Further examples might be considering individuals, normal sleep–wake cycles in order to individualize care (Mason and Redeker 1993) or when deciding which patients will share a hospital room.

As previously identified, enabling occupation may also require health practitioners to follow their clients out of the hospital to support their transition back to home, work and community settings, perhaps by training care givers in techniques and strategies to support occupation (Huijbregts et al 2000). In part, this shift to the community is necessitated, at least for children, by the finding that skills are experienced as more meaningful and receptivity to instruction and practice is enhanced when targeted skills are presented in natural settings where they are needed. In addition, natural settings have been found to offer greater opportunities to embed therapeutic strategies within child-initiated activities and routines, while still allowing the child to make choices, plan activities and take the initiative (Block and Davis 1996). Referring back to the notion of occupational self, it is clear that child-initiated occupations are more likely than therapist-initiated activities to enhance a sense of competence and to accord with the child's values and goals. I would suggest that this is also true for adults.

Activity worksheet 7

This final worksheet corresponds to the four questions discussed above. It asks you to reflect on your own practice in occupational terms.

In order to find out what occupations are important to your clients, you will need to ask them (or their care givers, if they are unable to report for themselves). Suggest two questions you might ask your clients. Use the actual words you might use when speaking to a client.

_____

_____

_____

_____

_____

_____

Think about two things that you do with or to clients that are part of your everyday practice. If you can, select two very different things. For example, one might be something you do to clients, and the other something you watch clients do for themselves. Or one might be part of your data gathering, such as interviewing or testing a client, and the other part of intervention. Describe each of these things as your clients might perceive them when they experience them for the first time. (Are they familiar and comfortable, or unfamiliar and threatening, casual or formal? Do they involve close contact with you? Are they painful, arduous, boring, and so on?)

_____

_____

_____

_____

_____

Activity worksheet 7 *cont'd*	Think about whether, at some stage in your care, your clients need your help to do something that they would normally do for themselves. For example, you may phone relatives to let them know where the person is, or position yourself next to the person to assist him or her to stand. Write down what it is that you do, and what you are responding to when you get ready to offer that assistance. Then describe how you know when the individual does not need your help any more.

_____

_____

_____

_____

_____

Write down one thing that your clients could do in your healthcare setting that would be a natural thing to do there, but is not currently available to them. Then record what it would take to make that occupation available. For example, can your clients get themselves a hot drink while they wait for you? What is needed to make that possible?

_____

_____

_____

_____

_____

This is the final Worksheet.

Summary

Pierce et al (1999) suggest that life satisfaction correlates with perceived health and participation, not with body structure or activity. That is, people will perceive that life is good if they are able to participate in occupations that are meaningful to them, despite ongoing or even life-threatening impairments of their body structure or function and difficulty in functioning on a day-to-day basis.

Acknowledging this raises fundamental questions about what health services are for. Some services directly address disease and injury. They are important for keeping people alive and limiting the residual impairment. Other services address people's ability to do things. SLTs work with people to resolve or manage problems that affect their ability to communicate. Occupational therapists teach skills and strategies that will enable people to do things despite impairments. These services and others have largely focused on those activities that increase people's independence and decrease the level of assistance needed from family, friends and the state.

Millie's story, which opened this chapter, reminds us that these interventions do not ensure that healthcare recipients return to good health. Millie, no doubt, returned home skilled in the management of her impairments. She may have been competent in the use of her wheelchair. But Millie was not prepared for new occupations. She did not return as a budding wheelchair athlete or an active job seeker.

Just as Mulley (1994) asserted, repairing and restoring the human machine is not sufficient to address depression, frustration or loss of quality of life, or the fearfulness Millie experienced. Rather, having a life worth living, a life that sustains long-term health, seems to relate to having opportunities to participate in the range of occupations considered normal for people who are healthy. Refocusing health practice towards occupational outcomes will be enormously challenging. Reframing our thinking to recognize the things that support or constrain clients' occupations will take time. My hope is that health professionals will accept the challenge and recognize the rewards that come with creating occupational practice for ourselves and others.

References

Arns P G, Linney J A 1995 The relationship of service individualization to client functioning in programs for severely mentally ill persons. Community Mental Health Journal 31:127–137

Badley E M 1987 The ICIDH: format, application in different settings, and distinction between disability and handicap. International Disability Studies 9:122–125

Baier M, Murray R, North C, Lato M, Eskew C 1996 Comparison of completers and noncompleters in a transitional residential program for homeless mentally ill. Issues in Mental Health Nursing 17:337–352

Bartlett D J, Palisano R J 2000 A multivariate model of determinants of motor change for children with cerebral palsy. Physical Therapy 6:598–614

Block M E, Davis T D 1996 An activity-based approach to physical education for preschool children with disabilities. Adapted Physical Activity Quarterly 13:230–246

Burton C R 2000 Re-thinking stroke rehabilitation: the Corbin and Strauss chronic illness trajectory framework. Journal of Advanced Nursing 32:595–602

Bussmann J B J, Stam H J 1998 Techniques for measurement and assessment in rehabilitation: a theoretical approach. Clinical Rehabilitation 12:455–464

Cardol M, de Haan R J, van den Bos G A M de Jong B A, de Groot I J M 1999 The development of a handicap assessment questionnaire: the impact on participation and autonomy (IPA). Clinical Rehabilitation 13:411–419

Christiansen C H 1999 Defining lives: occupation as identity: an essay on competence, coherence, and the creation of meaning. 1999 Eleanor Clarke Slagle lecture. American Journal of Occupational Therapy 53:547–558

Dekker J 1995 Application of the ICIDH in survey research on rehabilitation: The emergence of the functional diagnosis. Disability and Rehabilitation 17:195–201

Drummond A E R 1990 Leisure activity after stroke. International Disability Studies 12:157–160

Drummond A, Walker M 1996 Generalisation of the effects of leisure rehabilitation for stroke patients. British Journal of Occupational Therapy 59:330–334

Dubos R 1970 Man, medicine and environment. Penguin: London

Eklund M 1997 Therapeutic factors in occupational group therapy identified by patients discharged from a psychiatric day centre and their significant others. Occupational Therapy International 4:198–212

Enderby P 1992 Outcome measures in speech therapy: impairment, disability, handicap and distress. Health Trends 24:61–64

Folden S L 1993 Definitions of health and health goals of participants in a community-based pulmonary rehabilitation program. Public Health Nursing 10:31–35

Gooder J 2001 Older adults experience of rehabilitation. Unpublished master's thesis. Auckland University of Technology, Auckland, New Zealand

Guthrie S, Harvey A 1994 Motivation and its influence on outcome in rehabilitation. Reviews in Clinical Gerontology 4:235–243

Haley S M, Langmuir L 2000 How do current post-acute functional assessments compare with the activity dimension of the International Classification of Functioning and Disability (ICIDH-2)? Journal of Rehabilitation Outcomes Measures 4:51–56

Hill M 1994 Patricia's mother. In: Keith L (ed) Mustn't grumble. Writing by disabled women. Women's Press, London, p 142–148

Hocking C 2001 Implementing occupation-based assessment. American Journal of Occupational Therapy 55:463–469

Huijbregts M P J, Gowland C, Gruber R A 2000 Measuring clinically-important change with the activity inventory of the Chedoke McMaster Stroke Assessment. Physiotherapy Canada 52:295–304

John A, Enderby P 2000 Reliability of speech and language therapists using therapy outcome measures. International Journal of Language and Communication Disorders 35:287–302

Keith R A 1995 Conceptual basis of outcome measures. American Journal of Physical Medicine and Rehabilitation 74:73–80

Mason D J, Redeker N 1993 Measurement of activity. Nursing Research 42:87–92

Mulley G P 1994 Principles of rehabilitation. Reviews in Clinical Gerontology 4:61–69

Nixon S, Cott C A 2000 Shifting perspectives: reconceptualizing HIV disease in a rehabilitation framework. Physiotherapy Canada 52:189–197, 207

Peters D J 1995 Human experience in disablement: the imperative of the ICIDH. Disability and Rehabilitation 17:135–144

Pierce C A, Richards S, Gordon W, Tate D 1999 Life satisfaction following spinal cord injury and the WHO model of functioning and disability. Spinal Cord Injury: Psychosocial Process 12:121, 124–127

Piggot J 2000 Participation in home therapy programmes for children with cerebral palsy: a compelling challenge. Unpublished master's thesis. Auckland University of Technology, Auckland, New Zealand

Raaijmakers M F, Dekker J, Dejonckere P H 1998 Diagnostic assessment and treatment goals in Logopedics: impairments, disabilities and handicaps. Folia Phoniatrica et Logopaedica 50:71–79

Roulstone A 1998 Enabling technology. Disabled people, work and new technology. Open University Press, Philadelphia

Sim J 1990 The concept of health. Physiotherapy 76:423–428

Sinnott A, Mercer S 2000 The weightbearing shoulder and long-term paraplegia: a management issue. New Zealand Journal of Physiotherapy 28:36–41

Thoren-Jonsson A, Moller A 1999 How the concept of occupational self influences everyday life strategies for people with poliomyelitis sequelae. Scandinavian Journal of Occupational Therapy 6:71–83

Trigg R, Wood V A, Hewer R L 1999 Social integration after stroke: the first stages in the development of the Subjective Index of Physical and Social Outcome (SIPSO). Clinical Rehabilitation 13:341–353

Wilcock A A 1998 An occupational perspective of health. Slack, Thorofare, NJ

Wilkerson D L 2000 Perspectives from the field. Rehabilitation outcomes and accreditation. Journal of Rehabilitation Outcomes Measurement 4:42–48

World Health Organization 2001 International classification of functioning, disability and health. Final draft. World Health Organization, Geneva

Yaruss J S 1998 Describing the consequences of disorders: stuttering and the international classification of impairments, disabilities, and handicaps. Journal of Speech, Language, and Hearing Research 41:249–257

Additional readings and resources

Clark F, Ennevor B L, Richardson P L 1996 A grounded theory of techniques for occupational story telling and occupational story making. In: Zemke R, Clark F (eds) Occupational science. The evolving discipline. F A Davis, Philadelphia, p 373–392 (Outlines interviewing strategies to work with people to identify occupations which have been important to them in the past, as a basis for developing a vision of the activities they wish to pursue in the future.)

Davies S, Kaker S, Ellis L 1997 Promoting autonomy and independence for older people within nursing practice: a literature review. Journal of Advanced Nursing 26:408–417 (Discusses the tension between enhancing the autonomy of older people in continuing care settings by providing opportunities for occupation and managing the perceived risks involved in allowing people to do things unaided.)

Mozley C G 2001 Exploring connections between occupation and mental health in care homes for older people. Journal of Occupational Science 8:14–19 (Presents evidence that having opportunities for occupation is a key predictor of both survival and positive mood state in older people in continuing-care settings.)

Powell J, Bray J, Roberts H, Goddard A, Smith E 2000 Goal negotiation with older people in three day care settings. Health and Social Care in the Community 8:380–389 (Gives examples of the health benefits older people derived from participating in occupations offered in day-care settings.)

Raynes N V, Leach J M, Rawlings B, Bryson R J 2000 Using focus groups to seek the views of patients dying from cancer about the care they receive. Health Expectations 3:169–175 (Reports a study that asked people dying of cancer what sort of help they wanted and what kind of help was most important. As well as concerns about funding entitlements and being a burden on their families, participants identified a need for occupation.)

Using adult education theories: facilitating others' learning in professional practice settings

Lindy McAllister

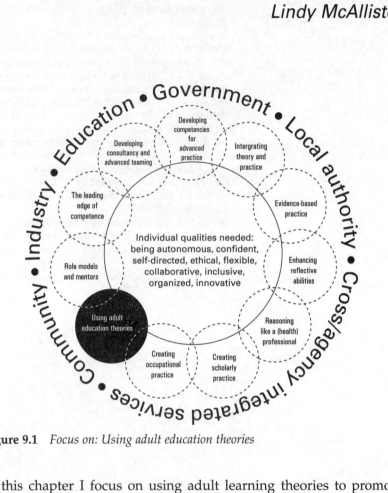

Figure 9.1 *Focus on: Using adult education theories*

Chapter outline

In this chapter I focus on using adult learning theories to promote advanced practice. I believe that adult learning theory has much to offer those charged with the responsibility for facilitating learning in others in the workplace. Adoption of adult learning approaches in the workplace can require a major shift in thinking about one's role as an educator, from transmitter of knowledge to facilitator of learning. However, the rewards for both educators and learners are great. A major tool in the implementation of adult learning approaches is reflection. This chapter overviews adult learning theory, provides a structure for reflection on practice, and describes some strategies which apply adult learning principles and reflection to the promotion of advanced practice in healthcare settings. The strategies described in this chapter—modelling of clinical reasoning, journalling, using critical incidents, story telling and working with a critical companion—are discussed in terms of how they can be used to promote development of self-knowledge and advanced practice in others and also in oneself. The chapter concludes with a description of advanced practice which places self-knowledge and awareness at the heart of professional artistry in healthcare practice.

Key words

Adult learning, reflection, critical incidents, story telling

Anticipated outcomes

As a result of reading this chapter, I anticipate that you will be able to:

- understand how adult learning principles can be applied to the promotion of advanced practice
- understand the importance of reflection in the promotion of advanced practice
- facilitate advanced practice in others and in yourself using a variety of reflective strategies suitable for adult learners.

Introduction

In discussing facilitating others to develop advanced practice, I am making the assumption that the people best placed to do this and most likely to be able to support this on an ongoing basis are colleagues at work. These will include one's senior clinicians, line manager, supervisors, colleagues (at all levels of seniority) and peers. (I am aware of the benefits of external mentors and formal supervision obtained outside the workplace, such as occurs in social work and family therapy, but that is not my focus here. Chapter 10 develops this aspect in practice.) Some of what I will talk about here will be the responsibility of everybody in a workplace; other aspects will be the responsibility of individuals designated to provide support to junior clinicians or who are in designated leadership or management positions, who have the ability to influence workplace culture.

As I will suggest in this chapter, being a facilitator of adult learning requires knowing yourself and using yourself as a tool to support others' learning. Adopting adult learning principles, and reflective and collaborative approaches to the facilitation of learning may require for some a radical shift in the nature of relationships within the workplace. If you are the supervisor or senior clinician responsible for the development and supervision of junior staff, adopting a different style of relating and sharing power can be extremely challenging, if not threatening. It means you cannot hide behind your authority or expertise, but must authentically engage with other learners as a co-learner. It means becoming a peer. This involves taking personal and professional risks, as you open your propositional knowledge, professional craft knowledge and personal practical knowledge (Higgs and Titchen 2000), expertise, thinking, and values up for observation, discussion and critique.

I believe that adopting adult learning principles to facilitate learning in others also requires the adoption of reflective practices. I will discuss a number of such reflective strategies in this chapter. I acknowledge that the adoption of reflective practice is resisted by many clinicians and managers. In workplaces dominated by increasingly technical–rational approaches to practice and management (Fish and Coles 1998), where time is scarce, reflection can be seen as a time-consuming practice, one with ill-defined processes and non-measurable outcomes. It cannot be denied that reflection takes time. However, reflective practice lies at the heart of the development of advanced practice (McAllister 2001), clinical expertise (Benner 1984) and professional artistry (Fish and Coles 1998, McAllister 2001, Schön 1987). Without reflection on practice, there can be no development of that practice. The acquisition of more knowledge and more technical skill is not sufficient for the development of advanced practice and clinical expertise. Additional knowledge and skill need to be applied and integrated into one's existing practice, and this application and integration must be evaluated through reflection and self-evaluation. Approaches to doing this are described in this chapter.

I am not for one moment suggesting that modelling reflection, and sharing the results of reflecting on one's practice, are easy tasks. Experienced clinicians will tell you that they dread exposing their practice, because they have long since embedded in their practice the propositional (theoretical) knowledge which might have once directed it. They have also developed their way of doing things (their professional craft knowledge), which may not reflect 'the evidence' or 'best practice', or may not yet have been empirically tested. In this era of evidence-based practice, to expose practice other than this can be risky. To do so will take a climate of trust, and genuine inquiry into practice. This needs to be modelled from the top, and encouraged from the bottom up.

In the sections to follow, I will summarize characteristics of adult learners and conditions which we know enable and support adult learning, and describe a range of strategies grounded in reflection and adult learning approaches, which can be used by individuals and colleagues to support the development of advanced practice in themselves and others.

Adult learning

Characteristics of adult learners

Knowles et al (1998) and Brookfield (1986) noted a number of key characteristics of adult learners. They concluded that:

- they are more self-directing, although they may choose dependence on the teacher in some circumstances
- their life experiences become a rich resource for learning
- they tend to learn better through experiential means, although they can use diverse learning styles
- their learning needs are more often determined by life circumstances at the time, e.g. the need to acquire job-related skills
- their learning becomes more problem-centred
- they want learning outcomes to have immediacy of application.

The desire for autonomy and self-directedness in adult learners forms a recurring theme in the adult learning literature (Brookfield 1986, Candy et al 1994). However, while adult learners like to exercise autonomy in their learning, they also like to learn interdependently with and from their peers (Lincoln and McAllister 1993), making the workplace a powerful venue for learning for adult learners.

Conditions which promote adult learning

Higgs (1992) distinguished between environmental conditions and decision-making/management factors which promote adult learning. She noted that environmental conditions conducive to adult learning are those which recognize the individuality of adult learners and provide acceptance, respect, trust and support for them. Such an environment provides freedom and autonomy for learners and enables effective interaction between learners. Authenticity and excellent interpersonal skills (Rogers 1969) are essential in the adult educator in order to create a supportive environment for adult learners. According to Higgs (1992), decision-making and management of learners' programs are shared between adult learners and educators in effective adult learning environments. Adult learners exercise a high degree of choice and control over deciding what is to be learned, how, when and where. They also become involved in evaluating their learning outcomes. Higgs suggested that adult learners and their educators often function as co-learners and jointly develop resources and strategies for learning and adult learners accept a high degree of responsibility for the evaluation and outcomes of their learning programs.

Roles and characteristics of educators in adult learning

Creating and managing conditions conducive to adult learning requires considerable awareness and management on the part of educators. Higgs (1993) suggests that educators of adult learners need to function as *managers* of learning programs, although this manager role will come to be shared with learners as their competence grows.

In pedagogical approaches to education, the role of the educator is normally that of teacher, information-giver and director of learning. The teacher controls what will be learned, when, where and how. The process of learning is teacher-focused and the learner's role is often passive. In contrast, Apps (1981, p. 133) lists eight characteristics of exemplary educators of adults, derived from the humanistic psychology literature. Adult educators:

> are concerned about learners, are knowledgeable in their subject, relate theory to practice and their fields to other fields, appear confident, are open to other approaches, present an authentic personality in the class, are willing to go beyond class objectives, and are able to create a good atmosphere for learning.

In essence, adult educators must function as facilitators. The distinction between facilitator and information-giver is fundamental in adult learning (Heron 1989). *Facilitation* can be described as a process of teaching in which the teacher endeavours to create a learning environment which is conducive to learning and aims to enable or empower the learner. Rogers (1969) perhaps best captured the elusive characteristics of facilitation in his seminal work on facilitation in education, when he described the qualities which facilitate learning as 'realness' of the facilitator, that is, truly being oneself, open and honest about one's own thoughts, emotions and perspectives; prizing, acceptance and trust of the individual learners; and empathic under-standing. Rogers stated that he did not believe that he could teach people anything of real value, but rather could facilitate their learning. He believed that teachers who effectively function as facilitators do so by:

> basing their work on the hypothesis that students who are in real con-tact with problems which are relevant to them wish to learn, want to grow, seek to discover, endeavour to master, desire to create, and move toward self-discipline. The teacher is attempting to develop a quality of climate in the classroom, and a quality of personal relationship with his students, which will permit these natural tendencies to come to their fruition (Rogers 1969, pp. 114–115).

In addition, Rogers believed facilitators should recognize their own limitations and be participative learners in the group. I fully support this view, as will be seen in the strategies I discuss later in this chapter.

Facilitating adults for advanced practice

We know that adult learners are motivated to learn by real-life needs and problems (such as those posed by working with new or challeng-ing client groups, or taking on new roles in the workplace), and that they learn best when they have autonomy over the nature and content of their learning, and can self-direct their learning. We also know that top-down change, involving directives to learn 'new things', imposed by management, rarely leads to significant or lasting change. However, when adult learners are encouraged to identify what they need to learn to manage change or to grow as people or clinicians, and are resourced and enabled to do that, real and lasting learning and therefore change can occur. We also know certain environmental con-ditions and decision-making factors lend themselves to the support of adult learning and adult learners in the workplace. These include the adoption of collaborative approaches to learning, authenticity and openness on the part of all involved in the learning environment, and the use of facilitation strategies, rather than directive teaching and information transfer approaches.

Adopting an adult learning approach requires a change of culture in many workplaces towards the adoption of a more egalitarian, reflective, and 'learning workplace' culture. Ideally, everyone in the workplace could function as a reflective practitioner (Schön 1987). Expert clinicians can assist this change of workplace culture by mak-ing explicit their reflections and clinical reasoning, including a consid-eration of the different types of knowledge they use (Higgs and Titchen 2000). Peers can support each other through engaging in story telling, recounting critical incidents and functioning as critical com-panions to their colleagues. These strategies for promoting advanced practice are discussed in the following sections of this chapter.

Modelling clinical reasoning

Clinical reasoning is a frequently discussed concept in the health pro-fessions (Higgs and Titchen 2000, Mattingly and Hayes-Fleming 1994, see Ch. 6). While we spend considerable effort developing the clinical reasoning abilities of students, my experience of professional settings is that we rarely attempt explicitly to develop this further with our colleagues. While we might make explicit our clinical decisions (e.g. in team meetings, in reports), we rarely make explicit the reasoning that lies behind those decisions (McAllister and Rose 2000). For competent and expert clinicians to do so would open up for discussion what lies behind the 'doing' component of professional practice (Figure 9.2), and begin to expose the experience, expertise, knowledges, assumptions, beliefs and values which underpin practice. Learners would be able to access what lies behind seemingly effortless 'expert' practice and truly learn from 'the experience' of their seniors. We know that 'sitting with Nellie', that is, simply 'observing', is not an efficient way to learn (Titchen 1998). Talking about what is observed and making explicit our clinical reasoning would help refine our own practice and highlight areas for continued personal and professional growth. It would also facilitate the growth towards expertise of others in our workplace.

Modelling clinical reasoning could happen in formal ways, such as in 'rounds' where clinicians explicitly agree to 'think aloud' about what they are doing and why, as they engage in assessments or treat clients, or in the presentation of case studies or formal tutorials. It can also happen informally, by simply talking with colleagues as one writes up case notes, or in the traditional 'lunch-room debriefs' (provided ethical behaviours are observed).

Facilitating the development of clinical reasoning in others

One of the editors told me about an on-going research project where she follows experts engaged in their practice, videoing what they do and asking them off-camera as they do it 'why did you do that? Why didn't you do this?' and so on, providing them with prompts to make explicit their reasoning. The clinical reasoning behind actions is subsequently explored as the clinician and the 'observer' review the videotapes.

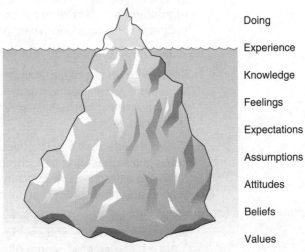

Doing

Experience

Knowledge

Feelings

Expectations

Assumptions

Attitudes

Beliefs

Values

Figure 9.2 *The iceberg of professional practice*

This concept could also be used within clinics between peers at any stage of development of clinical expertise, as part of an approved professional development activity, with appropriate informed consent from clients. A relatively short amount of videotape could yield hours of fruitful discussion of practice and enhance learning. The value of doing this with peers is that they may be more honest in exposing and examining their practice. The value of having experts working with novice clinicians is that the experts can use their higher levels of knowledge and skills to frame judicious questions and prompts which can help novices uncover their professional craft knowledge and identify areas and strategies for skill development.

Activity box 9.1

Using a peer to explore your clinical reasoning

1. Choose a peer at work with whom to do this exercise. It should be someone you trust and whose clinical work you respect

2. Obtain a portable video camera with a zoom function

3. Identify a client whose management you find in some way challenging—theoretically, practically or emotionally—and obtain his/her permission to video you working with him/her

4. Set the camera up close enough to get a clear view of you and your client, but far enough away so that your colleague's questions and comments off-camera do not distract you or the client. Your colleague sits beside the camera, out of view of the client if possible

5. Ask your colleague to suspend his/her assumptions about what you are doing and why, and instead identify any points of practice that might be of interest. Have him/her ask questions or make comments aloud (but quietly) as he/she watches you work, along the lines of 'I wonder why she did that'. 'Why are you doing it this way and not that way?' 'How is she feeling about what the client is saying/doing here?' These questions and comments will provide useful prompts for discussion when you review the tape

6. Video 15–30 minutes of your work with the client

7. Agree with your colleague that, when you view the tape, the aim is to explore your practice and help you understand what you are doing and why, not necessarily to critique it or measure it against 'best practice'

8. View the video with your colleague. Stop the tape whenever your colleague's questions or comments are heard and try to answer as fully, honestly and self-critically as you can. You can also stop the tape at any other point that seems important or relevant to you

9. Your colleague's role here is to help you get below the surface of what you are doing and saying. If, for example, you comment that 'I did x because of y', your colleague might respond with: 'But why

Activity box 9.1 *cont'd*	did you think that was important? Why did you choose to do *x* and not *z*?' 10. On another day, reverse roles with your colleague. You will learn from this experience in either role

Discussions about clinical reasoning might also help to uncover clinicians' preferred approaches to clinical reasoning and assist them to develop additional or more efficient modes. Experienced clinicians are reported to use the more efficient mode of pattern recognition in non-problematic or routine situations (Groen and Patel 1985) than less experienced clinicians, who may rely more on the slower mode of hypothetico-deductive reasoning (Higgs and Titchen 2000). Narrative reasoning (Mattingly and Hayes-Fleming 1994) offers yet another mode of clinical reasoning, allowing experienced clinicians to place clients in the context of their larger life story and reason about their current and future abilities and life needs. Sharing one's clinical reasoning with colleagues might highlight gaps and areas for development of clinical reasoning.

Both modelling and discussing their clinical reasoning are good examples of adult learning principles at work in that they demonstrate activities initiated by learners and not educators, they utilize real life learning needs and are problem-centred with the potential for immediate application (in this case, to manage clients better), they draw on previous life experience, and they involve learning with and from peers.

When clinicians cannot access their clinical reasoning or do not feel comfortable to share their thoughts with others, they could begin by reflecting privately on their work.

Reflecting on practice   Schön (1987) described two types of reflection: reflection-in-action and reflection-on-action. Reflection-in-action is reportedly harder to achieve and is more characteristic of experts (Benner 1984) and professional artists (Fish and Coles 1998). Reflection-on-action is more accessible to the majority of practitioners and can be promoted in a number of ways. The story of Daniel in Chapter 5 tells of ways this can be promoted. Journalling and the use of critical incidents can be used to promote reflection. The learning derived from the use of these strategies can be private, or shared with peers in formal or informal contexts in the workplace. Storytelling, by its nature a public act, can also be used to promote reflection and development of practice.

A structure for reflection   While direct experience is at the heart of professional practice, experience of itself is insufficient; there needs to be learning from experience. Boud et al (1985) suggested that reflection on experience is the key to learning from experience. Boud et al (1985) outlined three stages for reflection. Stage 1 involves the process of returning to the experience, recalling the events and emotions, 'replaying' the experience. Boud et al (1985) advise the learner to pay close attention to the details of what happened, rather than what the learner wished had happened. They advise against making judgements at this point.

Stage 2 involves paying particular attention to the emotions associated with the events. Positive emotions can enhance learning from an experience. However, negative emotions such as anger, embarrassment, or a sense of failure can pose barriers to learning. Such negative emotions need to be discharged in some way so that learning can proceed. Stage 3 involves re-evaluating the experience, through the processes of association, integration, validation and appropriation. Association is the linking of thoughts and feelings during the experience and on reflection. Integration refers to the synthesis of those thoughts and feelings into a whole new perspective. Validation involves testing out this new perspective against other opinions and experience. Finally, appropriation occurs if the new knowledge perspective becomes part of the learner. Different ways of constructing these abilities appear in several chapters, namely 2, 5–7 and 11.

These stages of reflection proposed by Boud et al (1985) can be applied to a range of learning contexts, including informal self-evaluation, formal performance appraisal, and journalling. In the next section I will discuss how these stages of structured reflection can be applied to journalling.

Journalling

Journalling is a form of writing to learn. It is not an exposition of what is already known. Rather, through reflective self-questioning and exploration of concepts and ideas arising from experience, journalling facilitates an 'ability to move progressively to higher levels of abstraction and conceptualisation' (Stockhausen and Creedy 1994, p. 77). As a result, new propositional knowledge, as well as personal and professional craft knowledges (Higgs and Titchen 2000), can be created, enabling the development of advanced practice. Nor is journalling a simple recounting of what happened. Holly (1997, p. 5), in advocating the keeping of professional journals, notes that:

> a journal is not merely a flow of impressions, it records impressions set in a context of descriptions of circumstances, others, the self, motives, thoughts, and feelings. Taken further, it can be used as a tool for analysis and introspection.
>
> It is a chronicle of events as they happen, a dialogue with the facts (objective) and interpretations (subjective), and perhaps most important, it provides a basis for developing an awareness of the difference between facts and interpretations.

I have learned through my own experience with journalling for personal professional development and as a means of promoting student learning that journalling is a powerful learning tool. However, many people find learning to write reflective journals challenging and question the value of reflective writing. People just beginning to journal often fall into the trap of stopping at the recounting of events, without moving into the stage of reflecting and interpreting. Some people complain that journal writing takes time, which they feel they do not have in the work-place. It is true that journal writing takes time, but then all professional development takes time. We are often keen to take time to attend conferences and workshops, but we resist taking time to reflect and write about our practice. I believe that the real reason why many people resist journalling is because it can be quite confronting. As Holly (1997, p. 14) noted:

> Habit, motivation, and sometimes our own biases and unrecognised needs move us to behave in ways that are uncomfortable when we question ourselves. We allow ourselves to be vulnerable when we question ourselves. Our humanness shows. We sometimes feel threatened by change and the discomfort that accompanies the cognitive dissonance arising from the difference between our image of ourselves and our behaviour.

Journalling need not be time consuming. Journal entries can be small and made irregularly (e.g. only once or twice a week). It need only take 5–10 minutes to make a journal entry once you are in the swing of it.

Because journal writing involves a style of writing quite different to our normal professional writing, some people find that they don't know where to start. The suggestions in Table 9.1, grouped into the

Table 9.1   *Suggestions for reflective journalling*

Stage 1 Return to the experience
- What was the setting?
- Who was involved?
- What happened?
- What preceded it?
- What followed it?
- What are the facts?
- What was my role?
- What did I do/say?
- Why did I do/say this?
- What was the flow of events?

Stage 2 Pay attention to the emotions associated with the situation
- What feelings and senses surrounded the experience?
- What were the negative emotions (e.g. anger, anxiety, embarrassment, distress, guilt, fear)?
- What were the positive emotions associated with the event (e.g. joy, pride, satisfaction, affirmation, love)?

Stage 3 Re-evaluating the experience through the processes of association, integration, validation and appropriation
- What were these emotions associated with?
- What was I thinking at the time? Afterwards?
- Do I still carry those emotions now?
- Are these emotions appropriate to the situation?
- What am I thinking and feeling now?
- What can I do to deal with them?
- What have I learned from this situation?
- What have I learned about myself as a person? My self as a professional? Others? The work setting?
- What might I be aware of if the situation recurs?
- How will I react and behave differently if the situation recurs?

---

three stages of structured reflection suggested by Boud et al (1985), might be helpful to those wanting to get started on journalling.

Journalling—a personal example

As I mentioned earlier, I find reflective journalling invaluable as a professional development tool. It can be useful at any stage of one's career. I have worked as a speech pathologist for 27 years, 18 of those in university settings as a clinical educator, lecturer and now head of a program. I do not journal every day but I do try to journal whenever I take on new challenges or find myself in emotionally demanding situations at work. I recently embarked on a project which took me right outside my comfort zone, personally and professionally. In September 2001, I accompanied 12 occupational and speech pathology students from Charles Sturt University on fieldwork placements in Vietnam. We hope to go each year to provide continuity of service to our host sites, and regular intercultural learning opportunities for our students. Although this was 'my project', one I had planned for 2 years and one I was deeply committed to in terms of learning, service and social justice, I was highly anxious about the experience. I had found Vietnam confronting enough as a tourist on a previous trip; now I was going there as a professional and as a facilitator of others' learning. I doubted my skills and abilities at almost every level. I decided that one way to manage my anxiety and to learn from the experience was to be at all times authentically myself with the students, to avoid being an expert (which I was not in this context) and to keep a professional journal, which I began in the days just prior to departure. Below are some excerpts from this journal.

Vignette 1   A personal experience of journalling

September 5 A pre-placement visit to the orphanage today. I reacted much the same way I did in 1999 at the sight of these severely physically disabled children lying in rows of cots: shock, pity and fear that I would not have the knowledge and skills necessary to do anything useful to help them, or to support the students to work with them. I stepped outside for a while to cry in private, and found a couple of the students there too, with wet faces and stricken looks. They were surprised to see me like this, but relieved too that it was somehow 'OK' to react in this way. I was pleased to be able to put my arms around their shoulders; I needed that physical reassurance as much as they did, I guess. My gut feelings that the girls would be upset by the severity of impairment of some of the children there and would need some time to adjust were right.

September 12 My first visit to the orphanage since the students began placement there on the 10th. I have been down at *xxx* with the students at the deaf school these last 2 days. I'm amazed at how independently the students have gone about finding out what is important to the teachers and carers and what they want us to do and show them. They have been spending time observing in the 'cot rooms' and the classrooms, have already met with the physios and key teachers, and identified some training needs and equipment needs. I spent some time working alongside them helping carers feed the children with severe physical impairment. I loathe this aspect of our practice; I find it messy and revolting; I'm ashamed to admit this but it's true. I've never worked in this area and I'm not at all sure of what is 'best practice'. But the students seem to be handling it with confidence and skill. Where did they learn to do this? I'm wondering what I can do to help the students. What's my role here?

September 13 I realized this morning that, although the students were all 'busy', they didn't have a clear sense of structuring what they were doing, or what their goals for this placement might be. I also realized that the occupational therapist and speech pathologist students had similar goals emerging, but hadn't shared these with each other. I spent most of today helping the students develop goals for this placement and to begin to plan as an interdisciplinary team. We talked about what the needs were as they had observed them and had them described to them by the staff (through our interpreters), what they could reasonably do to meet those needs in the 5-week period given staff knowledge and skills, resources, our knowledge and skills, what recommendations staff might accept and reject, what would likely make a lasting change, and so on. We developed a tentative timetable for who would go where when, so that all staff had some of our time and all the students got a range of experiences. I also spent some time listening to students' talk about team dynamics and suggesting ways they could deal with this. I was pleased to be of help here. I might not know much about physical impairments but I do know how to facilitate student thinking and learning, and how to help them frame up goals and develop plans. I really enjoy this role. Much to my surprise, I also really enjoyed going up to the 'cot rooms' and having the students teach me about positioning and feeding techniques. I was amazed at what the students have been doing, and how well they are coping with the culture shock—both of being in Vietnam and of being in this institutional setting. I'm very proud of them. I feel like this has been worth all the time and expense I've invested in getting this project off the ground.

My journal excerpt illustrates a number of adult learning principles at play. It conveys my perception of myself as a co-learner as well as educator, engaged in experiential learning. I am using my students as peers in this experience to support my learning, as well as functioning as an educator in supporting their learning. As a facilitator of others' learning, I am trying to be authentically myself with my student co-learners. There are clear life circumstances (e.g. change of cultures, a new professional setting) dictating my learning needs and I am using both reflection in and on action as a learning tool. The act of journalling is emotionally cathartic, and reflecting on my journal entries is affirming and consolidates my learning.

The journal entries quoted here are diffuse in their focus. They do not focus on any particular critical incident, which could have served as another way of structuring my journalling. However, discussing critical incidents has been my major means of conveying to colleagues the nature of the experience and its impact on my learning and the learning of my students since my return.

Critical incidents

Critical incidents have proved to be a powerful tool for exploring and promoting professional development in practitioners (Arthur 2001, Fish and Coles 1998), and in students and I am currently writing two papers for publication about this. Fish and Coles (1998, p. 71) describe a critical incident as a 'highly significant event with important consequences or—more likely—a commonplace event that occurs during routine practice'. It can be a routine event in our professional lives, but in my experience of asking students and practitioners to recount a critical incident, it is in fact more likely to be an event which we notice because it upset, puzzled, embarrassed, amused, pleased or affirmed us in some way. I agree with Fish and Coles (1998), however, that it is what we do with it that renders it *critical*. The event needs to be recounted or recorded, analysed, interpreted and appreciated for what it teaches us about ourselves and our practice. We can work with our critical incidents privately, recording them in our journal and reflecting on them in a structured way, or we can share them in written or oral form with colleagues in formal, scheduled settings such as professional development sessions, or informally, in private talk or lunchroom chatter.

Whether critical incidents are worked through formally or informally it helps to have a structure for exploring them. The suggestions provided by Fish and Coles (1998) for identifying and exploring critical incidents are helpful for deriving meaning from critical incidents. I have used these as a basis for developing guidelines for working with critical incidents with colleagues and students, and these guidelines appear in Table 9.2. I have found this structure for critical incident exploration helpful in both written critical incident work with students and oral incident analysis with colleagues engaged in professional mentoring. You can apply these guidelines in formal or informal contexts, using both written and oral recounts of critical incidents. Take time now to identify and think through a critical incident of your own, then talk it through with a trusted colleague at work.

Critical incident exploration is a powerful learning tool because the process taps into several adult learning principles. People typically initiate the sharing of critical incidents, hence they control the timing and manner of their own learning. Critical incidents arise from real-life experiences and real-life needs to resolve a tension of some sort. Their exploration and resolution typically involve sharing and discussing with peers, and general-life experience can be used as a resource for analysing and deriving meaning from critical incidents.

Although you can ask a colleague to produce a critical incident on request, for example for a professional development activity, critical incidents more typically arise spontaneously in our discourse. They often occur as part of a larger story or narrative. Story telling can be harnessed in the workplace for professional development and the promotion of advanced practice.

Story telling

My experience has been that when you get a group of health professionals together at work, for example at professional development events or lunch, or out socially, they love to tell stories. These stories

Table 9.2   *Using critical incidents to promote advanced practice*

Identify a critical incident

- Identify an aspect of your professional practice which seems to you important in some way, where working on it would enhance your practice. This could be an issue or recurrent problem, or it could be an actual incident or event which encapsulates and illustrates the issue or problem
- Identify to whom this event, problem or issue is important and why

Crystallize the event

- Reflect on the event, issue or problem, writing or talking about it in the first person to help capture the immediacy of the event, and the thoughts and emotions surrounding the event or issue. Try to hone in on specifics which illustrate the issue or problem of concern. This will help you recall your thinking and feeling about the issue or problem
- Reflect on the values and assumptions which underpin this incident and your reaction to it
- Reflect on the context in which the incident occurred. What are the systemic and environmental factors which contributed to the incident?

Clarify the nature of the problem or issue

- What is the real problem or issue illustrated by the incident?
- What is the nature of the problem or issue? Does it say something about you as a person? You as a professional? The nature of your discipline's practice? The setting in which you work?
- Is this a problem or issue concerned with being or doing? With knowledge, skills, assumptions, beliefs or values?

What are the lessons to be learned here?

- What do you personally need to understand, learn or do to resolve this issue or problem?
- What needs to change in the work setting? The system within which you work?

Identify what you might do to address the problem or issue

- What actions will you specifically take to address this problem or issue? This might include taking courses to improve your skill level or manage conflict in the workplace, committing yourself to regular reflection and self-assessment of your practice, reading up in a discipline area and agreeing to work regularly with a colleague to develop your clinical reasoning skills or ability to reflect in action so you can avoid problems such as those identified in the critical incident

are rich in detail and provide valuable insights into the knowledge bases, values, expertise and reasoning at play in professional practice. I had always enjoyed participating in this type of discourse, and was aware that I often came away wiser for having listened or participated in the story telling. However, my doctoral research, which used narrative inquiry approaches (Clandinin and Connelly 1986, 1994), and subsequent running of workshops for clinical educators to help them uncover their practice theory, has convinced me of the value of story telling as a professional development tool.

In my research with clinical educators (McAllister 2001), I observed for hours each day and interviewed at least once per day, clinical educators across the timespan of student placements. Once I knew my participants, and established a climate of trust, I would often commence interviews with the simple prompt of 'tell me the story of your day/week so far'. They would talk at length without the need for further prompting, often starting with a chronology of the day/week so far, but then focusing on something of interest to them, or a critical incident. They would tell story after story of the development and resolution of challenges experienced, for example with students on placements. As they talked, they were sometimes surprised by the feelings and thoughts that surfaced, occasionally making comments like 'I didn't know I thought that'; 'I'm surprised to hear myself saying these things'; 'I didn't know that about myself'; 'I wonder if . . .'; and often, later in the interview, things like 'I think I might now understand why . . .'.

My role was to encourage participants in their articulation of practice and self-exploration, by using verbal and non-verbal encouragers (e.g. mmm, or nodding), and asking the odd question to help them explore below the surface of what they were reporting. Using the analogy of Fish and Coles (1998) of professional practice as like an iceberg (see Figure 9.2), with only the visible 'doing' part of practice showing, I realized that what I was doing was helping them get below the waterline of their experience and explore the knowledge bases, values, assumptions, and so on which underpinned their expertise (or emerging expertise).

A number of participants in my doctoral research commented on how valuable sharing stories had been for them in understanding and developing their practice as clinical educators, and asked: 'couldn't we do this regularly as a professional development activity?' This inspired me to use story telling as a major learning process for clinical educators in workshops which were designed to help them uncover their practice theory as educators and to develop their practice further.

Using story telling to promote advanced practice

Storytelling has been used as a therapeutic tool in the form of narrative therapy (see, for example, White and Epstein 1990) and as a professional development tool (see, for example, Gersie and King 1990; Gersie 1997). The workshops I run for clinical educators use a structured workshop format, although of course the content differs from workshop to workshop depending on the stories participants bring to the workshop and the discussion amongst participants which these stories generate. The basic format is that we start off sharing stories of our experiences (in this case as clinical educators). The group discusses and explores these stories for what they can tell us about our practice as clinical educators, and lastly I take key elements identified in the discussion and relate them to propositional knowledge regarding the practice of clinical education.

The participants in these workshops are usually experienced clinical educators wanting to develop advanced practice in clinical education. I have however had clinicians about to take their first student, clinical educators with little educative experience, and even final-year students participate fully and fruitfully in these workshops. Although I have not run workshops in this format with clinicians focusing on practice with clients, the work of Titchen (1998) and feedback from workshop participants suggests this approach would work with clinicians also. This format could be used to explore many topics involved with professional practice, provided the facilitator had a knowledge of the topic, and excellent group facilitation skills. In Table 9.3 I have outlined in more detail the processes I use with story telling for the professional development of clinical educators.

Table 9.3 *Structure of story telling workshops used to promote advanced practice in clinical education*

1. This format works well with between six and 16 participants

2. When they enrol in the workshop, they agree to come with a story or a critical incident for sharing with the other participants. These stories or incidents can be in written or oral form, or captured on video and accompanied by some background information

3. After an introduction, the group establishes 'rules' for respecting and responding to what will be shared and treating it with confidentiality. I stress that what is to be shared will remain within the room, and not discussed in any identifying way outside the room. The aim of this stage of the workshop is to establish trust and engender a sense of safety for authentic sharing

4. I ask for our first volunteer to share his/her story. I invite him/her to tell his/her story free from interruption from the group, informing the group that, after the story is told, I will go round the group and invite each person in turn (including myself) to make one comment or ask one question. The purpose here is to flesh out the story, not to begin the analysis process

5. As the person tells the story, and during the group's initial response, I will begin to write key words or phrases on a whiteboard

6. Once everyone in the group has had a turn with one comment or question, I open the story up to discussion. Discussion of a story can last for up to an hour, depending on the complexity of the story, the openness of the storyteller, and the energy and imagination of the group, as the group with the storyteller dig deep into the story for what it says about our practice

7. My role in this stage of the workshop is both to model the sorts of questions and comments which will help explore rather than judge the story and practice embodied in it, and to record key words and phrases of the story and discussion. This stage is quite crucial for me as facilitator, as I am not only facilitating the discussion and monitoring group processes, but I am also continuing to note down words and phrases that will form the basis of my interpretation and summarizing later on. My aim is to help participants extend their focus past their actions and words to the knowledge and beliefs, emotions, values and assumptions which underpin what they do and say. I am in essence trying to help them get below the waterline of the professional practice iceberg (Fish and Coles 1998)

8. When we have mined the story as much as possible, I will make some short summary comments, thank the storyteller for his/her openness and courage, then invite another storyteller to share his/her story with the group, using the same steps. The number of stories shared in a workshop depends on the length of the workshop. In an all-day workshop, a group might share and thoroughly explore four or five stories

9. In the last session of the workshop, I attempt to relate what we have learned from the stories to theory of clinical education. I work with the key words and phrases on the whiteboard to help the group recall elements of the stories and points from our discussions. I relate these to both my theoretical model of the experience of being a clinical educator (McAllister 2001) and to the wider clinical education literature. My aim is to have them see that what they do as clinical educators is grounded in a whole range of professional craft knowledge and personal practical theories of clinical education, as well as formal educational theory. In valuing these knowledges and practice, participants are encouraged to further their propositional knowledge about their practice and to continue to reflect on and refine their personal and professional craft knowledge and practices as clinical educators (using the range of approaches outlined in this chapter, as well as formal professional development opportunities)

Telling and exploring stories is a powerful tool for the development of advanced practice knowledge and skills. It can also be quite an emotional experience for participants, as it can bring to the surface buried emotions, anxieties and self-doubt. Facilitators need to handle the emotional side of story telling skilfully, allowing it to serve its cathartic function, supporting participants who may have taken considerable risks in self-disclosure, and recognizing when they need to refer on for counselling or other appropriate support.

The guidelines I have provided for journalling, the analysis of critical incidents and sharing and exploring stories involve some level of structure and dedicated time. Some of the same principles can be applied in less structured ways, by functioning for our workplace peers as what Titchen (1998) described as a critical companion and Smith (1999) as a critical friend. Titchen's model of critical companionship arose from her naturalistic study of the facilitation of learning in nurses. The concepts and strategies she discussed are applicable to a range of health settings. Her strategies are grounded in adult learning approaches and lend themselves well to adoption by those charged with developing advanced practice in others. The brief summary below of her critical companionship model cannot do justice to the elegance and utility of her work, which is very readable and rich in examples of the educational strategies she discusses.

Critical companionship

Titchen (1998) described critical companionship as a metaphor for a relationship between an experienced and less experienced practitioner in which the more experienced partner functions as a critical companion on the less experienced partner's experiential learning journey. By providing constructive criticism and support, and acting as a resource, critical companions enable their colleagues to learn and to act more effectively in the workplace. Titchen (1998) identified four major domains in her model: the relationship domain, the rationality–intuitive domain, the facilitation domain, and the facilitative use of self domain. The key concepts in these domains are summarized in Table 9.4.

Titchen (1998) highlights the importance of relationship and the facilitative use of self, and in doing so is evocative of the work of humanists such as Rogers (1969). It also gives value to intuitive as well as rational perspectives on educating and learning, the lack of which in contemporary educational practice has been criticized by Fish and Twinn (1997) and Fish and Coles (1998). Titchen (1998) argued that using both rational and intuitive approaches requires and nurtures professional artistry in the critical companion as well as the practitioner.

The role of critical friends and critical companions

Titchen (1998) described critical companionship in the context of a formalized role of workplace educator. Few workplaces have such dedicated roles, but the principles of critical companionship can be applied in less formal ways, adopting Smith's (1999) concept of critical friends. Critical friends can be peers or colleagues in the workplace who by virtue of having built a trusting and open relationship are empowered critically to question their friends'/peers' practice and encourage them to do the same. Through thoughtful and sensitive questioning, they invite their friend/peer to reflect on something observed, reported, felt, or said (or not done or said, as is often the case in the workplace). They can invite their friend to debrief with them about a critical incident or shared story, or offer on-line comment and questioning as they work together as colleagues in the workplace. Those of us who have a critical friend in the workplace, perhaps established through years of successfully working together, know how invaluable and supportive such a relationship can be. My critical

Table 9.4 *Domains and key concepts in Titchen's (1998) critical companionship model*

Domain	Key concepts
1. Relationship	Constructing an effective relationship based on mutuality, reciprocity, particularity (knowing person in context and holistically) and graceful care
2. Rationality–intuitive	Using both rational and intuitive approaches, incorporating intentionality (self-aware thoughtfulness), saliency and temporality (deliberate timing of events and interactions)
3. Facilitation	Facilitating colleagues' learning, promoting consciousness raising, problematization, self-reflection and critique, and using articulation of craft knowledge, high challenge/high support, feedback, critical dialogue and role-modelling
4. Facilitative use of self	The actualizing domain, integrating domains 1–3 through attending to what is happening in self, interactions and environment

friend provides me with invaluable feedback on my handling of difficult people and situations in my management role, and engages me in conversations which help me critique my own decision-making processes. I sometimes find these conversations confronting and challenging, but I always find them helpful and empowering of continued personal and professional growth.

So far in this chapter I have discussed the principles of adult learning, and the characteristics of adult learners and their facilitators. I have suggested that the workplace is an ideal context for adult learning because the real and immediate needs of clients provide the motivations and foci for learning, and one's work peers as well as one's life experience provide resources for learning. A number of strategies which apply adult learning principles and are well suited to the workplace were then described. I have suggested that these strategies can be successfully used to promote advanced practice. But what do I mean by advanced practice? And how do strategies which use 'the self' and promote reflection on values, attitudes, and relationships, as well as knowledge and skills, relate to my vision of advanced practice? In the next section of this chapter, I provide a vision of advanced practice.

A vision of an advanced practitioner

This vision of advanced practice and an advanced practitioner builds on a model derived from my study of the experience of being a clinical educator (McAllister 2001). The feedback I have received from participants at workshops (see section on storytelling above) suggests this work is applicable to clinicians also, as a way of describing the experience of being a clinical practitioner. My study used phenomenology (Crotty 1996) and narrative inquiry methods (Clandinin and Connelly 1986, 1994) to explore stories of experience. Six major dimensions of experience arose from analysis of hundreds of pages of interview transcripts and fieldnotes of observations of the study participants at work. The themes were:

● a sense of self
● a sense of relationship with others

- a sense of being a clinical educator
- a sense of agency
- seeking dynamic self-congruence
- growth and development.

Each of these major dimensions, or themes, had sub-themes, as listed in Table 9.5. I will discuss these dimensions here as I believe they relate to successful clinical practice.

A sense of self

The core phenomenon in this study was 'sense of self', which influenced how one related to others, approached being a clinical educator, and took action in the workplace. Although not always apparent or on the surface, one's sense of self impacts on who and how we are at work. One of my study participants expressed that well in saying 'the most important thing you bring into your work is yourself'.

Having a sense of self includes having self-awareness and self-knowledge, self-acceptance and a self-identity, being aware of one's level of need to control people, time and events, and seeing oneself as a lifelong learner.

A sense of being in relationship

Who one is as a person in turns influences one's sense of relationship with others. This theme includes perceiving others as they truly are, not as we might wish them to be, being people-oriented rather than self-oriented, holding personal values, and actively seeking to implement those values and perceptions in relating to others.

Table 9.5   *Dimensions and elements of the model of the experience of being a clinical educator*

Dimension 1: a sense of self	**Dimension 2: a sense of relationship with others**
Elements	*Elements*
1. Having self-awareness and self-knowledge	1. Being people-oriented
2. Having self-acceptance	2. Perceiving others
3. Having a self-identity	3. Values in relating to others
4. Choosing a level of control	4. Seeking to implement values and perceptions in relating to others
5. Being a lifelong learner	
Dimension 3: a sense of being a clinical educator	**Dimension 4: a sense of agency as a clinical educator**
Elements	*Elements*
1. Understanding of role	1. Perceptions of competence and capacity to act as a clinical educator
2. Motivations for becoming a clinical educator	2. Creating and maintaining facilitative learning environments
3. Desired approaches to clinical education	3. Designing, managing and evaluating students' learning programs
4. Affective aspects of being a clinical educator	4. Managing self
	5. Managing others
Dimension 5: seeking dynamic self-congruence	**Dimension 6: growth and development: possible stages and pathways**
Elements	*Elements*
1. Bringing a higher level of attention to the role	1. Embarking on the journey of becoming a clinical educator
2. Drawing the selves together	2. Moving from novice to advanced beginner
3. Striving for plan–action congruence	3. Developing competence in the role
	4. Pursuing professional artistry
	5. Suffering burnout

A sense of being a clinician/clinical educator

How one seeks to relate to others in the workplace influences one's sense of being in the work role. This dimension includes how one understands one's work role, motivations for being in that role, desired approaches to fulfilling that role, and emotional aspects of practice. The desired approaches adopted by clinicians probably change with experience and confidence in the role, just as it did for the novice clinical educators maturing into their role in my study. New clinicians possibly rely more on what Higgs and Titchen (2000) have called propositional knowledge, that is, text book knowledge, or theory. With experience, clinicians develop professional craft knowledge, and bring their personal knowledge more fully into play in the clinical setting. What was interesting in my study of clinical educators, and I believe would apply also to clinicians, is that theory is only one factor guiding how they approach their work. Their desire to be true to themselves and to maintain empowering relationships with others in the workplace were equally important. The technical skill domain of practice was but one aspect of their work; emotional aspects were equally as important to them. They were essentially humanistic in focus, not technical–rational or managerial in orientation, despite attempts to impose this orientation by health services (Fish and Twinn 1997).

A sense of agency

The fourth interlinked dimension arising from my study was one's sense of agency. How one saw oneself, the types of relationships valued, and one's sense of being a clinician influenced one's sense of agency and the foci of that agency. How one perceives one's competence, capacity and confidence to act is an important aspect of this dimension, one which can be supported through professional development. The creation of supportive learning or therapeutic environments using adult learning principles is important, as is designing, managing and evaluating learning, or therapy programs. Managing self and others were also key sub-themes in this dimension. This self- and other-management was often directed towards containing possibly negative or relationship-damaging emotions and attitudes, as well as fatigue. This is mentioned in Chapter 1. Self-management was also directed towards using the self to facilitate learning and growth in others. Hence, this dimension has great applicability for those seeking to develop practice skills in others.

Seeking dynamic self-congruence

Enabling one's sense of self to be lived out authentically through relationships and actions in the workplace requires some meta-cognitive and meta-mood monitoring. I talk about this dimension as one of seeking dynamic self-congruence, that is, congruence between who one wants to be and who one actually is, or can be, in the workplace. This involves bringing into play what Torbert (1978) refers to as a 'higher level of awareness' to what one is doing, thinking and feeling, in order to draw the selves together (personal self, self in relationship and self at work), and to seek congruence between what one plans to do and what one actually does.

I have deliberately referred to this process as one of 'seeking' and of being 'dynamic' as one cannot always achieve congruence, nor is this achievement a steady-state phenomenon. It requires active cognitive and emotional awareness (Goleman 1995) and is, I believe, something that develops with experience in a role. Novice clinicians are often too immersed in the moment and too self-focused as they seek to survive in their new role (Christie et al 1985) to have much spare processing capacity needed to bring a higher level of attention to what they are about. Sustained high levels of attention are difficult to achieve, even for expert clinicians, because the complexity of the context, emotions and fatigue interfere with attention. Only when skills are deeply embedded in practice and one is able to be both self- and other-focused can this occur. I have argued (McAllister 2001) that this ability is a hallmark of professional artists. Nonetheless, peers and supervisors in the workplace can help promote the development of this ability.

Growth and development as clinician/clinical educator

Participants in my study were at different stages of growth and development. In describing these stages I borrowed terms from the work of Benner (1984), labelling them novice, advanced beginner, competent practitioner and professional artist. Chapter 2 goes into the stages in more detail. I found that each stage was characterized by varying degrees of senses of self, relationship, being, doing and becoming. I want to focus here on what characterized professional artistry in my study, as this is what I believe characterizes advanced practitioners and what they are striving for.

Advanced practitioners seek professional artistry

Professional artistry involves a commitment to the highest quality of work through the use of a range of practices, including reflection. Fish and Twinn (1997, p. 154) suggested that quality work in professional practice:

> encompasses not the pre-specified list of individual competencies that take no account of context, but a *repertoire* of skills, abilities, capacities, professional knowledge, personal attributes, personality and ability to work with other professionals, together with . . . flexibility, educational understanding, moral awareness and professional judgement.

Advanced practitioners as revealed in my study are individuals with a clear sense of self, self in relationships, and self as a practitioner, with the capacity and confidence to act in ways to manage the work environment, tasks and roles, self and others. They bring heightened levels of awareness to their work, as they seek to be true to themselves and to act congruently with their values and plans. They are able to exercise high levels of professional judgement and demonstrate professional artistry. My work with clinical educators striving for advanced practice suggests that they are open to self-exploration and exploration by others of their knowledge, practice, values and thoughts. They use reflection to explore and critique their own practice, and actively seek to support the practice of others in similar ways.

Conclusion

As noted earlier in this chapter, professional practice has been conceptualized by Fish and Coles (1998) as like an iceberg (Figure 9.2). What is visible is the 'doing' component, but beneath this (waterline) lies experience, knowledge, feelings, expectations, all overlaying assumptions, attitudes, beliefs and values. The invisible sense of self, self in relationship and sense of being (McAllister 2001) underpins the more visible sense of doing. 'Doing' congruently with the foundational values, beliefs, assumptions and attitudes requires a heightened level of attention. It is the invisibility and tacitness of much of what underpins professional practice, that makes it difficult to 'teach' and discuss. Adult learning principles and reflective strategies can be used to help clinicians surface and make visible their knowledge bases and professional judgements, and enable their growth towards advanced practitioner and professional artist status.

References

Apps J W 1981 The adult learner on campus. Follett, Chicago

Arthur N 2001 Using critical incidents to investigate cross cultural transitions. International Journal of Intercultural Relations 25:41–53

Benner P 1984 From novice to expert: excellence and power in clinical nursing practice. Addison-Wesley, Menlo Park, CA

Boud D, Keogh R, Walker D 1985 Promoting reflection in learning: a model. In: Boud D, Keogh R, Walker D (eds) Reflection: turning experience into learning. Kogan Page, London, p 18–40

Brookfield S D 1986 Understanding and facilitating adult learning. Open University Press, Milton Keynes, UK

Candy P, Crebert G, O'Leary J 1994 Developing lifelong learners through undergraduate education. Commissioned report no. 28. National Board of Employment, Education and Training. Australian Government Publishing Service, Canberra, Australia

Christie B A, Joyce P C, Moeller P L 1985 Fieldwork experience, part II: the supervisor's dilemma. American Journal of Occupational Therapy 39:675–681

Clandinin D J, Connelly F M 1986 Rhythms in teaching: the narrative study of teachers' personal practical knowledge of classrooms. Teaching and Teacher Education 2:377–387

Clandinin D J, Connelly F M 1994 Personal experience methods. In: Denzin N, Lincoln Y (eds) Handbook of qualitative research. Sage: Thousand Oaks, CA, p 413–427

Crotty M 1996 Phenomenology and nursing research. Churchill Livingstone, Melbourne, Australia

Fish D, Coles C 1998 Developing professional judgement in healthcare: learning through the critical appreciation of practice. Butterworth-Heinemann, Oxford

Fish D, Twinn S 1997 Quality clinical supervision in the healthcare professions: principled approaches to practice. Butterworth-Heinemann, Oxford

Gersie A 1997 Reflections on therapeutic storymaking: the use of stories in groups. Jessica Kingsley, London

Gersie A, King N 1990 Storymaking in education and therapy. Jessica Kingsley, London

Goleman D 1995 Emotional intelligence. Bantam, New York

Groen G J, Patel V L 1985 Medical problem-solving: some questionable assumptions. Medical Education 19:95–100

Heron J 1989 The facilitators' handbook. Kogan Page, London

Higgs J 1992 Managing clinical education: the educator manager and the self-directed learner. Physiotherapy 78:822–828

Higgs J 1993 The teacher in self-directed learning: manager or co-manager. In: Graves N (ed) Learner managed learning: practice, theory and policy. World Education Fellowship, London, p 122–131

Higgs J, Titchen A 2000 Knowledge and reasoning. In: Higgs H, Jones M (eds) Clinical reasoning in the health professions, 2nd edn. Butterworth-Heinemann, Oxford, p 23–32

Holly M L 1997 Keeping a professional journal. Deakin University Press, Geelong, Australia

Knowles M, Holton E, Swanson R 1998 The adult learner: the definitive classic on adult education and human resource development, 5th edn. Gulf, Houston, TX

Lincoln M, McAllister L 1993 Facilitating peer learning in clinical education. Medical Teacher 15:17–25

Mattingly C, Hayes-Fleming M (eds) 1994 Clinical reasoning: forms of inquiry in therapeutic practice. F A Davis, Philadelphia

McAllister L 2001 The experience of being a clinical educator. Unpublished PhD thesis. University of Sydney, Sydney, Australia

McAllister L, Rose M 2000 Speech-language pathology students: learning clinical reasoning. In: Higgs J, Jones M (eds) Clinical reasoning in the health professions. Oxford, Butterworth-Heinemann, p 205–213

Rogers C R 1969 Freedom to learn: a view of what education might become. Charles E. Merrill, Columbus, OH

Schön D A 1987 Educating the reflective practitioner. Jossey-Bass, San Francisco

Smith D L 1999 Facilitating reflective practice in the practicum. Unpublished keynote address to the staff of the Auckland College of Education and cooperating practicum schools

Stockhausen L, Creedy D 1994 Journal writing: untapped potential for reflection and consolidation. In: Chen S, Cowdroy R, Kingsland K et al (eds) Reflections on problem based learning. Australian Problem Based Learning Network, Sydney, Australia, p 73–85

Titchen A 1998 Professional craft knowledge in patient-centred nursing and the facilitation of its development. Unpublished PhD thesis. Oxford University, Oxford, UK

Torbert W R 1978 Educating toward shared purpose, self-direction and quality work: the theory and practice of liberating structure. Journal of Higher Education 49:109–135

White M, Epstein D 1990 Narrative means to therapeutic ends. New York: Norton

10 Role models and mentors: informal and formal ways to learn from exemplary practice

Linda M. Roth and Susan A. Esdaile

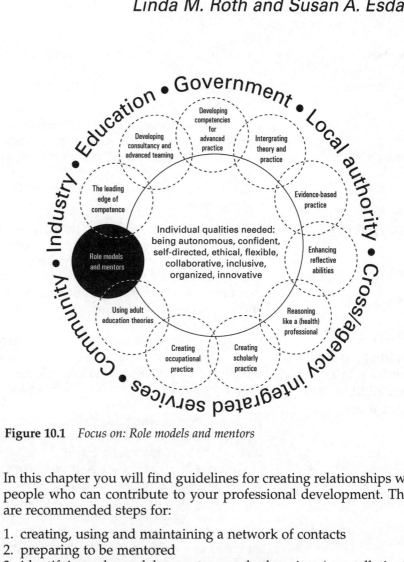

Figure 10.1 *Focus on: Role models and mentors*

Chapter outline

In this chapter you will find guidelines for creating relationships with people who can contribute to your professional development. There are recommended steps for:

1. creating, using and maintaining a network of contacts
2. preparing to be mentored
3. identifying role models, mentors, and others in a 'constellation' of developmental relationships
4. establishing and conducting mentoring relationships.

These skills are foundational for advanced practitioners. Your effectiveness as a professional requires that you stay aware of the changing context of your working environment and the larger environment of your profession. Ongoing networking and use of multiple mentors throughout your career will help you to grow continuously as a competent and successful practitioner. You will be able to satisfy your clients' needs, while also meeting your own personal and professional needs. As in Chapter 7, throughout this chapter we have included stories from the young healthcare practitioners we interviewed. Their stories illustrate how others in the beginning stages of their careers as health practitioners have used role models and mentors to help them develop as professionals. The questions we asked them are listed in Table 10.1.

Key words

Mentoring, multiple mentoring, networking, role model

Anticipated outcomes

As a result of reading this chapter, we anticipate that you will be able to:

- establish and maintain a productive professional network
- prepare effectively for mentoring relationships
- describe the traditional mentor–protégé process as well as the concept of a constellation or network of mentors
- create and maintain effective relationships that support professional development.

Introduction

We begin this chapter with an introduction to the benefits of networking as a career-long strategy for creating and nurturing collegial relationships. Your network provides a foundation from which to establish mentoring relationships of varying purposes and duration that can support your career advancement and provide both personal and professional satisfaction.

Networking: establishing and maintaining a constellation of colleagues

Picture yourself at a meeting of other professionals in your former school, college, or university setting, your current work setting, or at a meeting of your professional organization. There are 10 or 15 minutes before the session begins. You have settled into a seat and are reading through an agenda. Look around you and notice what other participants are doing. Some are sitting silently and keeping to themselves. Others quietly or animatedly engage in conversation with those around them. Networking begins in these very situations, when you have the opportunity for one-on-one conversations with new people whose work and interests relate to yours.

Networking can be defined as a procedure for establishing connections, securing information, and making problem-solving bridges out of shared experiences (Stevens 1995). Because it is essential to build and maintain a roster of professional contacts throughout your career, networking is an ongoing process, not something that is ever complete. This is one of your best tools for staying attuned to your career management process and for helping you to stay up-to-date in your profession. The most successful networking is a proactive approach to inviting colleagues into your life rather than waiting for someone else to make the first contact. That person sitting next to you at a conference may know excellent career development strategies that have worked well for her and could be useful for you. Or the man in front of you getting coffee on a break from a professional meeting may be able to put you in touch with someone who would be an excellent addition to your network. You will miss out on learning from others unless you initiate conversations with them. This is an important strategy for creating your professional support system. You can identify people within or outside your current employment environment who are potential colleagues, role models, and mentors. These are 'experts' who are doing, or have done, what you hope to accomplish yourself, and they can advise you from their experience. Importantly, you can reciprocate with these or other practitioners as your career progresses.

Healthcare practitioners naturally work in teams, which suggests that you may already have a network of current and former colleagues. In addition to people with whom you have worked, this may include fellow students and former teachers from your education and training experiences. To begin formalizing your network for yourself, use written records you already own, such as your personal and work telephone and e-mail directories and membership lists from professional organizations, or participant lists from conferences you have attended. Many professional organizations have formalized special interest groups, or SIGs, oriented around topics you may wish to pursue. For example, you may find a subset of people in a professional organization who focus their attention on patient–provider communication. If this is an important area of interest for you, you can find colleagues with whom to talk and even collaborate within that group. Consider also reviewing published directories from current and previous employers and from the college or university you attended. Make a list of names and contact information for each of the individuals you find who has potential as a career or psychosocial support resource for you. Stevens (1995) recommends that you 'list people who care about you, people who will support your decisions, people in positions of significant authority or influence, people who have expertise in helping others look at their careers'. He suggests that you indicate beside each person's name how that individual may help you, or what questions you would like the resource to answer. Remember that if this contact person cannot help you, he or she may be able to put you in contact with someone who can.

We asked the early-career practitioners we interviewed several questions. These are listed in Table 10.1.

One of the beginning practitioners we interviewed for this chapter shared a networking story with us. *Mary*, a 25-year-old physical therapist who has been practicing for 15 months, was interested in pursuing information to bring back to her colleagues on a wound care committee in the hospital-based rehabilitation unit in which she works:

> I've been researching about electrical stimulation and wound care. I went to a wound care course and I got new information that I wanted to add to. I attempted to contact one of the physical therapists who presented at the conference, but I couldn't reach him. There was a student at our facility who had given an in-service related to this, and I asked him where he got the information. He was able to refer me to one of the leading experts in wound care, a therapist who has done a lot with research in that area. This man was willing to give me resources, suggestions, and contacts and

Table 10.1   *Questions asked in the interviews for Chapter 10*

Our questions relate to two types of individuals who may influence people's careers: role models and mentors. First, let's talk about role models. These are people whom we admire and want to be like. We can learn from observing their behavior and by seeking their advice and counsel.

Question 1
I'd like you to think about one or two individuals who may have influenced your decision to pursue your profession. Can you name one or more people you would consider 'role models'?

Question 2
What experiences with [this person] caused you to see him/her as a role model?

Question 3
What sort of relationship, if any, have you maintained with this individual during your education/training and early work experiences?

Question 4
How do you expect your relationship to this person will continue through your professional career, if at all? (Repeat if more than one role model was mentioned.)

Question 5
Mentors are people who provide collegial support, feedback and advice. They may offer opportunities for entry into professional networks. I'd like you to think now about one or more individuals in your life currently whom you would consider a mentor.

Question 6
What sort of support does this person provide for you? Can you relate some specific examples? (Repeat if more than one mentor or coach was mentioned.)

to let me know about other courses coming up. I was a little intimidated because he is a big name. But wanting to know was my inspiration to contact him anyway. I would consider him a role model with respect to the current research. That is something I am thinking of doing in the future.

While *Mary*'s immediate network could not offer her the resources she needed, someone within that network linked her to someone who could. She also overcame her nervousness at contacting someone well known in her field; her need to know compelled her to initiate contact with an expert, and when she did, she found this man very willing to share.

Both of this chapter's authors have learnt to network to our advantage at professional meetings. Some organizations sponsor 'meet the experts' breakfast sessions in which noted experts in a field are available in an informal setting. One of your authors met and became collegial with several national-level colleagues using this method over the first few years of her career. As another example, one of us noticed a prominent researcher waiting in line for refreshments on break at a meeting. When approached and complimented about a recent publication, the researcher suggested that the two continue their talk over lunch. They ended up spending several hours in one-to-one conversation. This networking at a conference blossomed into an important collegial relationship.

While networking may seem a natural expression of many people's personalities, some people who are more introverted may find it awkward at first to initiate contact with a stranger, especially one who has more prestige in the profession. Our advice is to reflect upon the satisfaction you feel when someone compliments you. Similarly, you can provide that satisfaction to others when you express your admiration for their work. To cultivate your network base, Malugani (2001) offers the following advice:

1. When attending professional or industry meetings, set objectives for your career advancement before you go. These objectives should include not only the knowledge and skill gains you hope for, but also the connections with people you hope to meet who can impact your career.

2. Use your computer to expand your network online by joining chat groups, list-serves, and bulletin boards sponsored by your employer, professional association, or simply a group of like-minded professionals.

3. Use your network thoughtfully and judiciously. When making requests, keep them brief and personalized. Busy professionals who are interested in helping others appreciate a message that is written succinctly and specifically to them, noting how their expertise can benefit you in a specific situation. If you discover information that you know would be of interest to a network participant, send that with a brief introductory comment. Because of its richness in communicating information among professionals, this use of networking skills is sometimes called the 'invisible college' (Miller 1989).

4. Regularly review the members of your network. Compare this to caring for a garden which must be constantly groomed, and in which you periodically weed out your least helpful contacts and cultivate new ones.

5. Reciprocate: be a good giver and supporter yourself.

6. Always thank your contacts for each supportive act, by telephone, letter, or e-mail. Forgetting this important and considerate step can discourage future responses from those in your network.

Regarding this last point, advising people to acknowledge and thank those who provide information to them may seem too obvious. Alas, we've both experienced situations where we went to some effort to locate and send information that was never acknowledged. This made us reluctant to accept requests from or provide assistance to these individuals in the future.

What rewards will networking bring? You'll increase your interpersonal skills and self-confidence. You may discover possible areas of collaboration with fellow practitioners. You can keep up with trends and new information in your profession, and build your referral base for further career exploration. You may even discover new job opportunities. Because networking relationships are founded on trust, be certain to treat the individuals you contact with respect and handle information you receive in an ethical and professional manner.

Overview of the mentoring process

All of us relate to other individuals throughout our lifetimes. Both personal and professional relationships play an essential role in our growth and development. Parents and other family members are our first role models. As we grow older, we meet and learn about increasing numbers and kinds of people. We learn how to relate to others, negotiate our way in the world, and set the course of our lives through observing family members, friends, teachers, acquaintances and others, even those we 'meet' only through our reading, listening, or viewing of various media. For example, through the stories of their careers, Clara Barton and Florence Nightingale have inspired generations of nurses who never actually knew them. A personal story illustrates this: early in her career, one of us, had the good fortune to spend an afternoon in the archives of Edinburgh Castle, in Scotland. Among the correspondence being catalogued that day was a letter from Florence Nightingale to the general in charge of the British forces in the Crimea. She was writing on behalf of a young soldier, aged 21. He was the only source of support for his widowed mother. He had lost a leg, and had no skills to earn a living. Miss Nightingale was writing to ask the general to help him secure an apprenticeship as a boot maker. It was most impressive to find that Florence Nightingale's holistic approach to healthcare included vocational rehabilitation! As this anecdote reveals, some of our most influential role models may be people we have not met, but know from their own published work, or accounts of their work written by others.

Some of the people we observe in our youth may play strategic roles in helping us make decisions that will affect our future. A nurturing care giver may inspire us to want to dedicate ourselves to caring for others. A healing practitioner may make us want to be able to assist those whose ailments or conditions prevent them living life to the fullest extent possible. Alternatively, a negative experience with a harsh or careless practitioner may cause us to commit to behave in contrast, to strive always to be compassionate, competent, and professional in our work. Thus, we learn from observing behavior. Continually watching for and learning from role models allows us to pattern our behavior after those we admire and aspire to be like.

Beyond their capacity as role models, some of the people with whom we interact may take an active interest in our development, offering their advice, counsel, and support. These are individuals with whom we can develop a mentoring-type relationship. Traditionally, mentoring has been defined as 'an intense interpersonal exchange between a senior experienced colleague (mentor) and a less experienced junior colleague (protégé) in which the mentor provides support, direction, and feedback regarding career plans and personal development' (Russell and Adams 1997, page 2). In this conventional model, the protégé frequently is a young professional with high career aspirations. While either individual may initiate the relationship, the protégé may attract the mentor's attention through outstanding job performance or similarity in interests (Noe 1988). The two primary functions mentors serve are career and psychosocial support (Kram 1983). Aimed at facilitating and enhancing career development, career support typically includes sponsorship, exposure and visibility, coaching, protection, and challenging assignments.

Mentoring experts suggest a number of positive outcomes related to this career support function, including early career success, work satisfaction, career satisfaction, and number of promotions received (Young and Perrewé 2000). A mentor's psychosocial function enhances the protégé's sense of competence, identity, and work-role effectiveness through providing role modeling, acceptance and confirmation, counseling and friendship (Kram 1983, Russell and Adams 1997). Research on mentoring has indicated that people who are mentored perform better on the job, advance more rapidly within their organization both in salary and in position, report more job and career satisfaction, and intend to remain in the job longer than do non-mentored individuals (Eby et al 2000). In a study of nurses, dieticians, therapists, pharmacists, and other professionals at a large, private, general hospital, psychosocial mentoring was shown to benefit both the protégé and the organization, increasing job involvement and self-esteem at work and decreasing the likelihood that the protégé would leave the organization (Koberg et al 1998).

Multiple mentoring

In the mid-1980s, research by Kram (1985) demonstrated that mentoring is not solely a two-party partnership; rather, she showed that mentoring support is provided by a set or 'constellation' of development relationships with peers, subordinates, friends, family, and bosses. Building upon this work, Higgins and Kram (2001, p. 234) suggest one overarching term, 'developers,' to describe all of the individuals in a protégé's life who 'take an active interest in and will act to advance the individual's career by assisting with his or her personal and professional development'. These authors acknowledge that, often early in their career, individuals have one or two very special mentors. However, throughout their career, professionals rely on a much broader group of individuals for both career and psychosocial support. This research shows that the composition of one's entire constellation of developers is more important for long-term career advancement than any single mentoring relationship. Other researchers agree. Baugh and Scandura (1999) found that the use of multiple mentors may lead to greater commitment to one's organization, greater job satisfaction, enhanced career expectations, increased understanding about alternative employment, and lower uncertainty about one's work role. Rather than relying on one or two role models or mentors, then, it is wise to consider a constellation of developmental relationships with a number of individuals who can assist you to advance appropriately in your career.

Throughout this chapter, we will use the term 'mentor' in the generic sense, referring to the continuum of individuals with whom you as a protégé can create a short- or long-term developmental relationship. Horgan (1992) suggests that for your group of 'multiple mentors', you should cultivate a diversity of people, including experienced, well-established professionals as well as newcomers. These developers can help you through coaching, guiding, interpreting organizational culture, and supporting your professional growth in general. The close ties that characterize a traditional mentoring relationship may develop between you and some of these people, but the focus will likely be on the learning aspect of these experiences rather than on the interpersonal. There are many advantages of this approach. With a pool of multiple mentors, each can play a role suited to his or her strengths. For example, an early-career occupational or physical therapy practitioner may learn specific skills in neurodevelopmental rehabilitation from one mentor who may be either an occupational or a physical therapist. Additionally, the same practitioner may learn about the organizational culture of the unit from a senior nurse administrator, and then learn about searching databases to enhance evidence-based practice from still another professional, such as a pharmacist.

Thus you may accelerate your career development when your mentors have different jobs, perspectives, experiences, and areas of expertise. No one mentor need be burdened with the sole responsibility for mentoring; in fact, the responsibility will more clearly rest with you, as you manage your mentors as your developmental resources. Within this group, you will likely find one or more suitable role models whose styles match your own. Morahan (2000a) refers to this approach as a 'mosaic', recommending that developing professionals create their own 'advisory board' whose members can offer advice and skill development as needed.

Participating in mentoring relationships

As a new professional, your career plan should be based upon a strategy for continuous reflection upon your personal and professional strengths and needs for development. You can use the results of this assessment as a basis for seeking the assistance of others. Important tasks to complete on a regular basis are a review of your long-term career goals and shorter-term career objectives. In chapters 2, 5–7, and 9 of this book you will find excellent exercises to assist you in your self-reflection and goal setting.

Habits of self-management are key to profiting from mentoring. The first step in self-management is determining your goals as a practitioner. Research has shown that people who are mentored achieve greater job satisfaction and see themselves as successful when they set their own career goals (Murphy and Ensher 2001). Reaching these goals effectively requires that you stay aware of your career-growth-related behavior. To 'self-monitor', or pay attention to your behavior, you can use the journaling tools provided in Chapters 5 and 9. This process will allow you to reflect upon your current professional actions to see if there are differences between your current behavior and the standards you must meet in order to reach your goals. Furthermore, research has also shown that people who use positive 'self-talk' have higher job satisfaction (Murphy and Ensher 2001). Positive statements to yourself, such as, 'I am taking one step at a time; I am in control; I am learning something every day', can keep you on the path to success. Visualization, that is, picturing yourself as the successful professional you are striving to be, is another important strategy, as is purposefully creating positive beliefs and thoughts. People who use these behavioral self-management strategies report

Case study	While successful professionals proactively seek out developmental experiences that help them grow, sometimes we may miss these opportunities when they present themselves. For example, Lynn, a young respiratory therapist one of us knew, expected that any continuing education she might participate in should be paid for by her employer. However, due to funding cuts, the hospital had stopped supporting staff to attend professional conferences. Lynn felt that this was unjust, and remained adamant that she would not pay for her own continuing education or use vacation time to attend conferences. Some of Lynn's colleagues, however, disagreed with her actions. Although they would have preferred that their employer cover continuing education costs, they used vacation days and their own funds to learn new skills and keep up to date. To them, this was a necessary investment for their current professional practice and for future employability.
Activity	To assist you in reflecting upon your own behavior in past similar situations, consider writing a journal entry answering these questions: List two situations in which you have proactively sought out the help of others or invested your own time or funds in advancing your career. What were the results of each? Now, list two instances in which, as you reflect back, you missed an opportunity to invest in yourself or to learn from others. If you had the chance to relive those experiences, what would you do differently? How do you think you would you have benefited from behaving more proactively?

greater career success. Thus, self-management is an important foundation for reaching out for and benefiting from developmental guidance from others.

Once you have established both a baseline assessment of the knowledge and skills you would like to develop through relationships with others as well as a method for keeping your assessment up-to-date, it is time to focus on choosing individuals who help you meet the needs you have established. Often, these individuals are already members of your network, as described earlier in this chapter. Many sorts of developmental relationships can be helpful for beginning healthcare practitioners. These range from informal and sometimes short-term associations to formalized, intense, long-term partnerships with a more senior professional, along the lines of the traditional model of mentoring. To reiterate, throughout your career, you will benefit from a 'constellation of developers' (Higgins and Kram 2001), which can include family, friends, community members, professional peers, and senior colleagues. Seeking career assistance from a variety of developers can increase the information, resources, and opportunities available to you as you grow in your profession.

Participating in developmental relationships

Within your network of potential developers, people can play a number of roles, including:

1. peers
2. role models
3. coaches
4. sponsors
5. mentors.

Working with peers

Peers may be personal friends who are at a developmental level similar to yours. More often, peers are professional colleagues whose employment level is about the same as yours. Although they often have the same level of experience as you do, peers can still offer important and welcome support. For example, *Alex*, the medical technologist we interviewed, told us of a peer who helps him with a specific skill: 'He teaches me the computer aspects of my job. If I have computer problems he is always there so that I don't have to call the hospital's information technology people. He inspires me to go out of my range. He also talks to me about my family, calls my home if I am sick'.

Peers can serve as a sounding board as you talk through your thoughts and feelings about your life and work. With members in his or her own network, a peer may have access to organizational knowledge that is beneficial to you, and you may be able to reciprocate with information you have learnt through your own experience. Peers may have skills that are complementary to yours, and you may be able to teach or coach each other in areas in which one of you has more expertise.

Learning from role models

Role models are individuals who demonstrate for you how something is done. Professional or personal skills can be patterned after the performance of role models. We usually admire the actions of these individuals and learn by comparing our behavior to theirs, analyzing the gap in performance, and working to behave more like they do. One of the beginning practitioners interviewed for this chapter revealed that a role model whom she met before her college years influenced her career choice. *Lisa*, aged 23, had graduated with a Bachelor of Science degree in occupational therapy 4 months prior to our interview. While she was working part-time in home care, she was about to start working part-time in a special school as well.

> One great role model definitely influenced my decision to become an occupational therapist. I have a severely handicapped brother who attends high school. One time I went to visit his school. The program that this occupational therapist had started, the multitude of ideas that she was able to come up with, and the quality she exemplifies as a good professional helped me decide my career. I felt that occupational therapy would be something that I would want to do also. Just by watching her, I saw she was involved and engaged in what she was doing, working with the students and using her creative resources to come up with different projects, and then selling those projects at a fundraiser. She is

so dynamic and such a good professional. You can really tell she is happy doing what she is doing. I looked to her as a person that I wanted to exemplify and I wanted to follow in her footsteps. I am quite honored that this fall I will be working alongside her at the same school where I first met her.

One of *Lisa*'s first positions as an occupational therapist was to work in collaboration with the very therapist who was her role model. With role models such as this, learning takes place by observation and comparison. In some cases, we identify ourselves to role models as *Lisa* did. In other cases, we may admire them from afar. Role models can even be someone we have never met, but in whom we have identified something we want to emulate, as illustrated in the Florence Nightingale story shared at the beginning of this chapter.

Alex, the 25-year-old medical technologist with whom we spoke, told us of a senior technologist who was inspiring him:

In the blood bank, one of our senior technicians takes on a big workload, and she is also really helpful. When I have a question, she is there to help me out. She has been there 25 years and knows every procedure. If there are emergencies or if we are falling behind or have taken on too much, I will ask her help and she has no problem with helping. Lately I have compared myself to her; I will take on more work to see if I can do what she does. I have come close to reaching her level but I have not gotten there just yet.

Alex works with his role model on a daily basis and is measuring his progress in reaching her level. While the examples we have shared are typical, the absence of a role model can also contribute to our career decisions. *Alex* told us that his image of the sort of individual who was actually *not* in his current work environment could determine the direction of his career, because he felt an essential role was not being filled:

I am trying to decide whether to try to inspire more people to go into the field or manage the people who are already in the field. I will either get into a Master's of Business Administration program or go into education and maybe teach in the field. Right now I see some managers who are not motivational, and that inspires me. There is a manager who I see who is not very involved, and I want to be different from that and get everyone involved and excited, because morale at the lab is not great. If I get my business degree then I can go into management and fill the spot to become a manager and help people enjoy their jobs.

Alex does not see a manager whose behavior he wants to emulate; rather he sees a void in management and he is inspired to fill that void.

Training with coaches We seek out *coaches* when we need to focus on improving specific skills. Think about star athletes: their coaches provide very specific feedback that is essential for their performance. Because a coach can perform and recognize the level of performance you want to achieve, he or she can observe your actions and identify the critical areas in which you need improvement. He or she can then provide specific feedback in a skillful manner. Thus, the key to successful coaching is the coach's ability to create an enabling relationship with you that makes it easier for you to learn (Mink et al 1993). An effective coach helps you set and achieve performance goals at levels higher than those at which you are currently performing. Coaching is often a short-term task, involving day-to-day, hands-on involvement. Once you have practiced each component of a new skill until you have mastered it, the coach helps you put the entire sequence together. Application and reflection need to occur after each step. Working with a coach can enable you to perform new tasks, to do more than you were doing, learn something entirely different or even to perform at a higher level of complexity (Mink et al 1993).

Don, the radiation therapist whom we interviewed, has been in his current job for 2 years and has developed special skills in handling equipment. He described coaching less experienced colleagues and students. He also described some of the problems associated with effective coaching when there is a staff shortage.

> We have students all the time. I know most of the new stuff [equipment and techniques]. They always want me to teach the newer students because I am more familiar and better at it than the other people there.

> We are so busy that it is hard to slow our pace down to teach a newer person so that makes it hard. We always talk about [getting] everybody rotated so everyone can figure this out. We just do not have the time to slow down and teach everybody. Another guy and I, who learned in the beginning, were just kept on the machine for over a year, which they usually do not do.

Gaining advancement through sponsors

A *sponsor* is someone who is usually well connected among decision-makers within your organization, profession, or industry (Stevens 1995). In the course of his or her work, the sponsor has the opportunity and influence to say things about you to those in power that you cannot say yourself. This is someone who can open doors for you at work and/or within your profession. Like a role model, he or she can demonstrate how to behave as a professional in your organization, but a sponsor may also advise you in this area as well. Sometimes you will know that the sponsor is acting on your behalf, but many times this individual will speak to others about you and arrange opportunities for your development, such as adding you to committees or recommending your membership on task forces or special projects, without your knowledge of their actions. Sponsors sometimes have access to funding to support developmental opportunities outside your usual training or employment experience. For example, a sponsor may provide leave time and a travel stipend and thus facilitate your attendance at a conference or continuing education session.

Sponsors have more power within organizations than coaches, and they are motivated to perform this service for subordinates simply because they enjoy helping others or, in other cases, because they see some value for themselves or the organization as a result of your advancement. Sponsors can also be found during one's years of training. *Lisa,* our 23-year-old occupational therapist, found that faculty members in her bachelor degree program fostered her participation in local and regional professional organizations. Additionally, her program director allocated funds for student society representatives to attend the national conferences:

> As a junior in the occupational therapy program I was allowed the experience of working as a student liaison officer between our university's program and the state Occupational Therapy Association. That was a phenomenal experience because it allowed me a first look at the organization and at how occupational therapists can really promote this profession. I am also a member of the national organization, and that has afforded me the opportunity to go to several meetings that were held in a nearby city and talk with therapists who were working on a variety of studies. I watched them in action as therapists who were interested in promoting their profession and involved in the legal side of the organization. How do we promote the organization and have more therapists join? I had never thought about that. It really stressed to me the importance of organizations in terms of their promotion of the various health practitioners and how important that is.

Relating to mentors

As mentioned earlier, traditionally mentors are senior colleagues who provide support, direction, and feedback regarding career plans and personal development for less experienced junior colleagues, termed protégés, in the context of an intense interpersonal exchange (Russell and Adams 1997). This relationship is not seen as one-sided. It is built on the needs of both participants and both parties benefit. Protégés receive opportunities to learn and advance within their profession and connect with powerful and influential people. They learn how to work closely and effectively in collegial relationships and how to build their network of professional colleagues. While the protégé gains knowledge, skill, and confidence from working with the mentor, the mentor profits as well. Benefits include enhanced self-esteem through the recognition that comes as a result of being chosen to develop a more junior professional and enhanced status in the organization; revitalized interest in work through interacting with the protégé around professional topics and issues; satisfaction with the close relationship that can develop with the protégé; and fulfillment of one's own developmental needs for having an influence on the next generation (Murray 1991). Particular satisfaction can be prompted when questions posed by the protégé result in personal insights for the mentor that are only realized when the protégé's needs call them forth (Shea 1999).

Mary, the physical therapist who has been working for about a year, was fortunate to find a supervisor who acted as a role model, a coach, and a mentor.

> One of the supervisors that I work with was previously a team leader. She has been at the hospital for 9–10 years. She is one of my mentors. She sets a good example. She is always seeing patients and helping other teams out. She works weekends even though she does not have to. When I had my first students, she offered to help and be there to give advice. We sat down before they came and talked about ideas and she

Case study	*A reflection on the benefits of being a mentor*
	In my experience, the benefits of mentoring someone often come later, as we may be most effective when we are least aware of it. Early in my career, I taught a bright, enthusiastic student whom I supervised on her fieldwork placement at the hospital where I worked. Several years later, I met her at a conference. She had relocated to another country, now had a Master's degree, and planned to study for her Doctorate. I was delighted when she said that I had inspired her academic career by my early involvement in clinical research. We became friends and have collaborated on several projects and continue to do so. This is despite the fact that, 20 years on, we still have not managed to spend more than 2 months together in the same country!

gave me her suggestions. She is a mentor for me and also somebody that I want to be like, because she is very effective in what she does. She is a motivator, a good person to learn from and someone who I would like to be like. What I have been working on now is becoming confident in the intensive care unit. We have a list of competencies that we read through about using different equipment and what to be aware of in the unit. This supervisor and I have been going to the intensive care unit every opportunity we have, which has been good for me. We can treat patients together until I am ready for her to observe me and give feedback. Eventually I will be confident to treat more critically ill patients.

Initiating and maintaining effective mentoring-type relationships

Throughout your lifetime, your constellation of developers will include peers, role models, coaches, sponsors, and, in longer-term and more intense relationships, mentors. These individuals provide both career advice and emotional support. As mentioned earlier, we are using the term 'mentor' in a generic sense to refer to the continuum of individuals with whom you as a protégé can create short- or long-term developmental relationships.

Choosing a mentor

As you consider possible mentors, think of the individuals you admire and respect. As you consider each individual, ask yourself, 'Does this person believe in me? Can this person guide me as I move forward in my personal life and in my career?' You should be able to share your vision with a mentor and partner with him or her as you determine a path for reaching that vision. Your mentor needs to be a skilled listener who can clearly understand your current situation and also can frame your current experience in the bigger picture of your career path. A good mentor provides a mirror for you that extends your self-awareness so that you see yourself in new ways (Noe 1988). He or she expresses positive expectations for you and promotes your self-confidence. At the same time, a mentor must feel comfortable in challenging you to perform at your best and be able to provide accurate and supportive feedback when you stumble.

Our physical therapist, *Mary*, was fortunate to be mentored by one of her clinical instructors during her training:

> The physical therapist who influenced me the most was my clinical instructor with my last affiliation before I graduated. She helped me set realistic goals and focus on the areas I needed more exposure to. She helped me with clinical decision-making and she also showed me how to make therapy fun and functional at the same time. She taught me to approach each patient individually. Her guidance, example, and way of thinking were wonderful. She was open to communication and receptive to my feedback. She helped me develop my skills so that I was ready, and really felt ready, to practice on my own. She had the skills, knowledge, and experience to help me increase my confidence. She not only had skills as a role model and physical therapist, but she could also communicate; she was able to teach. I have maintained a relationship with her since then because we work in the same system. I have seen her through work-related activities, and I have also spoken with her and stopped by to see her to find out what is new and tell her what is going on. She has always made me feel like a colleague.

Characteristics that mentors of our interviewees share include commitment to and belief in their protégés, honesty regarding their skills and potential, and ability to coach the protégés to improve performance and progress along a productive and satisfying career path. Our beginning practitioners share some characteristics as protégés, too. They respect their mentors, are committed to their own professional development, are conscientious in working toward improvement, and appreciate their mentors.

Initiating a mentoring relationship

In some cases, people in your network who would like to mentor you will directly approach you because they see you as someone they would like to develop. If you work effectively, supervisors who can extend your opportunities to advance may note this. This situation is the ideal, but it may not occur. Do not wait for people to come to you; you can also approach potential mentors on your own or through an introduction by someone else. You might say, 'I have observed you for some time and I respect and look up to you. I am interested in developing in one [or some] of the areas that I've noticed you are really good at, and I am wondering if you would consider talking with me about establishing a mentoring relationship'. Many people are delighted to be approached as possible mentors and will agree. Others who are also interested may realize that their current time commitments preclude their working with you at this time. If so, you could ask them to reconnect with you at a time that is better for them. In cases in which you have a specific need that can be best addressed by working with a certain individual, Morahan (2000b) suggests that practitioners approach the potential mentor with a specific, time-limited request. For example, 'I am impressed with how you so effectively handle multiple, important projects simultaneously. Can you show me how you do it? I expect that I would need a few meetings, with me asking you for suggestions and then for feedback as I try out your advice'.

Conducting the mentoring relationship

As you begin working together, it is wise to establish and clarify roles and expectations so that both mentor and protégé agree on the purpose of your relationship and how you will work together. For example, you may start with a question such as, 'How will we both know that this relationship has been successful? What specific outcomes or accomplishments are we working toward?' Ask the mentor which communication method he or she prefers: face-to-face, telephone or e-mail, and decide how often each kind of communication should take place. You may also discuss confidentiality, the degree to which the discussions you have with each other are to be kept private. More specific details need to be established, too, such as: How often will you meet? For how long? Where? When? What will we do if a meeting must be canceled? Be certain that you each have the information you need so that you can contact one another in such a case. Finally, what do you expect will be the duration of your mentoring relationship? This will depend on what you expect to accomplish. Share goals and objectives from your career development plan that you would like to work on and determine which will be the focus of this relationship. In some cases a few meetings will suffice; in other cases a long-term commitment of a year or more can be negotiated.

To get the most out of each contact with your mentor, you will find it helpful to prepare goals or objectives for your sessions. To keep this list up to date, keep a running list of items to be covered with the mentor. During the time between your sessions, add issues or questions that arise. There may be a project you are working on about which you would like guidance. Or you may face a decision about which your mentor can provide a perspective. Because of his or her experience, the mentor will likely be much more able than you to see the larger context of your work and decisions.

At the beginning of each meeting, after some personal interaction, agree with your mentor on an agenda for the session. You will have one or more items you wish to discuss, and your mentor may add one or more, as well. If the list is long, prioritize what you want to be sure to accomplish during this meeting and what can be postponed, if necessary. Establish an ending time for the meeting if that is not already clear. Then discuss the items on your agenda point by point. Ask for information and advice, and also, ask for and be receptive to honest feedback about the knowledge, skills, and attitudes that you are developing with the help of the mentor. You need to know what current strategies are working for you and those that will benefit from change. After discussing each item, determine what you will be working on, if applicable, between this session and the next. Early in your relationship, it is a good idea to start modestly with manageable tasks that you both agree can be accomplished in the short term. Summarize orally at the end of the session what you have discussed and agreed to. Finally, on a regular basis, close your session with a question such as, 'Is there anything else you can provide feedback or advice about that I have not brought up?' This provides an opening for the mentor to comment on observations he or she may have made but has not had the opportunity to bring to your attention, or it may prompt the mentor to provide an additional opportunity for your growth.

As soon as possible after your meeting, schedule time for reflection. You want to maximize your gain from the session. You might answer questions such as: 'What did I learn today?' 'How can I apply this during the time before my next meeting with my mentor, so that I can update him or her about my growth, or ask for more assistance?' If your mentor agrees, follow up in writing with a summary of the meeting, including commitments you each made. This can be a basis for the agenda for your next meeting. An additional way to reinforce your learning is to share new ideas with a friend or colleague. The discussion will crystallize your thoughts and may also benefit your friend or colleague.

As your sessions progress, monitor the progress you are making toward the goals you set for this relationship. As you move toward meeting those goals, you can decide with your mentor to end the relationship or to continue and to work on additional development. When the relationship does end, be certain to thank the mentor. Writing a letter is an especially good way of conveying your appreciation. Not only will mentors appreciate your time and effort, but also they may find such letters to be valuable in documenting their own work to current and future employers.

In some cases, mentoring relationships that appeared to have good potential run into difficulties. A recent study (Eby et al 2000) described the responses of 156 individuals who reported having been protégés on an average of between three and four developmental relationships over the course of their careers. All had participated in at least one positive mentoring relationship. However, more than half reported at least one negative relationship. Reasons cited for classifying the experience as negative included:

1. poor matching of the mentor and protégé with respect to values, work style or personality
2. distancing behavior on the part of the mentor in the form of neglect, self-absorption or intentional exclusion
3. manipulative behavior, including tyranny and inappropriate delegation of the mentor's work
4. politicking, including sabotaging, taking credit for the protégé's work or being deceitful
5. incompetence, either interpersonally or technically, and dysfunctionality, meaning that the mentor had a bad attitude or was suffering from personal problems that interfered with the mentoring relationship.

These researchers recommend that you choose your mentors carefully, with an understanding of the potential mentor's motivations and true interest in developing you. Interacting with prospective mentors informally before committing to a mentoring relationship may help you to understand whether or not there appears to be a good match between the two of you. Working with multiple mentors both within and outside your organization is recommended, as well. Having more than one mentor within your employment organization may help you determine multiple ways of resolving conflicts between your own goals and those of your organization, and a number of contacts can increase your knowledge of possible career moves within your organization (Baugh and Scandura 1999). Related to this topic, it is important that you do not give up your responsibility for making your own decisions. This is your career, and no one will have more at stake than you. Your aims in a mentoring relationship are:

1. not to please your mentor but to learn from him or her
2. not to hide mistakes but to learn from them
3. not to conceal information but to share it
4. not to be protected but to be encouraged to take new risks (Noe 1988).

While there can be many reasons for a relationship to fail, once you notice that things are not working out, it is wise to take steps either to fix the relationship or to end it. You might consider asking another colleague for advice in confidence as you decide how to proceed.

The protégé can also create problems in a mentoring relationship. When a group of advanced practitioners talk about their current and past protégés, there are the success stories and enriched relationships that we are all pleased about. But, we also tell other stories. For example, there are times when we went out of our way to set up a meeting for a young colleague with someone we knew who was ready to assist him or her, but the protégé missed the meeting. Other times we have spent hours reviewing an article for a less experienced colleague who wanted to submit it to a professional journal, only to find that the person did not bother making the revisions. Make sure you do not miss future opportunities by shutting doors that were held open for you. We also think that sometimes people may be unrealistically concerned about not being 'used', and may be reluctant to do extra work when asked by their boss, or supervisor. Think carefully in order to determine whether you are really being exploited, that is, not given credit for your work, or whether by doing extra work you are in fact learning new skills and also building up your 'emotional bank account', thus investing in your future.

Some thoughts on mentoring and fee-for-service

In our discussion thus far in this chapter and in the literature that describes the mentor–protégé relationship, there seems to be an understanding that this is a voluntary professional service on the part of the mentor, and that your role is to respect the time and knowledge that your more experienced mentor is sharing. In contrast, however, in certain recent instances, mentoring has been offered in a fee-for-service arrangement. An example is Mentorlink, a funded program implemented by a group of occupational therapists, and managed by the professional organization, OT Australia-Victoria. Mentorlink's nine-member project management team offers courses for both mentors and mentees (*AAOT News* 2000a, b). The process involves a written mentoring/supervision agreement, and also offers a sample form for record keeping. Mentorlink has developed software in a CD format and provides a networking system that links individuals who wish to be mentors or mentees. These are all fee-based services. The definition of mentoring on which this project is predicated is as follows: 'Mentoring is the process whereby two occupational therapists, who have been deliberately matched, have regular dialogue on a range of issues with the agreed upon goal of having the lesser experienced/skilled occupational therapist grow, develop and address career development, where desired' (Marais-Styrdom 1999, cited in *AAOT News* 2000a, p 6). During 2002/2003 the OT Australia Mentorlink program was extended to encompass physiotherapists and podiatrists. There are plans to extend the program to other health professionals (AusOTNews 2002).

When a fee-for-service is introduced, the dynamics of the mentoring relationship will be changed. It may not be appropriate to call the less experienced person a protégé, and the term used is *mentee*. We believe that such programs as Mentorlink may be more like an organized supervision/counseling program than mentoring as described in this chapter. It also seems to be akin to the relatively new field of 'life coaching'. Yousey (2001), who works in private practice as a life coach, describes her work as 'helping clients clarify what matters most to them, measure where they are in relation to their goals, and take action to bridge the gap' (p 12). You may wish to explore employing such a paid coach at some point in your career, and some web-sites to assist you in such an exploration are included in the resources list at the end of this chapter.

Conclusion

You can accelerate your career growth and increase your personal and professional satisfaction by consciously focusing on building a network of colleagues from which you can choose potential mentors. Techniques suggested in this chapter and available from recommended resources can assist you to create, maintain, and assess the relationships you develop with colleagues. While such relationships serve a number of important functions with respect to career advancement, successful mentoring experiences can result in rewarding personal relationships that can last a lifetime. Both the mentor and protégé can achieve positive outcomes as a result of their work together. The mentor can take pride in success with helping a less experienced colleague to develop. The protégé likely will experience increased confidence and self-esteem resulting from the competence gained by working with the mentor. While you may benefit from mentors throughout your lifetime, in the near future, and perhaps even now, you yourself can serve as a mentor and gain the satisfaction of developing others.

Activities for further development

1. Contact two or three professionals whose work you respect and ask them to relate examples of their approaches to and experiences with networking as a career advancement strategy. Based on their responses and the advice provided in this chapter, what conclusions can you draw? List some networking strategies that can benefit you within the next 6–12 months. Share your results with current colleagues.

2. Reflect upon the colleagues in your current network. Are there peers with whom you could initiate a reciprocal coaching arrangement? Are there co-workers or professional colleagues a step or two ahead of you whom you could approach as mentors? Set a goal of establishing one or two such relationships within the next 6 months. Create your plan, including a method for tracking your progress, in your journal and share it with one or two colleagues. Plan to discuss what you learn with each other so that each of you can benefit not only from your own experience but also from the experiences of others.

3. Research the local, regional, national, and international professional organizations related to your current work. Have you joined the organizations that may prove most helpful to you in the near future? Do you have plans to attend meetings of these groups in order to network with new colleagues as well as to update your knowledge? Explore joining a special interest group, committee, or other section within a professional group in which you can begin to make a contribution and relate with colleagues beyond those with whom you regularly interact.

References

Australian Association of Occupational Therapists News 2000a Feature: mentoring and supervision. AAOT News 7:6–7

Australian Association of Occupational Therapists News 2000b Mentoring and supervision: elements of best practice. AAOT News 10:7–11

AusOTNews 2002 Victorian Mentorlink program extended. Australian Association of Occupational Therapists 9:7.

Baugh S G, Scandura T A 1999 The effect of multiple mentors on protégé attitudes toward the work setting. Journal of Social Behaviour and Personality 14:503–521

Eby L T, McManus S E, Simon S A, Russell JEA 2000 The protégé's perspective regarding negative mentoring experiences: the development of a taxonomy. Journal of Vocational Behaviour 57:1–21

Higgins M C, Kram K E 2001 Reconceptualizing mentoring at work: a developmental network perspective. Academy of Management Review 26:264–288

Horgan D D 1992 Multiple mentoring: all of the gain; none of the pain. Performance and Instruction July: 20–22

Koberg C S, Boss R W, Goodman E 1998 Factors and outcomes associated with mentoring among health-care professionals. Journal of Vocational Behaviour 53:58–72

Kram K E 1983 Phases of the mentor relationship. Academy of Management Journal 26:608–625

Kram K E 1985 Mentoring at work: developmental relationships in organizational life. Scott Foresman, Glenview, IL

Malugani M 2001 The importance of networking in healthcare: who you know may be as important as what you know. Online. Available at: http://healthcare.monster.com/articles/mentor. Accessed 30 May 2002

Miller N 1989 Personal experience, adult learning, and social research: developing a sociological imagination in and beyond the T-group. PhD thesis. School of Education, University of Manchester, Manchester, UK

Mink O G, Owen K Q, Mink B P 1993 Developing high-performance people: the art of coaching. Perseus Books, Reading, MA

Morahan P S 2000a How to be your own best mentor. SELAM News 3:13–14

Morahan P 2000b How to find and be your own best mentor. Academic Physician and Scientist November/December, 8

Murphy S E, Ensher J C 2001 The role of mentoring support and self-management strategies on reported career outcomes. Journal of Career Development 27:229–246

Murray M 1991 Beyond the myths and magic of mentoring: how to facilitate an effective mentoring program. Jossey Bass, San Francisco

Noe R 1988 Women and mentoring: a review and research agenda. Academy of Management Review 13:65–68

Russell J E A, Adams D M 1997 The changing nature of mentoring in organizations: an introduction to the special issue on mentoring in organizations. Journal of Vocational Behavior 51:1–14

Shea G F 1999 Making the most of being mentored: how to grow from a mentoring partnership. Crisp, Menlo Park, CA

Young A M, Perrewé P L 2000 What did you expect? An examination of career-related support and social support among mentors and protégés. Journal of Management 26: 611–632

Yousey J 2001 Life coaching. A one-on-one approach to changing lives. OT Practice 6:11–14

Further reading

Bolton E B 1980 A conceptual analysis of the mentor relationship in the career development of women. Adult Education 30:195–207

Covey S, Merrill A R, Merrill R R 1994 First things first. Simon and Schuster, New York

Ham J. 2001 As a support worker how do you undertake CPD? Occupational Therapy News 91:18

Jeruchim J, Shapiro P 1992 Women, mentors, and success. New York, Fawcett Columbine

Lacey K 1999 Making mentoring happen. Business and Professional Publishing, Warriewood, NSW, Australia

McMeekin G 2000 The 12 secrets of highly creative women. A portable mentor. Conari Press, Berkeley, CA

Parker M 1990 Creating shared vision: the story of a pioneering approach to organizational revitalization. Dialog International, Clarendon Hills, IL

Parnaby S 2001 Investing in a portfolio. Occupational Therapy News 9:11, 16

Phillips-Jones L 2001 The new mentors and protégés: how to succeed with the new mentoring partnerships. Coalition of Counseling Centers/The Mentoring Group, Grass Valley, CA

Senge P M, Kleiner A, Roberts C, Ross R B, Smith B J 1994 The fifth discipline fieldbook: strategies and tools for building a learning organization. Currency Doubleday, New York

Stevens P 1995 How to network and select a mentor. Resource Publications, California, USA

Wellington S 2001 Be your own mentor: strategies from top women on the secrets of success. Random House, New York

Zachary L J 2000 The mentor's guide: facilitating effective learning relationships. Jossey-Bass, San Francisco

Web-based resources

Australian Mentorlink Program: see OT Australia website	www.ausot.com.au
Coach University 800-48COACH	www.coachu.com http://healthcare.monster.com
International Coaching Federation (ICF) 888-ICF-3131	www.coachfederation.org
Mentoring Group Worldwide Mentoring	www.mentoringgroup.com/
Mentoring Institute Inc.	www.mentorin-u.com
National Mentoring Center	www.nwrel.org/mentoring

The leading edge of competence: developing your potential for advanced practice

Auldeen Alsop

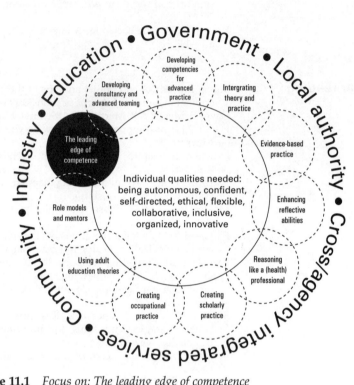

Figure 11.1 *Focus on: The leading edge of competence*

Chapter outline

This chapter takes a systematic approach to enhancing your understanding of continuing professional development (CPD). It introduces some definitions of CPD and outlines the stance now taken by many statutory or professional bodies with regard to competence maintenance. The chapter engages with the debates about competence and ethical practice, and elaborates on how your own competence and potential as a professional can be enhanced for advanced practice. The skills needed for learning are outlined as an essential feature of competence and its development. Your responsibilities as a practitioner to advance both your own professional skills and the profession itself are also addressed. Guidance is offered on ways in which you might achieve and maintain the status of an advanced practitioner and present the evidence of your accomplishments and learning in portfolio form.

Key words

Continuing professional development (CPD), competence, career development, portfolio

Anticipated outcomes

As a result of reading this chapter I anticipate that you will be able to:

- recognize the expectations of healthcare professionals with regard to CPD
- develop your potential as an advanced practitioner
- take steps to initiate your personal and professional development activity
- prepare a portfolio of evidence of your professional development.

Introduction

Everyone has the potential to develop. Attaining your qualification to practise in one of the healthcare professions exemplifies this. Your professional qualification confirms your ability to learn, to understand and to apply new specialist knowledge in a practice situation and to work therapeutically with different people who experience a wide range of health-related problems in their lives. The professional qualification you have also confirms your capacity to collaborate with your peers and to provide a sound, coordinated service to patients, clients and service users, in a range of organizational settings. It is important, in the first instance, to recognize this as a major personal achievement, and then to acknowledge that it is possible for this achievement to be extended in order to advance practice in both a personal and professional capacity. In this chapter I address ways in which you might recognize that potential and ensure that it flourishes.

Developing the ability to offer and provide best practice in healthcare should be an aspiration of each practitioner. It is a duty normally made explicit in professional codes of ethics and conduct, although it is anticipated that most professionals would expect to work in that way regardless of a written code. In many respects, best practice might be considered as a process as well as an aspiration and goal. It involves investigation, action, reflection, challenge to assumptions and change in behaviour. It is a process that entails constantly updating knowledge and refining practice in the light of experience and learning. For the practitioner, this represents a process of ongoing learning; for the public it represents confidence in being able to access appropriate, and up to date healthcare.

As illustrated in Chapter 1, practice has to change over time. There is no option. Contexts and environments in which health and social care are delivered change to reflect new professional, political, environmental, sociological and technological influences and each health practitioner must adjust practice accordingly. This involves being alert to changing circumstances and taking steps to maintain a level of competence that reflects contemporary need. It may involve keeping up to date with research findings and ensuring that they are evaluated for their usefulness in local practice, as described in Chapter 4. It may involve making modifications to practice in order to accommodate changes in other professionals' procedures, skills or availability. It may involve embracing new structures and organizational arrangements that demand a review of the behaviour that previously constituted professional practice in a given context. If you reflect back now to when you first qualified, it is almost certain that you will notice that practice has changed over time, even if you only qualified fairly recently.

Becoming an advanced practitioner, however, will make additional demands that will take you beyond the realm of merely remaining competent in a changing world. It will demand energy and a commitment to developing your potential to a different level. Initially it may be personally challenging for you, but it may ultimately bring you rewards and will almost certainly afford you an enormous sense of personal achievement and satisfaction.

For some practitioners, developing expertise in practice may be a natural progression occurring through hard work, through paying attention to detail, through reflecting on performance and modifying practice to accommodate insights from reflective experiences and from being proactive in novel and changing situations. But this needs to be recognized as professional development stemming from naturally occurring opportunities in the practice arena. This activity can make a significant contribution to your capacity to engage in advanced practice, but is unlikely, on its own, to lead to you becoming an advanced practitioner. Becoming an advanced practitioner means taking purposeful steps in career-planning, goal setting and in engaging in activity that will ensure your self-development and personal and professional growth over time. Ways to do this were discussed in Chapter 2 in particular, and elsewhere, as in chapters 7, 9 and 10. The coming sections in this chapter will address issues related to competence, your continuing professional education and development, and ways in which evidence of your development can be presented in portfolio form.

Lifelong learning

The notion of lifelong learning appears now to be readily accepted across the professions as a global phenomenon that has benefits for everybody. Lifelong learning principles stem from the concept of learning throughout the lifespan, not only as a need to secure the skills for seeking and continuing employment in a world of constant change, but also as a form of self-fulfilment and emancipation. The urge to learn and to be a master of our environment can lead to better control of our lives, the ability to make more informed decisions about our future and to having choice about how we engage in a working society.

Lifelong learning in a professional sense is also the responsibility of any practitioner, particularly those engaged in delivering a service within a health and social care system because of the responsibilities invested in those professionals. Those of us who practise as healthcare professionals have a duty to remain up to date and to deliver best practice that embraces ethical considerations of safe and effective practice for our clients. Our practice also impinges on our relationship with others with whom we work, so that teamwork, teaching and leadership also reflect best practice, and practice that evolves and improves over time through collaboration, dialogue and forms of inquiry. For those engaged in developing advanced practice skills, the concept of lifelong learning will need to be specifically targeted so that personal and professional qualities and skills are enhanced to meet the expanding and changing demands of contemporary practice.

There are various landmarks within a professional career and the first is that of attaining competence to practise in one's chosen profession. Competence on qualification serves as the foundation on which professional development takes place. This includes maintaining competence to practise and then developing breadth and depth of knowledge and skills to extend practice, to become a specialist in practice and to gain promotion. Each role within your profession and within your employing organization will make particular demands of you and you have a duty to ensure that you can continue to meet these demands as circumstances change. If you are seeking new challenges in terms of an extended role, a change in role or a new role on promotion, then efforts need to be made through the processes of life-long learning to prepare for these challenges. In each role, the elements of competence will be different according to the demands of the job and judgements about continuing competence will take these into consideration. The role of advanced practitioner will have particular requirements that span clinical practice, clinical leadership, research and education. The combined skills of these roles will contribute to competence in advanced practice.

Competence

Competence to practise in the profession of our choice is confirmed at the point of qualification. A structured, accredited program of professional education will have been completed and the newly qualified practitioner will be deemed to possess the qualities and characteristics of a competent professional. Eraut (1998, p. 129) offered a definition of competence as 'the ability to perform tasks and roles to the expected standard'. Those setting and judging that standard, however, have to be determined. Hager and Gonczi (1996) saw competence more specifically as a complex structuring of attributes needed for intelligent performance in specific situations, incorporating the idea of professional judgement. The context in which the tasks and roles are performed thus influences the performance so that, when the context changes, so does the nature of competence in that setting (Hollis 1997). Change occurs in the form of new developments, shifts in thinking and moves into new contexts of practice that constantly affect the way in which professionals work, and thus challenge a state of competence (Alsop 2001a). Sound professional judgements can therefore only be made if a practitioner remains alert to changing circumstances and engages in necessary professional updating. Improving and developing competence for advanced practice has to stem from a firm foundation of competent performance.

In order to progress towards acquiring a level of competence expected of an advanced practitioner it is necessary to have some concept of what advanced practice requires. Many references to these requirements are contained in this book. One summary might be that advanced practice requires:

- refined levels of critical thinking
- a sound theoretical understanding of practice in an area of special-ization, including knowledge of the evidence base for practice
- significant breadth and depth of knowledge, and higher-level clini-cal, research and/or technical skills in a particular area of practice
- well-developed skills of teamwork and clinical leadership
- sophisticated learning skills and the ability to examine and evaluate personal effectiveness
- an ongoing commitment to engaging in continuing education and professional development
- a commitment to advancing professional practice through inquiry and publication
- a commitment to the development of others through leadership, teaching, supervision, mentorship, professional dialogue and debate.

In summary, it can be seen that there is a wide range of responsibility associated with advanced practitioner status. Acquiring the necessary qualities means developing not only practice skills but also personal and interpersonal skills, and skills of learning, critical thinking, lead-ership, evaluation and research. Hidden in these responsibilities is also a requirement to be able to discriminate. Certainly, building on existing knowledge and developing new knowledge are crucial to remaining competent and to developing further competence as an advanced practitioner. However retaining obsolete knowledge is impractical (Eraut 1994). Skills of discrimination and judgement are needed in order to assess the relevance and currency of knowledge. For, as Barnett (1997) advised, discarding outdated knowledge and embracing new concepts are essential for accommodating change.

As an advanced practitioner, you will become a model and a resource for others. Therefore your professional development needs to be wide-ranging, in order that you may gain confidence as an expert in your area of practice, competence as a clinical leader and credibility as an advanced practitioner. This may seem a daunting prospect but acquiring skills is not going to happen overnight. This confidence, competence and credibility will develop over time, given a commit-ment to advancing your own expertise and to advancing professional practice.

Advancing your expertise: continuing professional development

Crist et al (1998) considered professional competence to be the out-come of thoughtful, self-directed professional activities that are shaped through careful evaluation of one's current knowledge, skills, abilities and individual learning needs in relation to future career and employment responsibilities. Codes of ethics and professional con-duct make it clear that the responsibilities of each practitioner include engaging in activity that ensures continuing competence to practise in the professional arena in which he or she works. This would normally demand a fairly systematic and regular approach to reviewing your personal competence in relation to your practice responsibilities and to establishing and pursuing a professional development plan in order to ensure your continuing currency of knowledge and skills in the workplace. Formal systems of appraisal or performance review might be avenues through which your professional needs are identified and your development plans are agreed with your line manager. This could be more difficult for you if you are working in an environment where such systems do not operate. You will still have a professional duty to maintain up-to-date practice but may not have the support for making this happen. However, you will still need to take steps to remain competent. This places a key responsibility on you to identify your learning and development needs, and plans and to make arrangements for achieving them.

CPD may take many forms, as will be discussed later, but the underpinning responsibility is for all practitioners to engage in some form of development at least to remain up-to-date in practice. This is the minimum required to sustain ongoing 'best practice' in line with contemporary standards of care delivery. This may demand not only the development of your professional knowledge and skills but also the evidence base for the practice in which you engage.

Therefore this is the baseline from which anyone seeking to develop advanced practice must work. It is the foundation for a more advanced, planned program of development activity that is going to extend knowledge and skills, and deepen understanding of practice in a personally selected and clearly defined area.

CPD has been variously defined. The definition now adopted by all the 'allied' health professionals in the UK, as stated in their CPD Strategy for the Professions Allied to Medicine consensus statement (1999, p. 8), is:

> the systematic maintenance, improvement and broadening of knowledge and skills and the development of personal qualities necessary for the execution of professional and technical duties throughout the practitioner's working life.

This is not a universally accepted definition. The Canadian Association of Occupational Therapists (2001), for example, refers to continuing professional education as that which allows therapists to remain abreast of current information, avoid information obsolescence and to provide an improved service to the public. It is said to assist individuals to maintain and increase competence in the rapidly changing fields of health and social service. Another view from Eraut (1994) maintained that CPD embraced continuing professional education. However, it could be argued that both development and education involve learning that will necessarily be at the root of any practitioner's ongoing ability to practise competently over time.

As outlined below, new legislative requirements for the state registration of health professionals in the UK have strengthened the need for the professions to agree a definition of CPD and to work towards establishing a national, inter-professional scheme for CPD that will meet with the approval of the new regulatory Health Professions Council in the UK. It is anticipated that evidence of CPD will eventually become mandatory for re-registration. Regulatory requirements in other countries such as Australia, Canada, New Zealand and the USA are all different, as has been illustrated in Chapter 1. In some countries, it is the professional body rather than a statutory body that dictates the terms of the CPD programs and monitors their execution.

UK policies

A series of documents has recently been published in the UK that set out the agenda for CPD in support of the government's quality improvement programme for the National Health Service (NHS). *Continuing Professional Development: Quality in the New NHS* (Department of Health 1999) provided details of the government's vision of CPD and summarized its intentions with regard to implementing CPD frameworks that aim to improve the quality of healthcare. *A First Class Service: Quality in the New NHS* (Department of Health 1998) had earlier established the government's plans for improving standards of healthcare delivery through a range of measures that addressed organizational, team and individual activity. This document (p. 42) provided a definition of CPD as:

> a process of lifelong learning for all individuals and teams which meets the needs of patients and delivers the health outcomes and healthcare priorities of the NHS and which enables professionals to expand and fulfil their potential.

Clearly, professional development was to be targeted specifically to address shortcomings and development needs, and to enable the NHS to meet its obligations to patients. Responsibility was to be placed on both individuals and organizations to ensure that professionals had the relevant knowledge and skills to deliver healthcare to the standards required.

The career aspirations of 'allied' health professionals were not to be ignored either, as the government then published its strategy for these professions (Department of Health 2000). This document sets out proposals for developing the leadership skills of a range of professionals operating at all organizational levels in the NHS and for creating consultant therapist posts by 2004. This document provided the impetus for promoting advanced-level practice. By 2001, new frameworks had also been proposed (Department of Health 2001) for the regulation of health professionals and the establishment of a Health Professions Council to complement the Nursing and Midwifery Council, which was also in formation.

Experiences in Australia and New Zealand

Current work in Australia undertaken by Susan Nancarrow and Julie Clark (work in progress) has sought to review systems used by various health and social care professions to assure standards of performance. This work has yet to be published but identified that, for all the professions examined (dietetics, occupational therapy, physiotherapy, podiatry, social work, speech pathology), the entry-level qualification to the profession was a Bachelor's degree. However, not all members of the different professions were required to be registered; the geographical area of their work often dictated whether this was a requirement. Of these professions, some had more advanced schemes for professional development than others, and there appeared to be no common currency of credit awarded across the different professions for development activity. The definition of accreditation used to assess the requirements was drawn from the International Society for Quality in Health Care, as cited by Tregloan (2000, p. 1).

> Accreditation is a self-assessment and external peer review process used by healthcare organizations to accurately assess their level of performance in relation to established standards and to implement ways to continuously improve the healthcare system.

Three broad themes relating to professional development were perceived as common across the different professions: continuing education, professional participation, and quality assurance. These themes provide helpful groupings of CPD activity, as follows:

- Continuing education includes attendance at conferences, education or training events and post-graduate study, publishing and presenting original work, undertaking research and reading discipline specific literature.
- Professional participation involves non-academic contributions to the profession through membership of boards or associations, mentoring and undertaking community service activities such as public lectures.
- Quality assurance activity includes, for example, audit, evaluating patient satisfaction, participating in a trial of a new product and peer review.

Hocking (1998) described the Cornerstone Programme in New Zealand that identified similar categories for occupational therapists to use when providing evidence in portfolios of ongoing competence to practise (Alsop 1998).

It is important to be aware of the regulatory, and accreditation systems in the country in which you work. Any development activity undertaken to advance practice may need to be recorded in a particular format or produced within a particular timeframe in order to demonstrate ongoing or developing competence in an area of practice.

The process of continuing professional development

As described in earlier work (Alsop 2000), CPD can take a number of forms. Essentially the process of CPD is much the same as any other process designed to bring about change and improvement as a process, or in the level of knowledge and capacity that is needed for its advanced practice. The CPD process, like the therapeutic process, or audit process, involves:

- assessing need
- defining goals
- planning to attain the goals
- implementing the plan
- evaluating the effectiveness of the process
- reviewing need and redefining the plan.

The most important requirement for developing the potential for advanced practice is having clarity of vision and direction. It is important to know the overall goal, even if the process of achieving it cannot be described. This is a professional journey leading to a high level of competence in a personally selected aspect of professional practice, where you will be known and regarded as having an extended, higher level of skill, than practitioners who have not developed in this area. You will have gained expertise in a combination of skills and techniques and be able to apply them in various contexts of practice. To achieve this, you need to think about where and how the relevant knowledge and skills might best be developed. For example:

- Will it be through continuing professional education leading to a higher academic award where others verify your knowledge and capacity to apply it to practice?
- Will it be through a carefully planned, systematic program of self-development using a variety of learning strategies, including learning from experience, where you, yourself, evaluate your personal progress towards this goal?
- Will it be a combination of both?

Academic awards

One particular question to ask yourself is: how important is it for the development of your higher-level knowledge and skills for advanced practice to be externally accredited A whole set of subsidiary questions that follow will help you to decide and plan:

- Do you need the academic award as evidence that you have attained a particular level of functioning?
- Do you need an advanced qualification to advance your career? To what extent will it help you in the future?
- Is there a local or national expectation that an advanced practitioner will have a Master's degree or other similar qualification?
- Do you, or would you, enjoy the academic challenge of study and all that it involves in terms of time commitments, meeting deadlines, addressing assessment criteria?
- On completion, will there still be gaps in your knowledge or experience that you will need to address?

If you refer to other chapters, particularly Chapter 2, you will see that you bring self-knowledge to this decision-making process. There are many higher degrees available at institutions all over the world from which to select the most appropriate to meet your needs. Higher degrees can focus on an area of profession-specific practice (e.g. sports medicine, hand therapy), a particular discipline (e.g. neurosciences, behavioural or social sciences), a clinical issue (e.g. health promotion,) a client group (e.g. older people, paediatrics), a context of practice (e.g. forensic services, intermediate or primary care) or an approach to practice (e.g. psychosocial interventions). There are also certificates, diplomas and degrees or equivalent awards available in subjects such as health service management, clinical leadership, research methodology, education and many more topics that would be suitable for those wishing to develop as advanced practitioners.

Distance learning now offers far wider scope than in the past and opens up many avenues of study at home, or abroad for those whose learning style and familiarity with information technology allow them to feel comfortable with this mode of learning. There is opportunity to work in one state or country and study in another. Countries such as Canada, Australia and the UK offer well-established programs through distance learning. For example, Dalhousie University in Halifax, Nova Scotia, the University of South Australia and the University of Exeter offer such programs where you can learn with a program based in a country other than your own.

It is also possible to participate in academic schemes delivered across two or more institutions or countries, for example the European Master's program (Runge et al 2000). Credit accumulation and transfer schemes (CATS) offer you the potential to negotiate your own, tailor-made, education program comprising units from a number of institutions in order to develop your expertise in a particular area. Accreditation of experiential learning from practice may also make a contribution to the credit requirements for a particular award.

University prospectuses and searches on the Internet provide the starting point for discovering what educational opportunities exist locally or at a distance that might go some way towards meeting your needs. As outlined in Chapter 2, in assessing your needs you need to take account of issues relating to learning styles and preferences, and to your ability, in order to access the programs of your choice. You should give considerable thought to how you like to learn. For example, ask yourself:

- Do I prefer to learn alone or with others?
- Do I need regular face-to-face contact with a tutor/instructor?
- Do I wish to study full time or part time?
- Do I prefer to study in the day or evening?
- Do I need a structured program or can I organize my own learning?
- Do I prefer taught courses or subjects, or to learn through conducting research?
- Can I travel or do I prefer to work from home?

You should also consider what access to resources you are likely to need, for example, library and learning resources, access to the Internet and e-mail. Many programs now make extensive use of electronic communication for conferencing and discussion, and e-mail communication. Fully online, internet-based courses are now available in many countries, so the choice is considerable in terms of what, where and how you wish to study.

Developing your expertise for advanced practice

In order to develop your clinical expertise it is first necessary to recognize what clinical experts do that is different from those who have yet to develop as experts. This may help us to understand the characteristics of anyone aspiring to be an advanced practitioner and expert in his or her field and what he or she must do to prepare for such a role. Maudsley and Strivens (2000a) suggested that clinical experts, acting in familiar territory, are noted for their problem-solving ability that involves generating multiple hypotheses, using well-developed knowledge retrieval processes, organizing data around scientific principles and incorporating experience in a more advanced way than novice practitioners. Guest et al (2001) reinforced the notion that skill in dealing with problems was the hallmark of dynamic experts and suggested that aspiring experts should strive to improve their understanding of practice-related problems through reflection, as illustrated in Chapter 5.

Guest et al (2001) proposed that the development and maintenance of expertise require extensive, sustained practice of the necessary skills. This demands not just time but quality time, specifically dedicated to the development of these skills. The development of expertise is dependent on the ability to make the most of experience and to address problems at the upper limit of complexity that a practitioner can handle. In contrast, the non-expert constricts the field of work so that it conforms only to those routines that the non-expert is prepared to execute (Bereiter and Scardamailia 1993). Those wishing to develop the qualities of an advanced practitioner must be prepared to work beyond the boundaries of their 'comfort zone' of practice in order to extend and deepen their knowledge and their capacity to operate at an advanced clinical level.

Gaining expertise also requires motivation to develop an understanding beyond that required for competent practice. Understanding is difficult to characterize (Maudsley and Strivens 2000a). Authors such as Hamilton (1990) have described it as a learning journey that involves states of intellectual upheaval where experiences are assimilated to arrive at understanding. This would suggest that understanding demands effort. It is not a passive, automatic or evolutionary process but one that expects assumptions and existing understandings and practices actively to be challenged and reformed into new frameworks for practice. As Maudsley and Strivens (2000a, p. 55) pointed out: 'developing expertise means moving from reliance on abstract principles to incorporating past experience, and from perceiving situations as comprising equally relevant pieces to seeing a whole in which only some pieces are relevant'. This ability to discriminate is seen as a characteristic of the advanced practitioner.

In order to become an advanced practitioner there will clearly come a time when you must take personal control, and set the direction of your learning and development. Learning can happen by chance but a clearly defined, systematic approach to advancing your knowledge and practice will enable you to develop in a way, and at a pace that is comfortable for you. Knowledge of your preferred personal learning style and how to use compatible learning methods to achieve your learning goals is important. Other chapters, such as Chapter 2 and Chapter 9, offer guidance on this. As Brookfield (1986) pointed out, successful self-direction in learning is only possible if you have an understanding of the learning process. Brookfield went on to suggest that professionals ought to engage in regular periods of reflection on their experience. They should explore with others their accounts of how they have managed ambiguities and contextual problems in their practice and become acquainted with new theoretical and technical advances in knowledge and practice. Chapter 9 offers ways in which these skills may be developed, Chapter 3 will assist you to select and apply a theoretical framework to your plans, and Chapter 7 will guide you in applying a scholarly focus.

Eraut (2001) also emphasized the need for participation, personally, and with others, in the learning process, but stressed that what came next was also important. There needs to be a plan for using or extending that learning in practice. Eraut draws on the work of Jennett, et al (1994) to describe three forms of self-directed learning:

- informal, ongoing activities for competence maintenance that can be part of the daily routine of practice, such as reading journals, having conversations, attending departmental events. These activities have no intended learning outcomes, although some new knowledge might ensue
- semi-structured learning experiences based on patient problems and decision-making in practice where learning is incidental
- formal, intentional, planned activities where there is some sense of what needs to be learned.

One way of thinking about the qualities of an advanced practitioner is to expect that these individuals are beyond the skill level of those required of a newly qualified practitioner. Higgs and Jones (1995) discuss the concept of proficiency and clinical expertise, where the characteristic of expertise is the ability to produce effectiveness and appropriateness in clinical outcomes. It is more a matter of the level of expertise and capability than anything to do with the number of years qualified. The way to attain this level of expertise is to develop skills of thinking and learning to an advanced state and to enhance the use of higher cognitive skills, particularly critical reflection, in practice. The capacity to make sense of experience and to learn effectively from it has consistently been said to be the basis of learning and professional development (Boud and Walker 1993; Schön 1987).

Competence to learn

Competence to learn has to be seen as integral to competence to practice. The following, developed from Alsop (2001b), summarizes the characteristics of learning as a feature of competence:

- being positive about learning
- being able to identify learning needs
- taking the initiative to learn
- knowing where to locate learning resources and how to use them effectively
- seizing learning opportunities as they occur
- being open to new methods and ideas as they emerge in practice
- evaluating new concepts and ideas for their usefulness to practice

- knowing how to question and reflect on practice
- being able and willing to evaluate one's own performance
- accepting and responding to constructive feedback
- knowing when and where to seek guidance
- evaluating personal progress and future needs.

Gratton and Pearson (1994) suggested that developing the capacity to learn from the widest variety of opportunities is a form of empowerment that enables individuals to be in greater command of their destiny. Practitioners clearly need to harness the skills of learning in order to advance their practice both in the sense of broadening their capacity for practice in different situations but also to deepen their understanding of practice in a defined area, so enhancing their particular expertise.

Maudsley and Strivens (2000b, p. 536) cited Cogan's (1953) contention that professional practices are refined by science and corrected by wisdom, a notion that holds true as much today as it did half a century ago, as human problems cannot all be resolved with scientific solutions. Complex and novel problems, uncertainty and variation can defy research-based theory, so practitioners must be prepared to exploit *knowledge-in-action* and *reflection-in-action* and solve their problems through wise, but essentially intuitive, processes. However, professional education does not always provide the means for practitioners to develop these skills to a level of sophistication for advanced practice. Wisdom tends to defy the education process, yet practising, refining and developing reflective and other learning skills can at least help. Anyone aspiring to have advanced practice skills must therefore ensure fundamentally that learning skills are given every attention.

Advancing your profession

Barnett (1994) argued that all practising professionals had responsibilities that extend beyond those that advance personal clinical competence to those that advance the profession itself. This involved not only being knowledgeable, skilful and ethical in practice, but also offering insightful thoughts about practice, creating knowledge through one's own practice and developing and transforming practice over time. It required practitioners to be alert to, and proficient in examining society's changing demands, to form views about a profession's needs, to have a vision for advancing practice, and to take steps to shape and change practice. These are clearly higher-order responsibilities that require the development and effective use of the ability to think and practise critically and to take a critical stand in the changing world of practice. Practitioners should not just accept the status quo, but should have the confidence to challenge policy (Taylor 1997) and to enter into a wider public debate about uncertainties in practice (Brookfield 1995).

This may be daunting to those who have only just qualified and have only just embarked on their professional career journey. But Barnett (1994) was clear that advancing the profession was as much a responsibility as advancing oneself. For many practitioners, this is unlikely to come naturally or to take effect at the start of their career. However, advancing professional practice can be deemed to be integral to professional practice (Barnett 1994). The point at which each practitioner assumes this responsibility may vary, and could relate directly to each person's level of confidence in the work that he or she does.

Confidence, it seems, is the key to challenging professional practice. It demands the ability to feel comfortable with uncertainty and about taking steps to respond to uncertainty in the light of others' contradictory arguments and counter claims (Barnett 2000). As Barnett observed, this demands courage and a certain amount of resilience. Anyone who takes such steps may be challenging long-standing traditions and long-held beliefs, challenging that which has been tried, but not necessarily tested in practice. In today's climate that 'testing', that evaluation of professional practices, that determining of 'best practice', has to take place. Those wishing to develop advanced practitioner skills are likely to be the individuals who undertake these activities and collaborate in research in order to help the profession to develop its knowledge base, defend its practice and thereby stand up to public scrutiny.

Advanced practice will require individuals to develop inner strength to be able to cope with contradictions and to manage uncertainties. They will not just deal with change, but will also instigate change on the basis of advancing the profession. These qualities may not be in place in the early stages of a career, but can develop over time. Small steps taken in search of 'best practice' through reflective practice, service audit and small-scale evaluation studies can all help with informing practice and with self-development. Engaging with the research agenda needs to be a longer-term goal that can be attained over time, initially by participating in activities such as journal clubs to critique and debate literature, conducting literature searches and reviews or becoming involved with others' research, either as a respondent or in a research role. Debates such as these are explored in Chapters 1, 5 and 7. Becoming involved with such activities can enable you to build your confidence as well as a repertoire of skills to draw on in the future. In summary, the responsibilities of an advanced practitioner extend beyond those aimed exclusively at developing oneself. They embrace a wider public responsibility for engaging actively in practices that will help the profession as a whole to move forward.

Presenting the evidence of your professional development

Increasingly, professional bodies are recommending to their members that they keep a record of their achievements and evidence of their capacity to practise in their profession, and of the activities in which they have participated for professional updating, development and improvement. These records may be subject to formal scrutiny for renewing professional registration and ongoing licence to practise. Historically, such activity would have gone unrecorded but, with the increasing demands of accountability, evidence of professional development is now being required. One way of presenting this evidence is in portfolio form.

The word portfolio comes from two Latin words (*portare* and *folium*) meaning to carry a leaf or leaves. By custom and practice, artists have tended to carry samples of their work in a portfolio in order to demonstrate their creative skills and professional ability to prospective employers. Other professions have now adopted the term and expanded the way in which a portfolio has come to be used, although the original intention remains the same. It is a folder in which work is placed that demonstrates the owner's personal and professional capacity in a designated field of practice. Brown (1995, p. 2) offered a definition of a portfolio as:

> a private collection of evidence which demonstrates the continuing acquisition of skills, knowledge, attitudes, understanding and achievement. It is both retrospective and prospective, as well as reflecting the current stage of development and activity of the individual.

Brown (1995) went on to suggest that each portfolio should be personal, reflecting the individuality and uniqueness of each person's life. This is a really important point as a question frequently asked is 'what should my portfolio look like?' While some general recommendations might be made, the question cannot readily be answered because each practitioner will have a different career history, different professional interests and skills and different aspirations. You can see already that the retrospective element of your portfolio will be evidenced by your career history (perhaps your curriculum vitae or CV). Your current stage of development will be demonstrated with evidence of your current clinical interests, professional capabilities, and technical skills, and the prospective element could be in the form of an outline of your aspirations, details of personal and professional goals and plans for their achievement. So there is nothing difficult about starting, or maintaining a portfolio—it just takes time.

The one thing to address, however, is the tension between what Brown refers to as a 'private' collection of evidence and the 'public' scrutiny of that evidence for verification of ongoing competence. Someone has to be the judge of your competence in order to register you, to award you a licence to practise or, as in Australia, to grant you personal accreditation. The evidence will need to be provided to an authorized person so that this judgement can be made. However, only those empowered to make the judgement need access to the material that forms the evidence, and you will have selected that evidence purposely from all the material in your private portfolio. The rest of the material remains 'private' since you do not have to release everything for scrutiny. Only the salient pieces of evidence that demonstrate your ongoing ability to practise in the context in which you are, or wish to be, working will be important. Commonly, while each practitioner's portfolio will need to be kept up to date and ready for scrutiny, most countries are adopting a system of sampling so that a percentage of portfolios annually are reviewed from each profession.

Whatever stage you are at in your professional career, be it newly qualified or established practitioner, you will have accumulated a range of material that indicates your qualities, skills and abilities. You may already have aspirations of becoming an advanced practitioner so your portfolio will reflect your goals and plans. You may already have developed your practice from initial qualification, in which case your portfolio will contain evidence of achieving relevant goals. For example, you might have evidence that you have:

- undertaken some relevant continuing education
- achieved a higher degree
- engaged in some research
- carried out a literature review
- presented a paper or a poster at a conference
- published an article
- carried out a work-related project and prepared a report
- explored and reviewed the management of a particularly complex case with which you were involved
- written some protocols for practice
- prepared some literature or a video for clients, carers, students
- undertaken some teaching or facilitated the learning of others
- carried out a critical review of a service or made a case for a new service
- been a member of a working group to develop practice.

There are so many ways in which you might have developed yourself and your practice. Evidence of the work that you have undertaken will be key. If you are focused in what you are doing and plan to develop your skills as an advanced practitioner then you will almost certainly aim to undertake some of the above activities.

Assembling your portfolio

The contents of your portfolio can be assembled in whatever way you choose. The material is yours and the way in which you wish to display it is up to you. There may be guidance offered by a professional, statutory or academic body that should be heeded, particularly if the portfolio is to be assessed for a licence or award from that body, but otherwise the contents and the way in which they are presented will be unique to you and will reflect your individuality.

As has been suggested elsewhere (Alsop 2002), material might include tangible references to your past experiences from external sources, such as testimonials, certificates of learning or other evidence of achievement. Other material could include your own personal reflections on events, incidents or experiences that demonstrate your learning. Critical analyses of situations serve to enlighten and offer evidence of your critical thinking and personal learning. As Crist et al (1998) pointed out, preparing a portfolio can be a learning process in its own right.

On the practical side, a neatly presented and well-ordered portfolio can impress. Different sections can demonstrate different aspects of your professional life. Your employment and professional experiences may be separate from evidence of your academic achievement. A separate section might indicate the clinical aspects of your role and include your reflections, your learning and your observations about the application of this learning to your practice. Similarly, another section may deal with roles such as supervisor, manager, leader, educator, researcher or project worker, and hold the evidence that pertains to the development of relevant skills in that role. It will be a combination of this evidence that lends itself to demonstrating your capability as an advanced practitioner.

The dynamics of portfolio preparation

All of us work in a changing context of practice and, like a picture, a portfolio can only represent a snapshot in time. The time that is portrayed in your portfolio always needs to be the present time, which means that your portfolio must be continuously updated. Redman (1994, p. 42) remarked that a portfolio 'is a living, growing collection of evidence that mirrors the growth of its owner'. Hence it must evolve over time and be seen as a dynamic, rather than static, entity that reflects your professional updating and development. Change means just that. Documents and your own personal insights and other evidence can be constantly added to your portfolio, but if the portfolio is to act as a display of evidence of your current capability, rather than just a historical record of your achievement, then the evidence in your portfolio needs to be reviewed periodically and decisions need also to be made about what might be withdrawn. Your portfolio will thus be a changing profile of you that reflects developments over time but also your current capability. The selection of evidence for submission to a regulatory or awarding body must be taken from material that is current and that accurately reflects the present state of your competence.

Structuring your portfolio

Starting to put together a portfolio is often seen as the greatest hurdle to overcome, so the best way of tackling this task is to start with the facts. In other words, start with what you know. A CV is one of the first things to prepare. It should be concise, up-to-date, accurate and dated, and give details of your qualifications, employment and more recent professional activities. Some people add a summary of learning or achievements in each role undertaken most recently. This would indicate your capability rather than just the experiences you have had. The CV also acts as a prompt so that you can think in more detail about the roles that you have held in your professional life and can reflect on what learning has taken place in those roles. Sometimes it is a useful exercise to list the roles that you currently hold. Some possibilities might be:

- clinician
- care manager
- manager
- supervisor
- researcher
- mentor
- educator
- author
- project worker

- representative
- committee member
- consultant
- expert
- facilitator.

When you have listed the roles in which you currently engage, then think back over the last 2–3 years and note down any professional development activity that you have undertaken in support of each of those roles. These are exercises that can help you to think more clearly about what you have done, what you have experienced and what you have achieved. It may be quite easy for you to list any qualifications that you have gained but you also need to think more widely about the less formal activities that have provided learning opportunities for you. Some of the informal learning opportunities might include:

- making visits to specialist centres
- shadowing other people (including patients, clients)
- undertaking project work
- engaging in audit activity; service evaluations
- in-service training (undertaken by yourself or made available to other people)
- participating in learning sets
- participating in special interest activity
- organizing training, conferences or other events
- publishing or preparing literature to support clinical activity
- teaching, giving talks, making presentations
- making videos
- participating in journal clubs
- undertaking literature searches and reviews
- undertaking voluntary work.

These are by no means definitive lists (see Alsop 2000 for other activities) but they should encourage you to think carefully about what you have done, either on your own or with other people. You may decide to review each of these roles and make a judgement about whether you perceive yourself to be competent, proficient or expert in each role or still at the novice stage. In doing this, you would also need to have a view about which level of expertise is necessary for the job that you are doing so that you can assess how far you have developed and what your priorities are for further development. Clearly, maintaining competence in specific roles or domains of practice will be essential for your continued employment, whilst other areas of personal interest may be less urgent and can be developed over time. In preparing your portfolio and development plans, however, you should always set them in the context of your overall career goals.

Another way of documenting what you have learnt is to write up some of the more challenging clinical cases with which you have been associated, taking all necessary steps to maintain confidentiality, of course. These may have involved investigations, research, collaboration with others, new methods of assessment or new approaches to problem-solving. You will not record every case, but those that make particular demands, are unusual or have led to new learning are the ones that will be particularly significant. A series of studies or stories could form the backbone of your portfolio. Personal reflections on learning from these cases can demonstrate evidence of your engagement with clinical scenarios and the way in which advanced skills are being developed. (See Chapter 5 for a detailed, reflective example.)

Your professional development plans

Your portfolio ought not only to contain evidence of your past achievements and current capability but also be an indication of your professional development needs and plans. You should have available your current job description and a self-assessment of your development needs undertaken in relation to the job that you are doing. Your development priorities should reflect the need for you to keep up to date with practice and help you to develop greater depth or breadth of knowledge in the clinical area in which you work. The self-assessment may be part of a performance review or appraisal that you have had with your line manager. Your development plans should address areas of clinical expertise, leadership, management and supervisory skills and any specific needs or intentions with regard to evidence-based practice, research and education. All these areas should be addressed so that you can develop the wide-ranging skills necessary for advanced practice.

Type of portfolio

Given the increasing use of technology these days, software packages exist that you can use to record your past professional development activity and your future plans. The various screens will prompt you to record a range of data that can then be drawn on for various purposes. The electronic versions lend themselves to maintaining and updating portfolio records and are likely to be particularly attractive to an increasing number of professionals, as practitioners' skills in the use of information technology increase. However, the actual hard evidence of professional development still has to be stored methodically so that it can be called into use at any time. Hence many people still opt for a manual version of the portfolio so that materials and records can be maintained together and can be transported easily for presentation at interviews or other events.

Dos and don'ts

This section offers you advice on how you might present a professional portfolio.

Do:

- structure your portfolio into sections that best reflect your career, roles, achievements and professional development needs over time
- include an index and cross-reference material as necessary
- present material clearly, concisely, neatly and professionally
- be selective in what you present

- ensure that any criteria set by a professional, statutory, licensing or academic body, and that you are aiming to meet, are addressed accordingly
- present the evidence in the context of your professional needs and goals
- demonstrate self-evaluation, reflection and personal awareness
- indicate what you have learnt from the various experiences in your career
- indicate how the learning is to be applied in your practice
- include your future visions, goals and development needs
- attribute any work that is not your own
- present the portfolio in such a way that it allows others to make sense of it.

Do not:

- breach any confidentiality
- include casual comment or unprofessional remarks
- include informal notes or materials that will lower the standard of presentation unless they are set in the formal context of how they contribute to the evidence
- make claims that are not supported by evidence
- put everything into a portfolio.

Do make judgements about what is important. It is essential to remember that this portfolio reflects you as a person as well as your professional development. The quality of its presentation is important as it gives other people an impression of how you work and present yourself. A portfolio should be something of which you are proud and that portrays you in the best possible light.

Ownership

This is your portfolio. It belongs to nobody else. This means that you can determine what is to be included, how it should be presented, where it is to be kept and who can have access to it. Sometimes there can be tensions about ownership and access if the portfolio (manual or software version) has been purchased by, for example, an employer or manager. It is as well to have an agreed protocol about ownership, storage and access if the portfolio is maintained in work time and for any purposes associated with work practices, for example, performance review.

Sometimes it is agreed, or you might wish to determine, that some sections can be made available for public scrutiny whilst other, more private, sections and evidence are retained separately for presentation only to a select few, at your discretion.

Concluding remarks   This chapter has explored ways in which you might develop your knowledge, skills and overall competence to practise over time and attain a level of confidence in your own ability that will allow you to be judged as an advanced practitioner. It has set the expectations with regard to your CPD into national policies (e.g. in the UK) that now generally require practitioners working in health and social care to demonstrate evidence of their ongoing and developing competence to practise. The chapter has set out various ways of developing this competence through formal educational programs, informal learning and work-based activities. It has also presented guidance on how the evidence of your professional development might be presented in a portfolio. Becoming an advanced practitioner is an incremental process undertaken over time. However, by systematically taking active steps and by using personal strategies that facilitate your learning and development, your status as an advanced practitioner will be confirmed.

References

Alsop A 1998 Maintaining competence to practise. British Journal of Occupational Therapy 61:331

Alsop A 2000 Continuing professional development: a guide for therapists. Blackwell Science, Oxford

Alsop A 2001a Competence unfurled: developing portfolio practice. Occupational Therapy International. 8:126–131

Alsop A 2001b Perspectives on competence. British Journal of Therapy and Rehabilitation. 8:206–212

Alsop A 2002 Portfolios: portraits of our professional lives. British Journal of Occupational Therapy 65:(in Press)

Barnett R 1994 The limits of competence. Society for Research into Higher Education and Open University Press, Buckingham

Barnett R 1997 Higher education: a critical business. Society for Research into Higher Education and Open University Press, Buckingham

Barnett R 2000 Realising the university in an age of supercomplexity. Society for Research into Higher Education and Open University Press, Buckingham

Bereiter C, Scardamailia M 1993 Surpassing ourselves: an inquiry into the nature and implications of expertise. Open Court, Chicago, IL

Boud D, Walker D 1993 Barriers to reflection on experience. In: Boud D, Cohen R, Walker D (eds) Using experience for learning. Society for Research into Higher Education and Open University Press, Buckingham, p 73–86

Brookfield S 1986 Understanding and facilitating adult learning. Open University Press, Milton Keynes

Brookfield S 1995 Becoming a critically reflective teacher. Jossey-Bass, San Francisco

Brown R 1995 Portfolio development and profiling for nurses, 2nd edn. Quay, Dinton, UK

Canadian Association of Occupational Therapists 2001 Position statement continuing professional education. Online, Available at: www.caot.ca. Accessed 25 May 2002

Cogan M L 1953 Towards a definition of profession. Harvard Educational Review 23:33–50

CPD strategy for the professions allied to medicine: consensus statement 1999 Occupational Therapy News 7:8–9

Crist P, Wilcox B L, McCarron K 1998 Transitional portfolios: orchestrating our professional competence. American Journal of Occupational Therapy 52: 729–736

Department of Health 1998 A first class service: quality in the new NHS. Department of Health, London

Department of Health 1999 Continuing professional development: quality in the new NHS. Department of Health, London

Department of Health 2000 Meeting the challenge: a strategy for the allied health professions. Department of Health, London

Department of Health 2001 Establishing the new health professions council. Department of Health, London

Eraut M 1994 Developing professional knowledge and competence. The Falmer Press, London

Eraut M 1998 Concepts of competence. Journal of Interprofessional Care 12:127–139

Eraut M 2001 Do continuing professional development models promote one-dimensional learning? Medical Education 35:8–11

Gratton L, Pearson J 1994 Empowering leaders: are they being developed? In: Mabey C, Iles P, (eds), Managing Learning, Routledge, London, p 87–104

Guest C B, Regehr G, Tiberius R G 2001 The life long challenge of expertise. Medical Education 35: 78–81

Hager P, Gonczi A 1996 Professions and competencies. In: Edwards R, Hansen A, Ragatt P (eds) Boundaries of adult learning. Routledge Open University, London, p 246–260

Hamilton D 1990 Learning about education: an unfinished curriculum. Open University Press, Buckingham

Higgs J, Jones M (eds) 1995 Clinical reasoning in the health professions. Butterworth-Heinemann, Oxford

Hocking C 1998 The cornerstone programme: ensuring ongoing competence to practise in New Zealand. In: Book of abstracts. 12th International Congress of the World Federation of Occupational Therapists. Session C1.13. Montreal, Canada: WFOT

Hollis V 1997 Practice portrayed: an exploration of occupational therapy clinical skills and their development. Unpublished PhD thesis. University of Exeter, Exeter, UK

Jennett P, Jones D, Mast T 1994 The characteristics of self-directed learning. In: Davis D A, Fox R D (eds) The physician as learner—linking research to practice. American Medical Association, Chicago, Il, p 40–65

Maudsley G, Strivens J 2000a Science, critical thinking and competence for tomorrow's doctors. A review of terms and concepts. Medical Education 34:53–60

Maudsley G, Strivens J 2000b Promoting professional knowledge, experiential learning and critical thinking for medical students. Medical Education 34:535–544

Redman W 1994 Portfolios and their development: a guide for trainers and managers. Kogan Page, London

Runge U, Fitinghoff H, Josephsson S et al 2000 A European Master of Science programme in occupational therapy. British Journal of Therapy and Rehabilitation 7:374–376

Schön D 1987 Educating the reflective practitioner. Jossey-Bass, San Francisco

Taylor I 1997 Developing learning in professional education. Society for Research into Higher Education and Open University Press, Buckingham

Tregloan M L 2000 Health service quality assessment: defining and assessing healthcare standards; an international picture. Healthcare Review-online. Online Available at: www.enigma.co.nz/hcro_articles/0006vol4no6_002.htm. Accessed 25 May 2002

12 Consultancy and advanced teaming: promoting practice beyond the healthcare environment

Gwilym Wyn Roberts

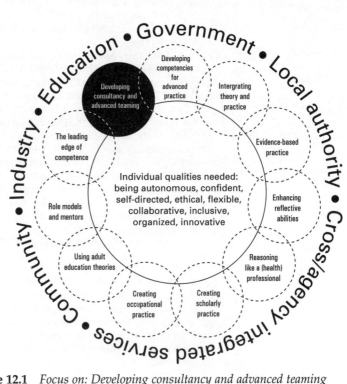

Figure 12.1 *Focus on: Developing consultancy and advanced teaming*

Chapter outline

This chapter offers some guidance for practitioners who are moving towards higher-level practice and consultancy work within the statutory, voluntary and private sectors. The aim is for individuals to consider key elements and influences which allow such a transition. Environmental factors, strategies for improving effectiveness, and continuous quality improvement initiatives are explored in this context. Integrated into the discussion is the role of health professionals as *lifelong learners*, a commitment towards continuing professional and personal development as a means of deepening knowledge and skill. Inherent in key factors that need to be considered is the potential role for health workers to be employed as consultants within private and corporate industry to provide expert advice on organizational development.

Key words

Advanced and higher-level practice, consultancy, lifelong learning, organizational structures

Anticipated outcomes

As a result of reading this chapter, I anticipate that you will be able to:

- understand the nature of higher-level practice and consultant work
- write a rationale for developing consulting work in your area of health
- understand the importance of organizational effectiveness
- outline the knowledge and skills required for consultancy work
- identify the core function of a consultant health professional.

Introduction

During the latter part of the 20th century many healthcare workers were inspired to consider developing their specific expertise and advancing towards independent work at consultancy level. They started to develop confidence in recognizing their own capabilities to be seen as equal partners with medical practitioners in healthcare delivery. The move towards degree status for pre-registration practitioners and, the development of a much higher research profile, combined with new career opportunities, away from traditional work-places inspired many healthcare workers to consider independent work. The number of practitioners further expanding their continuing professional development (CPD) to become higher-level experts in specialized areas influenced a new, and more realistic understanding of the progression of becoming consultants. There has been an increase in the number of these individuals entering private practice either within corporate industry or as independent practitioners. An example of the above is the advent of a new type of consultant nurse announced by the UK government in 1999. Among the motives for this development of an enhanced professional role was the desire to:

- improve career pathways in clinical practice
- reward clinical leadership in terms of pay and autonomy
- develop new innovative services
- retain and make best use of high-level clinical skills.

As a result, there emerged a growing willingness amongst the health professions to recognize that there may no longer be a need to hide behind the *jack-of-all-trade* image, and that professions other than nursing and medicine may well have the capability of also being masterful, advanced-level professional practitioners. No one profession deserves to dominate over the others. There is an argument that the uniqueness of all professions demands a healthy balance of breadth and depth of knowledge. This said, in mastering specific aspects of professional skills and knowledge, can health professions aspire to be seen as consultants, experts and higher-level practitioners both within and outside the health and social care arena?

In the UK, factors such as the National Health Service (NHS) White Paper *The New NHS: Modern and Dependable* (Department of Health, 1997), the *National Service Framework* [NSF] *for Older People*

(Department of Health, 2001a) and subsequent legislation have led to what some may argue to be profound changes in the provision and delivery of health and social care and the way in which experienced staff develop their careers. Emerging clinical outcomes guidance, with imperatives for consistent best practice and patient-centred care, are challenging current models of service delivery, and encouraging the development of higher-level practice at consultant level, resulting in new and often contemporary ways of doing things.

The vision of continuous quality improvement and the introduction of clinical governance (College of Occupational Therapists 1999) does rest on a clear commitment to evidence-based practice, research and the use of specific outcomes and protocols. This requires appropriate development of the workforce through education and training, CPD and lifelong learning. Worldwide, there have been moves to strengthen agreements for professional self-regulation, reinforcing individual professional responsibility and accountability for practice. This will apply equally to professionals working within statutory services as to individuals working within the private and voluntary sectors. In addition, *A Strategy for the Allied Health Professions, Meeting the Challenge* (Department of Health 2000) identifies new career development opportunities as consultant health professionals as a priority for the UK government. Lifelong learning and CPD can only be seen as an integral aspect of becoming, and continuing to be a consultant practitioner.

While the context being referred to lends itself to a health service, one could strongly advocate the same for the development of expertise and higher-level practice in social care. Historically, the UK healthcare system has been seen as separate to the social care sector. Within this, potential organizational and managerial barriers often appear too great to allow such developments to occur at the same pace. As intermediate care becomes streamlined into the UK, health and social care culture and higher-level practice within local authorities could equally become an exciting and viable career opportunity for social care employees. New opportunities for allied health consultant work have created renewed enthusiasm and encouragement to pursue careers at consultant level, by maximizing on the knowledge and skills required for such positions. As a result, a growing number of independent consultant professionals are employed in this capacity as an effective way of readdressing a variety of problems, for example, lengthening waiting lists that have arisen as a result of chronic recruitment and retention dilemmas.

Understanding consultancy work

The development of a consultant role, for health professionals, may also be influenced by external forces. Organizations and professions that do not respond to triggers such as new legislation or the expectations of clients/service users may soon decline and subsequently cease to exist. However, in addition to bringing about change in the internal environment, practitioners and managers alike may influence factors external to the organization. For instance, they may influence current government vision/policy regarding what constitutes a *mod-*

ern healthcare system. Involving and empowering service users, professional bodies, including health professionals, and others working in healthcare, have been given the opportunity to lobby the media, politicians and policy- and decision-makers at all levels. This in turn has led to the publication of a Department of Health definitive definition of a *consultant allied health professional* (AHP). This may help to identify some baseline expectations and features of such a position (Department of Health 2001b p. 2):

> A consultant AHP is an expert in a specialist clinical field, bringing innovation, influence to clinical leadership and strategic direction in that particular field for the benefit of patients. The consultant will play a pivotal role in the integration of research evidence into practice. Exceptional skills and advanced levels of clinical judgement, knowledge and experience will underpin and promote the delivery of the clinical governance agenda. This will be by enhancing quality in areas of assessment, diagnosis, management and evaluation, delivering improved outcomes for patients and extending the parameters of the specialism.

The document goes on to state that (Department of Health 2001b):

> Consultant posts provide the opportunity to retain clinical excellence and mature skills within the service. They will sit within a range of models of practice and service configurations. While the focus of the consultant posts will be the delivery and practice of clinical care, the development of more detailed job descriptions will be undertaken at local level, tailored to meet local needs and based on local circumstances. This ensures that AHPs can develop through a range of opportunities and routes, either as specialists or generalist practitioners to consultant level in the acute, community and intermediate care settings. This approach gives services the flexibility to meet their specific needs within the local community.

It is clear from these statements that the underpinning area of expertise of consultant health practitioners is often a clinical and/or managerial profile. This is an important factor to remember when exploring consultant work in areas outside health and social care (Roberts and Cusack 2001). The Department of Health (1997) definition followed on from the guide published in 1995, which was based on a three-year research study commissioned by the department, entitled *Exploring New Roles in Practice* (Department of Health 1995). When the study was commissioned, many professions began to consider the proliferation of new roles. This report highlighted several distinct—though interrelated—aspects of planning that needed to be considered. They were:

- planning future career pathways for individuals
- reviewing innovations and role development
- succession planning.

In addition, the professions identified a need to consider other interrelated aspects of developing new roles at a higher practice consultant level in the following fields:

- clinical expertise
- education/teaching, clinical and higher education
- research/evidence-based practice and practice evaluation
- management.

Many believed that, even if better educated and more experienced individuals were to be attracted into innovative roles, some reassurance would be needed that they were making the right career decisions. Also, it may be relevant to note that very able practitioners with high levels of ability and interests would be attracted by the challenge of new roles. However, they may run the risk of disillusionment if there is nowhere for them to progress in their career after a reasonable period in a given post.

Towards a new paradigm of working

Professional identity and professional regulation is an area of concern which often dominates debates about professional role innovations. Practitioners often tread a careful line between developing advanced expertise within a specialized area while retaining a sufficiently wide knowledge base and the credibility to function effectively in broader terms within a given organization (Senior 1997). With this in mind, professions may need to consider strategies for improving this dilemma by streamlining consultant levels and organizational effectiveness, whether in health, social care or the private sector. In addition, individuals and groups may need to focus on developing processes that support the achievement of identified business goals. There are no universal prescriptions for the development of these strategies; however, the following generalities may assist the process, on the understanding that they would have to be turned into specifics in accordance with the assessment of the particular needs of differing business environments. These are:

- clearly defined goals and strategies to accomplish them
- a value system that emphasizes performance, productivity, quality, customer service, teamwork and flexibility
- strong visionary leadership owned by everybody
- a powerful management team
- commitment to CPD and lifelong learning
- a well-motivated, committed, skilled and flexible workforce
- effective teamwork throughout the organization, progressing beyond the win/lose conflict and culture
- continuous pressure to innovate and grow
- the ability to respond fast and effectively to opportunities and threats
- the capacity to manage, thrive and facilitate necessary change
- a sound financial base and good systems for management accounting and cost control
- services tailor-made for local communities and service needs
- career development and CPD requirement and needs.

In order that practitioners improve their personal and organizational effectiveness, there may be a need to progress rapidly in ever less bureaucratic and ever more entrepreneurial directions, cutting out unnecessary layers of the hierarchy and forging closer collaborative ties with colleagues. Pursuing a level of excellence may increase the number of demands made upon both consultants and managers. Good relationships, effective communication and the flexibility to combine resources are most important. Historically, many would argue that health professionals have had to work within a disempowering culture in which obstacles to develop expertise have been firmly entrenched. Such obstacles have included lack of career opportunities, inflexible mind-sets around the validity of some academic qualifications and lack of credible professional profiles, especially for professions with fewer members. In this sense, a new paradigm for consultants may need to be considered—one in which consultant practitioners are:

- placing increased emphasis on the *soft* dimensions of style and shared values
- operating as networks rather than hierarchies
- moving from the status-driven view that consultants think, and workers do as they are told, to a belief in consultants as facilitators with workers empowered to initiate improvement and change
- placing less emphasis on vertical tasks within functional units and more on horizontal tasks and collaboration across units
- focusing less on content and the prescribed use of specific tools and techniques and more on *process* and the holistic synthesis of techniques
- changing the *military command* model to a *commitment model*
- increasing professional credibility and status through promoting a new culture around evidence-based practice and research.

Within this new paradigm, those holding positions may need to be prepared to work across a range of new service delivery structures and be expected to influence decision-making. As health workers, they may function autonomously, working within the ethical framework provided by their own profession's code of ethics and professional conduct, ensuring they only practise in those areas in which they are safe and competent. Therefore, as consultants their autonomy will be exercised to the very highest level, and as such they can be expected to have clinical practice responsibilities beyond their immediate management structure.

By virtue of the recognized higher level of knowledge and skill expected from consultants, a significant element of expert clinical practice will involve working with patients, clients and communities. In addition, consultants should be required to provide an exceptionally high level of clinical expertise and be recognized as making a distinguished contribution to their respective professions. Dependent on the local service requirement, there may be an emphasis on one or more of the other supporting functions, for example, service and practice development, or education and professional development. However, in order to demonstrate evidence of working at consultant level, the Department of Health

(2001a) guide may give directions on what may be required to demonstrate a high level of understanding and be integrated into specific roles.

Expert clinical practice: the core functions

In identifying the core functions of expert clinical practice in the statutory, voluntary and private sectors, the Department of Health (2001a) described the indicative features of a consultant health professional. Included are some key elements such as taking responsibility for and management of a complex caseload. In addition, the following features were also identified:

- demonstrates advanced knowledge, skills and experience within specific specialist or generalist areas of practice
- is recognized as a national and/or international expert within his or her own specialty service or field, ensuring that locally endorsed standards are evidence-based to reflect the very best available practice
- is responsible for ensuring that ethical and moral dimensions of practice are adhered to
- exercises the highest degree of personal professional autonomy, involving highly complex facts or situations, which require analysis and interpretation of statistics and data, leading to the implementation of a treatment or management strategy for clients
- creates and develops protocols of care, and designs patient care pathways with the aim of providing best practice examples to others
- is responsible for delivering a whole system patient-focused approach which is not rooted in a uni-professional perspective
- promotes and demonstrates best practice; most particularly, facilitates the integration of the most up to date research theory into practice through an advanced level of clinical reasoning and decision-making across a spectrum of practice
- is responsible for facilitating and promoting a learning culture within the organization, enabling others to develop to their full potential within the specialist field.

From this, one can identify how individual consultants might maximize on their own capability towards higher-level practice at consultant level. This said, other functions might also be expected, in particular areas of management and leadership. Consultants may well be identified as having to be effective leaders—individuals who are able to motivate and inspire others to deliver the optimum quality of care while reaching organizational goals within the specialist field and beyond it, including other staff groups and organizations.
Other features may include being a person who:

- is an acknowledged source of expertise, who develops innovative practice and service delivery models, and ensures that they are applied throughout the specific organization
- has the ability to process complex, sensitive or contentious information leading to the development of strategic plans, which will drive change within and across organizations and specific partners.

Within the UK, consultants will be expected to contribute to a quality strategy, including influencing and delivering in relation to clinical governance agenda. Clinical governance is being defined as:

> a framework that encompasses a full range of quality activities, building first upon what is already being carried out. These combine to improve the overall quality of care for clients. They include, for example, the use of evidence-based practice, standards for practice, clinical guidelines, clinical audit, complaints procedures, risk management, incorporating clients' views, training and continuing professional development (Sealey 1999).

Within this context in particular, the Department of Health (2001a) has expressed clearly its vision that consultants will drive practice, service development, research and evaluation. Individuals at this level will be expected to ensure that high-quality patient-centred services are based on best available evidence. Other features may include:

- evaluating the provision of clinical services leading to new development and/or redesign
- response to identification of gaps in the evidence base
- taking the initiative to facilitate and/or undertake research and development programs which enhance the evidence base of the service, and make an impact outside the organization
- establishment of research partnerships within the higher education sector.

To maintain and develop these features, consultants may well be expected to develop a portfolio of career lifelong learning, experience and typically formal education, usually up to or beyond Master's level. Additional indicative features may guide consultants to promote and facilitate the development of a learning environment to enable others to achieve their potential, particularly by encouraging and supporting reflective practice. This may encourage the service to become one which continuously improves and develops. Also, some undertaking of education/facilitation and research may be expected. As a result, consultants may be required to have the skills to enhance the links between practice, professional bodies and academic research institutions. Finally, providing education in a specific field of clinical expertise nationally and internationally by lecturing or through publishing research in professional journals may also be a key feature and form an integral avenue for lifelong learning.

Risk-taking and resilience

The best lifelong learning consultants and leaders seem to have high standards, ambitious goals and a real sense of mission in their lives. Such goals and aspirations spur them on, put their accomplishments in a humbling perspective, and help them endure the short-term pain associated with growth and change (Machon 2000). However, consultants as lifelong learners do have to take risks. They often have to push themselves beyond their 'comfort zones' to try out new ideas. This way of working may not be inherent within the statutory health and social care environments; however, it may be argued that it is an approach that is well established in corporate and private industry. While others might be seen as having become set in their ways, consultants in these environments are often seen as being experiential in their attitude and approach to learning.

Risk-taking inevitably produces greater success and greater failures. Lifelong learners reflect on their experiences to educate themselves. They may not sweep failures under the carpet or examine them from a defensive position that undermines their ability to make rational conclusions. They actively solicit opinions and ideas from others, and build on some things that have not worked out well. They do not make assumptions that imply *they know it all* or that *most other people have little to contribute*. Just the opposite—they believe that, with the right approach, they can maximize on learning from others. They appreciate that careful listening may help give accurate feedback on the effects of some actions. From listening, lifelong learners are equipped to give honest and objective feedback. Without direct feedback, learning may become ineffective. The more volatile economic environment, along with the need for more effective leadership and lifelong learning, is producing careers that look quite different from those which were typical of the latter part of the twentieth century.

Future health workers will have to continue to be part of a dynamic, and evolving workforce, aligning themselves to change with changing needs and expectations. Already we are seeing fewer people doing one job the same way for long periods of time. Workers who learn to master more volatile career paths along consultancy routes are seen to become more comfortable with change generally and thus better able to play more useful roles in organizational transformations. They more easily develop whatever leadership potential they have. With more leadership, they are in a better position to help their colleagues advance in the transformation process. They are able to achieve significantly improved, meaningful results while minimizing the painful effects of change.

Those practitioners attempting to grow, to become more comfortable with change and to develop leadership skills are typically driven by a sense that they are doing what is right for themselves, their families, their profession and their clients and service users. That sense of purpose acts as a catalyst to spur them on with renewed inspiration during difficult periods. Those people who are at the top of enterprises today and who encourage others to leap into the future, who have helped them to overcome their natural fears and who thus expand the leadership capacity in their professions and organizations provide a profoundly important service for society in general.

In considering the further development of consultancy and the advancement of knowledge and skill, there is a need for even more self-awareness, self-pride, independence of thinking and determination. Holding all of these together will demand a high level of professional resilience—professional resilience that protects us against hierarchical and organizational barriers such as deeply ingrained mind sets around capabilities and career opportunities. A commitment to enhance group facilitation skills, for example, by pursuing formal and informal training will provide individuals with credible resilience to combat deliberate and/or non-deliberate barriers to embracing health-care practitioners in the consultancy arena. Inevitably, credibility often comes as a result of reputation and evidence of experience. This may be achieved through a commitment to developing a CPD portfolio with evidence of reflective practice focusing on expertise and an advanced level of knowledge and skill. Practitioners become more confident with experience, and experienced consultants become more credible with confidence in their own abilities.

Antonovsky (1979), a medical sociologist, came to the view that the key challenges facing us when progressing and deepening knowledge and skill at consultant level are dependent on three elements:

- meaning—the sense that the challenge is worth the investment of energy and attention
- comprehensibility—the confidence that we will be able to find some order and understanding in the situation
- manageability—the confidence that the resources required are accessible and manageable.

These qualities of resilience make it possible to stay afloat in a profes-sional world of stormy turbulence and uncertainty. So, rather than allowing stormy turbulence to overwhelm us as healthcare workers, as resilient professionals we should try and value it, accept it and make the most of it.

In considering an outcome-based framework to facilitate lifelong learning, consultancy and CPD, consideration can be given to embed-ding it in a humanistic and holistic philosophy such as the one pre-sented by Fish and Coles (1998), in which they recognize that:

- professional knowledge and advanced clinical practice are created in and during practice
- knowledge and expertise are developed through critical analysis and reflective activity
- the application of theory to practice and theorizing from practice are central to developing a higher level of competence to practice
- CPD enables practitioners to develop expertise and advanced prac-tice skills through a process of continual change within practice.

A move towards mastery at this consultant level demands a balance between professional and personal mastery. Personal mastery explores the very craft of the practitioner where the individual practi-tioner models ideal personal and professional practice through a deepening self-awareness and one's purposeful action. The shift is not only one of deepening, and advancing technical and clinical experi-ence, but also of effective clinical reasoning, where the professional consciously uses the self as an instrument in service, respecting the therapeutic power of one's presence and relationships (Machon 2000). Cultivating this attitude of continuous personal growth and learning, guided by both self-awareness and alignment with one's deepest qual-ities and values, results in the choice to take purposeful actions that produce the results one ideally wants from life.

Activity box 12.1	A helpful exercise might be for you to list your own personal value and belief systems, and reflect on the way that these might have changed as you developed through life into new situations. You might also need to reflect on some work ethics issues that you have experienced, and reflect on ways in which your personal desires have been compromised by these. End the exercise with a statement of intent, highlighting meaningful and purposeful actions that can be achieved to cultivate personal and professional growth.

Integrated into this attitude of continuous growth is the question of the extent to which we value ourselves and the process of being *in service* of the other. A factor often missing within most employing cultures is time for reflection and time to appreciate and value our own and others' contribution to service. At an organizational level this attitude in turn cultivates a community of shared practice. Hagedorn (1995) highlighted that we not only bring personal and professional values to the process of consultant work—we also have values as individuals, and a need to be valued by others. She goes on to refer to therapists as agents for change and a gateway to resources and information. But, most importantly, she attached value to the concept of *the therapist*, and saw that valuing oneself as a skilled therapist is not egocentric, but another aspect of maturity.

Higher-level practice and extended-scope practice

Another dimension to consider is the way in which higher-level practice is often blurred by the parallel process of extended-scope practice. Often, advancing one's own level of knowledge and skill to a higher level is closely linked to extending one's own practice to skill areas that are historically associated with other professions. For example, a physiotherapist with expert qualifications, working within a specialist rheumatology team (in the UK), may be required to administer pain-relieving medication. It is important to emphasize effectiveness within an individual's scope of practice. Safety and risk limitation also need to be implicit, as essential knowledge for practice. Recognizing the limitations of an individual's scope implies that development in one area of practice will be balanced by dilution in other areas of professional work.

Activity box 12.2	Within either your CPD portfolio or your reflective diary, list your current skill base in relation to your desired work. Against this, list areas of interest that can be developed that lie outside your view of your skill area. It is important that you feel a real desire to develop these additional skill areas. Draw out a realistic action plan delineating how these can be achieved and for what purpose. Highlight your aspirations for developing advanced skill and knowledge in the area, and state the desired job opportunity (realistic or not). If it is not realistic, ask yourself why not? And what can be done to achieve it?

Being identified as expert consultants puts another level of responsibility on practitioners to be recognized as change agents with high levels of problem-solving skills. Historically, healthcare workers have often seen themselves as real-life problem-solvers. There may be a tendency to focus on what is wrong or what is missing in the daily life of our clients and to see everything through that filter or frame. However, there may be a danger in some instances that the filter or frame is our unconscious set of assumptions. Society tends not to be aware of our frame of reference, and may sometimes fail to notice that we disregard some information that may not fit our reality. Health practitioners have had many years of practising the art of problem-solving and being exhorted to be part of the solution. As practitioners develop knowledge and skill at a higher level, and as they *fine-tune* the advanced level of clinical judgement, they might also need to consider a clinical and organizational culture in which they look for what works and find ways to do more of that. There seems to be an obsession with learning from mistakes instead of appreciating successes and inquiring more robustly why success has occurred. The primary focus is on what is wrong or broken, since society often looks for the problem. Framing management in healthcare with more emphasis on managing quality (Wheeler and Grice 2000) is presenting a more positive accentuation.

With this in mind, aspiring to, and developing appreciative inquiry skills is an exciting philosophy for change within the work environment. This applies equally to leadership skills, because a major assumption of appreciative inquiry is that in every organization something works, and change can be managed through the identification of what works, and the analysis of how to do more of what works. Might this be the fundamental basis upon which clinical governance and benchmarking is built? And yet organizations often develop cultures in which work appears only to nurture problems and then carries out the often time-consuming and costly exercise of solving those problems. If consultants own what they do well and share it with confidence, then there is no reason to expect that there are any magical answers to change.

Organizational changes

Within most areas of work, it is important to understand specific triggers for organizational changes and the way in which other professions and society in general view the emerging role of health professionals as consultants. First, there has been what can be termed the temporal environment, which encompasses the longer-term historical influences in the structure and role identification of health practitioners. Second, external environment influences may include factors associated with changes brought about by political/legal, economic, technological and socio-cultural developments such as a change in government policy and new legislation. Third, internal triggers may be identified as changes in people such as their attitudes, values, and beliefs, the scale of activities and organizational tasks, the organizational strategy and structure, services, reward systems or use of technology. Working with organizational change may enable consultant health practitioners to expand their area of expertise in human resource work and senior management in both the public sector and also within the private sector, including corporate industry.

Case study	Richard is an occupational therapist with a Master's degree in counselling. He is employed by a major pharmaceutical company to assist the human resource management team to facilitate change in organizational culture. Because of his qualifications, and background in working within community mental health, he is seen as having expert skills in facilitation, communication and leadership styles.

Consultants and organizational development

Within a culture of change, healthcare workers as consultants need to be familiar with organizational development (OD) and knowledgeable in applying the principles of OD. Senge (1999) described OD as a planned, systematic process in which applied behavioural science principles and practices are introduced into an ongoing organization, directing the goals and effecting the implementation of organizational improvement, greater organizational competence, and greater organizational effectiveness. The focus is on improving the effectiveness of organizations—or, to put it another way, effecting total system change. The orientation is on action. The aim is achieving desired outcomes as a result of planned activities. It concentrates on *how* things are done as well as *what* is done. It is concerned with system-wide change. The organization is considered as a total system and the emphasis is on inter-relationships, interactions and interdependencies of different aspects of systems operations. The organization transforms inputs and outputs and uses feedback mechanisms for self-regulation. While this belief has been inherent within private and corporate industry for some time, voluntary and statutory service organizations are only now beginning to integrate OD principles into their systems. Consultants working at this level talk about *client systems*, meaning that they are dealing with the total organizational system.

Consultants working with OD awareness and growing skills may have the following assumptions and values:

- Most individuals are driven by the need for personal growth and development as long as their environment is both supportive and challenging.
- The team, especially at the informal level, has great importance.
- Perceived satisfaction and the dynamics of satisfied teams have a powerful effect on the behaviour of team members.
- Improving the quality of working life is an important aim.
- Organizations can be more effective if they learn to evaluate their own strengths and weaknesses and make choices about progress and change.
- Managers often do not know what is wrong and need special help in diagnosing problems, although the outside *change consultant* ensures that decision-making remains in the hands of the client.

Consultancy at this level may involve helping clients to generate and analyse information that they can understand and, following a thorough diagnosis, act upon. The information will relate to organizational processes such as inter-group relations, interpersonal relations and communications and/or cross-functional changes. The job of a change consultant is to help the organization to solve its own problems by making it aware of organizational processes, of the consequences of these processes, and of the mechanisms by which they can be changed. As I reflect on the concept of the change consultant, I realize that it is a further evolutionary step from the consultant practitioner that involves the development of facilitative skills—skills developed by individuals working beyond their own specific role and across organizational boundaries. As a result, individuals are able to work through themselves as instruments of service, through the *other* and teams and, finally, through the organization, with awareness of the organizational system. Therefore, I can see a continuum of development that extends from the practitioner to the consultant practitioner, to what I would now call the facilitative consultant practitioner—in essence, the organizational change agent.

The challenge for healthcare workers as consultants is to be able to make the transition from the public sector to new areas such as the private and voluntary sectors. I would suggest that, as consultants grow and develop skills around interface working and systems knowledge, they naturally extend their interest and potential work application to other organizations and sectors. In this context, the consultant will need to develop a deeper awareness of personal vision and organizational change strategies. This approach will ensure that consultants respond strategically to new demands and continue to function effectively in the dynamic environment in which they operate.

Making a difference through understanding the dynamics of change

Organizations that aim to manage change, maximize their use of consultant expertise. This can become a major factor that drives and perpetuates success and growth. Every change presents a new opportunity to increase efficiency or to grow and build the business. But all too often, change fails, as organizations and professions fail to rise to the challenges it brings. Why the full potential of change cannot be fully realized lies in the heart and nature of change. For change is a dynamic paradox, that is realized through considering both the drivers of change and the resistances to change (Senge 1999). However, the consultant practitioner cultivates a personal awareness of both the drivers of change (purpose/direction) and the resistances to change (personal limitation). Therefore, he/she can model this awareness of how the full potential for change can be realized within him or herself and for others, whether individuals or teams. The resistances to change may be manifest as fear, anxiety and unwillingness within established institutions or professions that resist this potential for change. Within the current political climate of change in health, social care and higher education, health practitioners can rise to this challenge in the knowledge that their unique contribution is central to the government's change agenda. As highlighted above, consultant practitioners who can model personal and organizational change can be more fully realized as change agents.

Experts in organizational development, such as Senge (1999), Morgan (1997), Senior (1997) and Dixon (1994), indicate that change efforts of the past decade have tended to appear under many banners, including:

- Total Quality Management (TQM), with an emphasis on the flexible, team-based organization where employees are asked to dig beneath the surface of recurring problems and uncover the forces producing them
- Business Process Re-engineering, where the primary emphasis is on the design of technical 'business systems' as the key to change, and a belief that effectiveness comes about by transforming prevailing organizational mind-sets and political patterns
- right-sizing/restructuring, where the focus is on evaluating the effectiveness of the workforce by re-aligning responsibilities and re-structuring the system accordingly
- OD, with an emphasis on efficiency and productivity in the interest of all, and a belief that we can live full and satisfying lives if we fulfill our personal needs through the organizations that dominate the contemporary scene.

In most cases, the primary drivers of the proposed changes for health practitioners are the demands of an evolving marketplace, such as:

- service user involvement
- self-regulation
- the emergence of new technologies
- new legislation
- swings in the economic cycle
- the rapid movement to a global economy.

Why change may fail

The causes of failure to change are varied, but most reasons may come from lack of awareness of the importance of resistance or barriers within the professionals and/or professions themselves. Consultants may need to be aware of potential difficulties, and act appropriately, using their expert skills and knowledge. Common barriers are described below.

Understanding change

Change is a journey, not a destination. Change is a dynamic paradox that demands an understanding or resistance as well as drivers for change. Here, the error is to view change as a single event that is progressed through specific drivers only.

Lack of planning, preparation and change management

Management may suffer from tunnel vision, looking only to the end result and oblivious to the steps required to get there.

Program change has lack of vision

If you don't know where you're going, how can you expect to get there? Other important questions are: what does success look like? And how will you know when you get there?

Goals are set too far in the future

Enthusiasm cannot be sustained for a 10-year plan if there is no recognition of short-term achievements. There has to be a strategy for setting short-term goals and action plans.

The quick-fix option

Change is complex. It is organic. It is a continuum, and means more than a quality poster or a management message in a newsletter,

Poor communication

It is essential that communication is clear, direct and immediate. Giving information gradually is risky; the grapevine may get there first.

The legacy of previous change

Failed change initiatives have an impact on future change initiatives. The result of years of streamlining and right-sizing may be a sceptical, risk-averse culture incompatible with the innovative spirit central to change.

'The way we do things around here'

This assumes, wrongly, that success will always be realized. Having enjoyed success in the past, managers may believe it is because of, not in spite of, the way they do things. They may fail to realize that success stemmed from other sources, for example, a wide-open marketplace, a product idea or new models of practice.

Following some basic principles, consultants can at least help ensure that change is not doomed to failure from the start. For example, consultants working at this level may need to guide organizations and individuals in the following aims.

Be clear about the kind of change required

One of the impediments to change initiatives arises when the change is ill defined and not clearly articulated. The specific change needs clear definition, of its nature, size and scope. For example, major shake-up versus moderate process improvement; slow versus rapid roll-out. Each involves different implications for the company. Decide which is best from a customer, competitive, and corporate viewpoint.

Plan

Planning makes work conscious, and therefore enhances its potential for realization. Therefore, schedule—do not skip—steps that must occur throughout the process. Set out clearly defined objectives and responsibilities; focus on the detail.

Set short-term goals

Define the steps that need to be taken to complete the change—the war will only be won by winning the battles along the way. Reward achievement, and if goals are not met, focus on improvement, not fault-finding.

Prepare employees

Tackle CPD before initiating the change program in order to give staff the confidence and ability to clear the raised hurdles. Reward the engagement with change and the modeling of new values.

Communicate

Walk the talk—ensure communication is two-way. For example, establish feedback sessions, anonymous comment or suggestion slips, open dialogue and identify how information should be cascaded.

Deal with the domino effect

Be aware that things are interconnected; changing one thing has an impact on others. For example, reward systems, the organization structure, and sign-off procedures may require adjustment to facilitate change.

Perhaps the greatest challenge facing the workplace is for all practitioners aspiring to advanced-level practice, and in particular consultant work, to sensitize their thinking, and their ways of knowing to the interplay of forces that shape the world. These issues are also discussed in Chapter 1. Complexity reveals itself when we look at our historical situation and examine some of the great myths about health, social care, and private work. These myths seem to underlie many of the professional debates of our time. As healthcare workers, this time of crisis presents us with an opportunity. We may now be able to see that, inherent within the paradoxes, is the opportunity for a new synthesis which may be emerging from the tensions in our times. Philosophically, there may be a belief that there is a need for such a synthesis and integration.

Summary

Consultancy and expert practice are on a path paved with paradoxes—apparent contradictions that hold hidden opportunities, which stand as sentinels, guarding the approaches to wider fields. Only when we have discovered their hidden reconciliation do we reach a true point of balance in our professional and personal life. We may see this point of balance as our new horizon, an apex midway on the scales, only attained through long experience of trial and error. It offers a steady vantage point. Through long experiments, weighing, testing, trying, leaving, alternating and reassessing, we might emerge at last as serene professionals, empowered to work at an advanced level as consultants in our own right (Roberts 2001).

My intent through this chapter has been to illustrate the probable continuum of practice, skills and competencies that can emerge and be realized by health practitioners as they progress from practitioner to consultant practitioner, to what I have called the *facilitative consultant practitioner*, or change agent. This continuum cultivates a deeper scope of working while honouring the specific depth of individuals' first-chosen specialized training. This broadening scope includes skills to work beyond their specialism to extend across personal, professional and organizational boundaries. The next stage is to develop *systems* awareness, so that individuals can be instruments of service to themselves and through others to groups and teams, further reaching outward to cultivate communities of practice and learning, within the organization. The maturity of consultants lies in their ability to hold and work with paradox. The paradox of change requires us to live with the consciousness of both drivers and resistances to change. The paradox of experience requires us to honour both specialism and scope or breadth, and, in so doing, holding the paradox, embracing it and realizing its generative and organic potential.

References

Antonovsky J 1979 Health, stress and coping. Jossey-Bass, San Francisco. Cited in: Stamp G (2000) Resilience in turbulence. Paper presented at the Bloss Southern Africa Spring School Conference (handout). Bloss, South Africa

College of Occupational Therapists 1999 Position statement on clinical governance. British Journal of Occupational Therapy 62:261–262

Department of Health 1995 ENRIP report. Exploring new roles in practice. Department of Health, London

Department of Health 1997 White paper. The new NHS: modern and dependable; a national framework for assessing performance. Stationery Office, London

Department of Health 2000 A strategy for the allied health professions. Meeting the challenge. Stationery Office, London

Department of Health 2001a A national service framework for older people. Online. Available at: http://www.doh.gov.uk/nsf/olderpeople.htm. Accessed 25 May 2002

Department of Health 2001b Health service circular. HSC 71/21. Department of Health, London

Dixon N 1994 The organisational learning cycle. How we can learn collectively. McGraw-Hill, London

Fish D, Coles C 1998 Developing professional judgement in healthcare. Butterworth-Heinemann, Oxford

Hagedorn R 1995 The Casson memorial lecture 1995. An emergent profession—a personal perspective. British Journal of Occupational Therapy 58:324–331

Machon A 2000 Personal mastery workshop. College of Occupational Therapists National Conference, Keele University, England.

Morgan G 1997 Images of organisation. Sage Publications, London

Roberts G W 2001 The Casson memorial lecture 2001. A new synthesis—the emergent spirit of higher level practice. British Journal of Occupational Therapy 64:493–502

Roberts G, Cusack L 2001 Consultant therapists—core functions. Occupational Therapy News 9:12–13

Sealey C 1999 Clinical governance: an information guide for occupational therapists. British Journal of Occupational Therapy 62:263–268

Senge P 1999 The dance of change. Nicholas Brealey, London

Senior B 1997 Organisational change. Financial Times management. Online. Available at: www.ftmanagement.com. Accessed 25 May 2002

Wheeler N, Grice D 2000 Management in healthcare. Stanley Thornes, Cheltenham, UK

Epilogue

As an ending to this text, we decided to share with you some of our own *favourite good housekeeping tips* for advanced practice. Every advanced practitioner, like every experienced cook, has these. No doubt you will add your own and collect many more from your colleagues. Here are some of ours:

- Be efficient, but not over-efficient. Going too fast may mean missing some important clue or detail along the way, especially when it comes to understanding the politics and interpersonal aspects of an organization. If detailed instructions are pending, wait till they come. You may think they are coming via snail mail, and you are in the fast track, and have no time to waste. However, jumping the gun may land you in a big ditch, and digging yourself out will take longer in the long run. Always reflect first, before you speak, write or act.

- Do not try to compartmentalize your life, thinking you can keep your work, leisure, personal life, and studies in neat little areas that do not spill over into each other. Life is a tapestry. Yes, the flowers, people, animals, are all separate and distinct; they have their place, colour and shape within the whole picture. But when you turn the tapestry over, the threads are all woven in, connecting and strengthening the whole. Often the wrapping up, running the threads back through, occurs outside the frame of the actual activity. Thus, you make notes for implementing important issues at work when you are at home and you make a call to take care of some family matter during a break at work. If you don't take care of these loose ends, they have a way of unraveling, weakening the whole fabric of the tapestry and making your life stressful.

Working towards advanced practice is not about achieving an easily defined goal or, having once reached that goal, ceasing to seek further development. In fact, there is no end point. Advanced practice is about establishing a proactive outlook on your work and constantly re-evaluating and re-prioritizing what you are doing. This will allow you to respond to the changes in practice demands, the shifting health status of the people with whom you work and the never-ending social changes that occur constantly. It will enable you to drive changes in practice, not just respond to them. We believe that it is most important always to make good use of the challenges that change offers. Take opportunities when they present themselves to you and do not wait until you feel completely proficient. By that time the job will have changed. Have confidence and learn as you go.

This is all from us at this time. Now it is up to you to create your own trajectory and make it an exciting, meaningful and productive journey, as you take off to create a never-ending story that is your successful career as an advanced healthcare practitioner.

Gillian Brown, Susan A. Esdaile, Susan E. Ryan

Index

Note: As the major subject of this book is Advanced Healthcare Practitioners, entries under this term have been kept to a minimum, and readers are advised to seek more specific entries. *Abbreviations*, CPD - continuing professional development

A

Abstractness, of theory, 70
Academic awards, CPD, 268–269
Academic disciplines, 172
Academic educators, 165–166
    shortage, 174
    see also Adult educators
Academic institutions
    continuing professional development via, 269
    linking, scholarship of integration, 164
    see also Universities
Accountability, professional, 163
Accreditation, 267
Accreditation in Occupational Therapy
    (AccOT)(Australia), 14
Achievement period, of career development, 166–167
Action learning, 113–114
    components, 113
Action research, 180–183
    function and uses, 181–182
    goals/objectives, 182–183
    holistic understanding, 180
    implementation, 182–183
    model, 181, 182
Active learning, reflection and, 136–137
Activists, 42
Activity, reduction in stroke survivors, 195
Adolescence, 36
    career development initiation, 36
Adult educators, 219
    authenticity, 219
    characteristics needed, 219–220
    dimensions/elements of model of
        experience, 234
    as facilitators, 217, 219–220, 220
    growth and development as, 236
    roles, 219–220
    sense of being, 235
    story telling workshops, 230
Adult learners, characteristics, 218–219

Adult learning, 218–220
    conditions promoting, 219
    critical incidents, 228, 229
    facilitators, 217, 219–220, 220
    story telling, 228–232
    see also Journalling; Reasoning, clinical;
        Reflection in practice
Adult learning theories, 16, 66, 216–238
    adoption of principles, 217, 220
    for distance education program, 83–84
Advanced beginners, 33
Advanced practice, 24, 53, 151
    clinical reasoning as key, 151
    development of competencies, 30–63
    expertise development, 269–271
    goals, 268
    'housekeeping tips,' 300
    requirements, 263–264, 267–268, 273
Advanced practitioner, 236
    alternative terms for, 2
    definition, 2, 31, 32–35, 53
        critical thinking role, 34–35
        mastery, excellence and leadership, 33
    demands of, 262
    how to become, 49–53, 54
        see also Career-paths; Competency;
            Reasoning
    as new career role, 2
    non-clinical areas of competence, 3
    requirements, 3, 263–264, 267–268, 273
    roles and responsibilities, 3, 262, 263, 264
    transition from 'novice' to 'expert,' 33–34
    vision of (characteristics), 233–236
Advertising, consumer behaviour and, 75, 76
Agency, sense of, 235
Allied health professional, consultant, 285
    opportunities, 284
    see also Consultants
Allied health sciences
    continuing professional development, 265, 266
    use of term, 171

Ambiguity
  management, 271
  tolerance for, 49
American Occupational Therapy Association,
    practice guidelines, 80–81
American Physical Therapy Association,
    practice guidelines, 80
Application models, 78
Applied behavioural science, 182
Applied science, 68–69
Applied scientists, 68–69
Appraisal of evidence, 101–102
  checklist, 102, 103
Apprenticeship model, 148
Artistry, professional, 154–156, 155,
    236
Attention levels, 236
Audit, evidence-based, 112, 113
Australia
  continuing professional development,
    266–267
  professional standards and quality
    framework, 10
  regulatory procedures, 11
  work salience and values, 39
Authenticity, adult educators, 219
Autobiography, writing, 183
The Autobiography Box (Bouldrey), 183
Autonomy, professional, 9, 166, 174
  adult learners, 218–219, 220
  consultants, 287
Awareness
  'higher level,' 235–236
  self-awareness, consultants, 290,
    291–292

B

Bachelor-level programs, 174, 266
Bandura's Self-Efficacy Theory, 86–87
Belief systems, on illness, 15
Benchmarking, 7
Benchmarks, 7
Benchmark Statement (QAA 2001), 123
'Best evidence,' 102, 104, 105
'Best practice,' 273
  continuing professional development and,
    265
Boud's retrospective model, 124, 223–224
Brainstorming, 20
Bureaucracy, 287
Burnout, risks, 23
Business Process Re-engineering, 296

C

Canada
  regulatory procedures, 11
  work values, 39
Canadian Association of Occupational
    Therapists
  continuing professional development,
    265
  practice guidelines, 79–80
Canadian Model of Occupational
    Performance, 79–80

Career
  commitment to chosen field, 36
  definition, 36
  landmarks, 263
Career development
  acceleration by mentors, 246
  continuum from practitioner to consultant,
    295
  early, interviews, 166–170
  elements affecting aspiration attainment, 37
  establishment and achievement periods,
    166–167
  lifelong process, 36
    see also Lifelong learning
  new opportunities for consultants, 284
  professional evolution paradigm, stages,
    171
  relationships/people influencing, 248–257
  theory, 35–37
  see also Career-planning
Career-paths
  to become an advanced practitioner, 49–50
  fictitious healthcare practitioners
    (examples), 31–32
  multiple interests and, 52
  patterns (linear, expert, spiral and
    transitory), 49–50
  strategies for progression, 2
Career-planning, 30, 35–41, 53
  advanced degrees and, 51
  balance between roles, 38
  choice and personality influence, 43–45, 173
  consultants and, 285
  decision-making, 37–39, 53
    impact of values on, 47, 173
    Salience Inventory, 47–48, 173
  elements to consider, 35, 183
  health and social care trends, 41
  lateral shifts, 41, 50
  mentoring and self-management, 246–247
  need for proaction, 167
  preparing to 'ladder up', 40–41
  staying or moving on, 39–40
  websites, 63
  see also Career development
Career profiles, fictitious practitioners, 54–61
Case studies, evidence-based, 107–108
Causal propositions, 71
Centre for Evidence-based Medicine (CEBM),
    104–105
Centre for Evidence-based Physiotherapy, 94
Challenging, of professional practice, 272, 273
Change consultant, 294, 298
Changes, 295–298
  paradoxes, 298, 299
  see also Organizational change
Children
  career development initiation, 36
  care givers' long-term influence, 244
  self-initiated occupations, 211
Choice(s)
  forced, 41, 49
  levels (Gouws'), 37–38
Client-centred practice, 92
  see also Evidence-based practice (EBP)
Client systems, 294

Clinical governance, 284, 289
  definition, 289
Clinical problem-solver model, 148
  see also Problem-solving
Clinical reasoning see Reasoning
Coaches, training with, 249–250
Coaching approach, 136, 137
  criteria for success, 250
Coaching approach, reflection, 141
Codes of ethics/conduct, 261, 264
Collaboration
  action research, 180–181
  in discovery area of scholarship of
      practice, 163
  importance, 164
  occupational practice, 204
  scholarship of integration and, 164
'Comfort zones,' 289
Commitment
  professional, 166
  Salience Inventory, 47–48
Commitment model, 287
Common healthcare framework, 7
Communication, for effective changes, 297
Community approach, occupational practice,
    211
  consequence of, 204–205
Community care, 6
Compact disks (CDs), 164
Competence, 263–264
  attaining and maintaining, 263, 277–278
  continuing, forces driving, 9
  to learn, 271–272
Competency
  broadening areas of, 52–53
  development, 30–63
  leading edge and development, 260–281
    see also Career development; Continuing
        professional development
  portfolio of, 50
  in reasoning see Reasoning
Competent clinician model, 148
Competent practitioners, 34
Complaints, management, 20–21
Complementary and alternative healthcare,
    professional development, 3
Comprehensibility challenge, to consultants,
    291
Concepts
  Bandura's self-efficacy theory, 86, 87
  broad vs specific, 76
  'buying,' 76
  definition, 70–71
  example, 71–72
Conceptual model, 73
'Constellation of developers,' 247
Constructs
  connecting with reflection, 120
  definition, 71
Consultant allied health professional, 285
Consultant nurses, 283
Consultants, 282–299
  challenges and elements of, 291
  change consultant, 294, 298
  continuum of development to, 295
  credibility, 291

description, 287, 288–289
  core functions of expert practice,
      288–289
  Department of Health, 285, 287–288
  educational role, 289
  extended-scope practice, 292–293
  goals, 289
  increase in number, 284
  as leaders, 288
  leadership potential, 290
  lifelong learning, 289
    maximization, 290
  listening and feedback, 290
  managerial profile, 285
  nature of work, 284–286
  new career opportunities, 284
  new paradigm of working and, 286–293
  organizational change and, 293, 294–295
  organizational development, 294–295
  paradoxes affecting, 298
  professional resilience, 290–291
  risk-taking, 289–290
  roles and functions, 284–286, 287, 289
    Department of Health description, 289
  self-awareness, 290
Consultant therapist, 2
Consumer behaviour, 76
Consumer of theory see Theory
Continuing competence, forces driving, 9
Continuing education, 267
Continuing professional development (CPD),
    14, 16, 260–281, 264–266, 283
  academic awards, 268–269
  allied health sciences, 265, 266
  definitions, 265, 266
  expertise development, 269–271
  identification of needs, 265
  legislative requirements, 265–266
  plan, establishment, 264–265
  portfolio, 273–279
    assembling, 275–276
    contents, 275, 276–277
    definition and characteristics, 274
    do's and don'ts, 278–279
    dynamics, 276
    ownership, 279
    practical aspects of presentation, 275–276
    'private' evidence vs 'public' scrutiny,
        274
    sampling system, 274
    structure, 276–277
    types, 278
    updating and changing profiles, 276
    write-ups of cases, 277–278
  presentation, 273–279
  process, 267–269
  reasons for, 14
  resources and access to, 269
  responsibility for, 265, 266
  themes and activities, 267
  see also Expertise; Professional
      development
Cornerstone Programme in New Zealand,
    267
Covey's quadrants system, 23
Credibility, consultants, 291

Credit accumulation and transfer schemes (CATS), 269
Crisis period, 171
Critical appraisal, of evidence, 102
Critical companionship (Titchen's), 232–233
Critical friends, 232–233
Critical incidents, 228
  exploration and sharing, 228
  guidelines, 229
Critically appraised papers, 107, 108
Critical questions, prerequisite to evaluating, 35
Critical thinkers
  learning to become, 35
  qualities, 34–35
Critical thinking, 34–35
  in CPD portfolio, 275
Cultural issues/interactions, 15–17
Curriculum vitae (CV), 274, 276

D

Databases, 100
Debriefing, 129
Decision-making, 30, 149
  careers, 37–39
    see also Career-planning
  consultants and, 287
  ethical, strategies, 156
  experience use of, 93
  learning, 152
  public involvement, 5
  Straker's hierarchy of evidence, 104
  see also Reasoning
Declining continuum in development, 36–37
Deductive thinking, 66
Degrees, 283
  advanced, 51
  Bachelor-level programs, 174, 266
  graduate, 50–52
  Master's see Master's degrees
Delineation models, 78
Demand-driven systems, 4
'Developers' (mentors), 245, 247
  see also Mentors
Development
  career see Career development
  competency, 30–63
  see also Professional development
Developmental levels, 36–37
Developmental relationships, 248–257
Developmental tasks, cycling/recycling, 36
DHNet, 18
Disability, 190, 213
  measures of performance, 201
Disablement model, 80
Discovery, in scholarship of practice, 162, 163–164, 171, 172–173
Disempowering culture, 287
Disillusionment, 286
Distance education, 83–86, 269
Doctoral programs, 51
Documentation, integration of learning, 169

E

Early-career practitioners
  interview questions, 242
  networking, 241–242
  scholarship of practice, 166–170
Education
  of academic staff, 165
  adult educators/learning see Adult educators; Adult learning
  continuing, 267
  distance technology, 83–86, 269
  e-learning programs, 17
  enhancement, academic educators and, 165–166
  evidence-based culture development through, 109, 110
  facilitation in, 219–220
  fast-track syllabi, 16
  graduate, importance, 50–52
  international differences, 16
  leadership in, 177
  post-baccalaureate entry-level, 174
  re-framing goals/outcomes to extend reasoning, 152–153
  role of consultants, 289
  shifts driving quality changes, 18
  shortage of educators, 174
  teaching area of scholarship of practice, 165–166, 177–178
Educational theory, for distance education program, 83–84, 85
Educators see Academic educators; Adult educators
E-learning programs, 17
E-mail, 18, 164
Emotional intelligence (EI), 41–42
Empirical relevance, of theory, 70
Empiricism, theory relationship, 68
Employees, benefit reduction, 4
Empowerment, 285
Entrepreneurial qualities, 16, 287
Environment
  conducive to adult learning, 219
  for healthcare practitioners, 1
  trigger for organizational changes, 293
Establishment continuum, in development, 37
Establishment period, of career development, 166–167
Esteem, loss, 201
Ethical dilemmas, 176
Ethnic minorities, recruitment, 14
European Master's Program, 269
Evidence
  appraisal, 101–102
  'best,' 102, 104, 105
  experience and reflection as, 106–107
  hierarchy see Hierarchy of evidence
  nature of, 102–108
  search strategies for, 99–101
Evidence-based audit, 112, 113
Evidence-based case studies, 107–108
Evidence-based culture, development, 109–112

Evidence-based medicine (EBM), 90, 91, 95
  definition, 91, 94, 95
Evidence-based nursing (EBN), 95
Evidence-based occupational therapy
    (EBOT), 94
Evidence-based physiotherapy (EB PT), 94
Evidence-based practice (EBP), 90–117, 218
  benefits, 112
  definition, 91
  development, 95
  dilemmas, 92
  evidence types for and evidence-based
      questions, 105
  integration area of scholarship of practice,
      164
  'jigsaw' model, 106
  limitations/barriers, 93–94
  nature of evidence, 102–108
  obstacles to development, 109
  process and stages, 95–96
    appraisal of evidence, 101–102
    evidence source and search strategy,
        98–101
    identification of problem/questions,
        96–98
  reluctance to use, 93–94
  resources, 99
  skills, 96
  utilization and changing practice, 109–114
    activities for, 110–111
    development of practice, 112–114
    essential factors for, 114
    evidence-based culture development,
        109–112
    journal clubs, 111–112
    skills required, 110
    support for, 109–110
Excellence, 33
  pursuit, 287
Exemplary practice, learning from, 239–259
Experience/experiential learning
  articulation of and method to use, 107
  as evidence for decision-making, 93,
      106–107
  learning from in early career development,
      168
  reflection on experience and, 223–224
  uses and advantages in decision-making,
      107
Expert career pattern, 50
Expertise, 151
  concept, 271
  development, 269–271
  levels and knowledge/reasoning, 153
  maintenance, 270
  motivation to gain, 270
Expert performers, 50
  definition, 34
Expert practice, 24
  consultants, 287
  core functions, 288–289
  outcome of qualitative studies, 185
  see also Advanced practice; Advanced
      practitioner
Experts, clinical vs development of, 269–270
Expert status, 50

Exploring continuum, in development, 37
Exploring New Roles in Practice (Department
    of Health 1995), 285
Extended-scope practice, consultants,
    292–293
Extraversion Types^R, 44

F

Facilitation
  for action learning, 113
  in critical companionship model, 233
  definition, 219
  in education, 219–220
Facilitative consultant practitioner, 295, 298
Facilitators
  of adult learning, 217, 219–220, 220
  group work (reflective), 141
Falls prevention program, development, 86–87
Fawcett Hill's learning through discussion,
    178–180
Feedback, direct, consultants and, 290
Fee-for-service arrangement, mentoring and,
    256–257
Financial aspects of healthcare, 4, 147
Finland, Internet use, 17
Fitness level, 195
Flow charts, 67
'Follow me,' reflection in action, 136, 137
Frame of reference, 74
Free-flow writing, 130

G

Globalization, health/social services, 147, 148
'Global Village' concept, 18
Goals, business, 286
Goodall, Jane, 162
Gouws' levels of choice, 37–38
Governments, healthcare re-organizations, 2
  factors driving, 4–5
Graduate degree, importance, 50–52
Graduates, new, 33, 36, 172
  early-career development, 166–170
    see also Early-career practitioners types,
        147–148
Grand theories, 72
Greeks, ancient, philosophy, 67
Group facilitation skills, 290–291
Growing continuum, in development, 37
Guidelines, practice, 79–81, 165
  American Physical Therapy Association, 80
  Canadian Association of Occupational
      Therapists, 79–80
  evidence-based, 112
Guide to Occupational Therapy Practice, 80–81
Guide to Physical Therapist Practice, 80

H

'Habits of mind,' 165
Habitual action, 135
Hall of mirrors, 136, 137
Handicap
  intervention outcome measures, 201
  measures, 207

Health
    definition, 195, 207
    occupation as outcome *see* Occupation, as
        health outcome
    occupation relationship, 191, 193–196,
        206
        two-directional, 195
Health Belief Model, 73
Healthcare
    career trends, 41
    changing features, 147, 261, 272, 284
    common framework and features, 7
    costs, 174
    factors driving changes, 4–5, 261
        public role, 5
    financial aspects, 4, 147
    globalization, 147, 148
    management, 293
    management of quality needed, 293
    modern system, 284–285
    pace of change, 5–6
    rationing, 4
    re-organization by governments, 2
    universality, principle, 4
Healthcare organizations, funding, 4
Healthcare practitioners/professionals
    changing roles, 6–7, 285
    changing within/between disciplines,
        6–7
    evolution of theory and, 68–69
    expansion in numbers (UK), 14
    fictitious (examples)
        career profiles, 54–61
        career structure, 31–32
    inter-relationship with clients, 7, 8
    motivation, 173
    numbers, 171
    overlap between, 7
    reasons for concern over client's
        occupations, 191, 193–207
    responsibilities *see* Responsibilities
    shortages, 6, 15–16, 174
        UK, 16
Healthcare profession, joining, 146–147
Health professional model, 148
Health Professions Council (UK), 265
Hearing loss, occupations limited by, 207
Hearing science, clinical/professional
        reasoning, 150
Hierarchical propositions, 71
Hierarchy of evidence, 94
    alternative (Straker's), 104
Higher-level practice, 282, 292–293
History, theory and practice, 67–69
Holistic paradigm, 73, 291
Holistic treatment goals, occupational
        practice, 204
Honey and Mumford's Learning Styles
        Questionnaire (LSQ), 43
Hospitals
    client transition to home/work,
        210–211
    occupations/activities supported,
        210–211
Howerton's 'success circles,' 51
Humanistic and holistic philosophy, 291

I

Ideas, procedures for investigation, 19, 20
Impact on Participation and Autonomy, 207
Impairments, 192
    occupational difficulties, 196
Individuality, CPD portfolio, 274
Individualization of interventions
    occupational goals and, 198–199
    rehabilitation, 202–203
Innovation
    importance, 164
    role development and, 285, 286
Integrated profession, model, 171, 172
Integration, in scholarship of practice *see*
        Scholarship of practice
Intellectual debate, 176–177
    methods, 176
'Interactional professional' model, 152–153
Intercultural interactions, 15–17
Inter-disciplinary work, 16
Intermediate care, 284
*International Classification of Functioning,
        Disability and Health (ICF: WHO 2001)*,
        189, 192, 197, 198
    activity and participation categories, 192
    limitations, 204
    standard terminology adoption, 199
    support for occupational practice, 203–204
International developments, advantages and
        applications, 17–19
International differences
    continuing professional development,
        265–266
    cultural issues/interactions, 15–17
    education, 16
    regulatory procedures, 10–14
International Society for Quality in Health
        Care, 267
International Work Importance Study, 173
Internet
    continuing professional development via,
        269
    DHNet, 18
    educational resources, 18, 19
    usage, 17–18
    see also Websites
Interpersonal skills, adult educators, 219
Inter-subjectivity, of theory, 70
Intervening, 138
Introspection, 135
Introversion Types^R, 44
Intuitive approach, in critical companionship
        model, 233
Intuitive Types^R, 44
'Invisible colleges,' concept, 18, 243

J

Joint experimentation, reflection in action,
        136, 137
Journal clubs, 111–112, 166, 180
Journalling, 224–227
    personal example (of author), 226–227
    suggestions for approach, 225
    time requirement, 225

Journals
  critically appraised papers, 107, 108
  letters from readers, 176
JP scale, 43, 45
Judgement
  professional practice, 154, 155
  reflective *see* Reflective judgement
Judgements, professional, 263
Judging Types^R, 44–45, 45
Jung's views on mental functions, 43

K

'Knowing in action,' 136
Knowledge, 173
  about self *see* Self-knowledge
  acquisition, 33
  forms, 149
  non-propositional, 149
  personal, 149
  professional craft, 149, 153, 218, 235
  profession's body of (discovery phase),
    172–173
  propositional, 149, 218, 224, 235
  reasoning integration, 149–151, 153
  scholarship as product, 171
  in scholarship of practice, 162
Knowles' educational theory, 83–84, 85
Kolb's Learning Cycle, 121

L

Lateral shifts, 50
  careers, 41
Law and ethics, 175
Leaders
  attributes, 177
  consultants as, 288
Leadership, 9, 33
  in education, 177
  management *vs*, 177
  need for, 2
  potential, consultants, 290
Learning
  active and reflection, 136–137
  adult *see* Adult learning
  capacity for, 272
  competency for, 271–272
  control over what is to be learned, 219,
    270–271
  of decision-making, 152
  from exemplary practice, 239–259
  informal, types of opportunities, 277
  lifelong *see* Lifelong learning
  maximization by consultants, 290
  from mistakes, obsession, 293
  participation in, 271
  process, 219
  reflective, 122
  from role models, 248–249
  self-directed, 156, 270–271
Learning programs, managers, 219
Learning style preferences, 42–43
  questionnaire, 43
Learning through discussion (LTD), 178–180
'Learning workplace' culture, 220

Legislative requirements, CPD, 265–266
Leisure activities, decreased participation
    after stroke, 195
Leisure rehabilitation, 196
Licensure (L) system, 14
Life, satisfaction, 212
Lifelong learning, 36, 156, 262–263, 282
  consultants and, 289
  principles, 262–263
  risk-taking by consultants and, 289
Linear model, career pattern, 49–50
Listening, by consultants, 290
Literature (professional), importance,
    173–174
Litigation, 5
Locus of control, 48–49
  definition, 48
  external, 48
  internal, 48, 49

M

Maintaining continuum, in development, 37
Manageability challenge, to consultants,
    291
Management
  of complaints, 20–21
  healthcare, 293
  leadership *vs*, 177
  of organizational change, 295
  of power, 19–22
  of quality, emphasis needed, 293
  of self *see* Self-management
  of stress (work-related), 23–24
  of time *see* Time management
Managerial profile, consultants, 285
Managers, learning programs, 219
Master's degrees, 16, 43, 51
  entry-level for professions, 174
Mastery, 33
  consultants, 291–292
Medical dominance, of healthcare
    professions, 22
Medical technologists, 167
  early-career, 166
Meetings
  action research, 182–183
  for development of evidence-based
    practice, 97
  learning through discussion (LTD) and,
    178–179
  networking at, 242
  objectives for networking, 243
Memoir, writing, 183–184
  definition and process, 183
  steps, 184
Mental illness, residential program and
    outcomes, 208
Mentee, definition, 257
Mentoring, 258
  communication method for, 254
  conducting, 254–256
  definition, 244
  difficulties, 255, 256
  duration, 254
  fee-for-service arrangement and, 256–257

Mentoring (*contd*)
  'mosaic' (multiple), 246
  multiple, 245–246, 247, 255
  participation in, 246–247
  process, 243–245
  self-management and self-monitoring, 246
  sessions
    agenda for, 254
    closure and feedback, 254–255
    goals and objectives, 254
    progress assessment, 255
    reflection after, 255
Mentoring-type relationship, 244
  aims of, 256
  conducting, 254–256
  difficulties, 255, 256
  initiating and maintaining, 252, 253
  negative, 255
  participation in, 246–247
Mentors, 251–252
  benefits, 245, 251
  choice, 247, 252–253, 255
  functions, 244
  multiple, 245–246, 247, 255
  questions about, 242
  roles and clarification of, 254
  use of term, 252
Metacognition, 138, 151
  as component of reasoning, 154
Meta theories, 72
Mezirow's types of non-reflective action, 135
Microbiology, 172, 173
Military command model, 287
Model(s), 73
  action research, 181, 182
  application, 78
  apprenticeship, 148
  Boud's retrospective, 124, 223–224
  clinical problem-solver, 148
  commitment, 287
  competent clinician, 148
  conceptual, 73
  critical companionship, 233
  delineation, 78
  disablement, 80
  dynamic, 73
  health professional, 148
  integrated profession, 171, 172
  'interactional professional,' 152–153
  'jigsaw,' evidence-based practice, 106
  linear, career pattern, 49–50
  military command, 287
  personal, 78
  PICO, of clinical questions, 98
  professional, 78
  reasoning, clinical, 149
  reflective judgement, 123–124
  reflective practitioner, 148
  role *see* Role models
  scientist practitioner, 148
  as two-dimensional representation, 74
Modern healthcare systems, 284–285
Motivation
  in early-career development, 170
  to gain expertise, 270
  of health professionals, 173

  for rehabilitation, 191, 196–197
  theories, 84–85
Multidisciplinary health, 189–215
Multi-disciplinary teams, 22
  reflection in practice and, 138–140
Multi-disciplinary training, 52
Myers-Briggs Type Indicator^R (MBTI), 43–45, 183

N

Narrative inquiry approach, 229, 233
Narrative reasoning, 223
Narrative therapy, story telling, 230
National Committee of Inquiry into Higher
    Education, 5–6
National Health Service
  consultants and, 285, 286–287, 289
  CPD policies, 266
  White Paper, 91, 109, 283
Natural philosophers, 68
Netherlands, regulatory procedures, 12
Networking, 239, 240–243, 257
  advice, 242–243
  definition, 240
  formalizing, 241
  proactive approach, 240
  rewards, 243
The New NHS: Modern, Dependable
    (Department of Health 1997), 91, 109,
    283
New Zealand, continuing professional
    development, 266–267
Nightingale, Florence, 244
Non-propositional knowledge, 149
Non-reflective action, 135
Noticing, 138
Novice practitioners, 33
  transition to advanced practitioners, 33–34
Nurses, consultant, 283
Nurse specialist, 2
Nursing
  clinical/professional reasoning, 150
  evidence-based, 95

O

Observation of practice
  in discovery area of scholarship of
      practice, 163, 169
  inadequate for learning, 221
  skills, importance, 170
Occupation
  challenges of clients, 193, 194
  definition, 190
  frequency and quality of performance, 197
  as health outcome, 191–192, 196–197
    consequences of occupation, 202–203
    individualization of interventions,
        198–199
    occupational goals, 197–199
    occupational language/outcomes,
        199–200
    occupational practice, 200–202
  importance, reasons, 190–193, 193–207, 213
    as health outcome *see above*

Occupation (*contd*)
  health relationship, 191, 193–196, 206
  meaning to life/motivation, 191,
    196–197, 205
  important, identification, 207–208
  motivation for rehabilitation, 191, 196–197
  reasons for health professionals' concern,
    193–207
  role in everyday life, 190, 191
  self-initiated and therapeutic, 208, 211
  understanding of clients focused on, 197
Occupational practice, 173, 189–215
  consequences of, 204–205
  consequences of occupations and,
    202–203
  discrepancy between client/therapist'
    goals, 207
  ICF support, 203–204
  outcome measures, 204–205
  skills for, 207–212
    client readiness for occupation, 209–210
    nature of intervention, 208–209
    occupations enabled by practice setting,
      210–212
    occupations important for clients,
      207–208
  strategies for development, 200–202
  see also Occupation
Occupational science, 173
'Occupational self,' concept, 209, 211
Occupational Therapist Registered (OTR),
  10
Occupational therapy, 212–213
  bibliography of theory-based articles,
    77–78
  clinical/professional reasoning, 150
  distance education program, 83–86
  early-career development, 167
  education (US), 174
  evidence-based, 94
  falls prevention program development,
    86–87
  frame of reference, 74
  goals, 198
  levels of theoretical information, 78
  scholarly debate, 176
  Sweden, 17
  therapeutic nature, 208
Organization, as total system, 294
Organizational change, 293–295
  clarity over type, and goals, 297–298
  consultants and, 293, 294–295
  drivers and resistances to, 295, 296
  as dynamic paradox, 295, 296
  dynamics, 295–298
  ill-defined, 297
  management, 295
  as opportunity, 295
  reasons for failure, 296–297
  triggers, 293
Organizational change agent, 295, 298
Organizational development (OD), 294–295,
  296
  definition/description, 294, 296
Organizational effectiveness, 286–287
  improving, 294

P

Paradigms, 72–73, 171
  acceptance stage, 171
  new, for working and consultants, 286–293
  professional evolution, stages, 171
Participation
  in continuing professional development,
    271
  Salience Inventory, 47–48
Part-time employment, 4
Pattern recognition, 223
PEDro, 94, 95
Peer discussions, 156
Peer learning experience, 156
Peers, 217, 220
  clinical reasoning exploration, 222–223
  as critical friends, 232–233
  working with, 248
Perceptive Types[R], 44–45, 45
Personal control
  learning, 219, 270–271
  professional development, 156–157, 270–271
Personal effectiveness, 286–287
Personality style and preferences, 43–45, 173,
  183
  MBTI types, 44–45, 183
Personal knowledge, 149
Personal mastery, consultants, 291–292
Personal models, 78
Personnel management, approaches based on
  personality styles, 45
Pew Health Professions Commission, 6
Phenomenology, 233
Philosophers, 67
Physical therapy
  consequences of occupation consideration,
    202–203
  early-career development, 167
  education, 174
    leadership conceptualization, 177
Physiotherapy
  clinical/professional reasoning, 150
  evidence-based, 94
PICO model of clinical questions, 98
Planning
  career *see* Career-planning
  new roles and, 285
Podiatrists, goals, 198
Portfolio, professional, 141
  consultants, 289
  CPD *see* Continuing professional
    development (CPD)
  definition, 274
  reflection, 132
Portfolio of competencies, 50
Power
  definition, 19
  management, 19–22
  personal, 19
  politics, understanding, 22
  viewpoints in health literature, 21
Practice
  integration with theory *see* Theory–practice
    interconnection
  professional *see* Professional practice

Practice guidelines *see* Guidelines, practice
Practice theories, 72
Practice wisdom, 154
Practitioners *see* Advanced practitioner;
    Healthcare practitioners/professionals
Pragmatists, 42
Prayer, 176
Preferences
    functions and attitudes, 43–45
    inclusion in theory–practice connection
        framework, 82, 85
    personality style and, 43–45, 173, 183
Preparadigm period, 171
Prioritization of work, 23
    time organization and, 23
Proactive approach
    career-planning, 167
    networking, 240
Problem-framing, 139
Problem-orientated culture, 293
Problem-solving, 139, 152, 270
    negative emphasis of, 293
Profession
    advancement, responsibility for, 272–273
    body of knowledge, 172–173
    characteristics (scholarship of integration),
        173–175
    members of, 146–147
    uniqueness of each, 283
Professional accountability, 163
Professional artistry, 154–156, 155, 236
Professional autonomy *see* Autonomy,
        professional
Professional behaviour, 145
Professional commitment, 166
Professional competence, 3, 9
    in reflection, 123
Professional craft knowledge, 149, 153, 218,
        235
Professional development, 262
    administrative, 167
    identification of needs, 265
    personal and journalling role, 224
    plan, establishment, 264–265
    plans for, 278–279
    scholarly, 166–167
    taking control, 156–157, 270–271
    wide-ranging, need for, 264
    see also Career development; Continuing
        professional development (CPD)
Professional evolution paradigm, stages, 171
Professional identity, 286
Professionalism
    features, 147
    self-interested, 166
Professional journals, writing *see* Journalling
Professional judgements, 263
Professional mastery, consultants, 291–292
Professional meetings, networking *see*
        Meetings
Professional models, 78
Professional organizations
    involvement for advanced practitioners,
        51–52, 176–177
    networking, 241
Professional participation, 267

Professional performance, mastery,
        excellence and leadership, 33
Professional practice
    challenging of policies, 272, 273
    'doing' component, 221
    iceberg concept, 221, 230
    wisdom and science in, 272
Professional practice judgement, 154, 155
Professional reasoning *see* Reasoning
Professional regulation, 286
Professional resilience, consultants, 290–291
Professionals, 145
    demands and challenges, 262, 263
Professional self-regulation, 9, 284, 294
Professional standards *see* Standards
Proficiency, concept, 271
Proficient practitioners, 34
Propositional knowledge, 149, 218, 224, 235
Propositions, 71
    Bandura's self-efficacy theory, 86, 87
    'buying,' 76
    types, 71
Protégés, 257
    mentors for, 244
    roles and clarification of, 254
Psychosocial functions, mentors, 245
Public
    healthcare changes driven by, 5
    involvement in decision-making, 5
Public accountability, 9
Public health, action research model, 182
Purpose, sense of, 290

Q

Qualifications, professional, 261
    vs academic, 10
Qualitative propositions, 71
Qualitative studies, of expert practice,
        outcomes, 185
Quality, management, emphasis needed, 293
Quality assurance, 175
    continuing professional development and,
        267
Quality Assurance Agency (QAA), 123
Quality of evidence, 35
Quantitative propositions, 71
Questions, in evidence-based practice, 96–98

R

Radiation therapy
    coaching and, 250
    early-career development, 167, 168–169,
        170
Rational approach, in critical companionship
        model, 233
Rationing, healthcare, 4
Reasoning, clinical, 145–160
    clinical approaches, 150
    discussing, 222–223, 223
    exploring with peers, 222–223
    extending competence in, 151–157
        ethical decision-making strategies, 156
        expertise development, 153
        metacognition and self-evaluation, 154

Reasoning, clinical (*contd*)
   professional artistry, 154–156
      re-framing goals/outcomes, 152–153
      self-directed learning, 156
   facilitating development of, 221–223
   as key to advanced practice, 151
   knowledge integration, 149–151, 153
   modelling, 220–221, 223
   models, 149
   modes, definitions, 150
   narrative, 223
   reflective, theory–practice interconnection, 81
   requirements, 152
   scholarship of practice and, 163
   teaching, 152
   see also Decision-making
Recruitment, ethnic minorities, 14
Reductionistic orientation, 73
'Reflection in action,' 136, 137, 141, 163, 223
   challenges, 138
   scholarship of practice and, 163
Reflection in practice, 118–144
   after mentoring sessions, 255
   case history, 119, 120–122, 124–126, 127–129, 130, 131–132, 135–136
   definitions, 119, 122
   in early career development, 168
   environmental/organizational factors supporting, 126
   as essential component, 123, 217
   experience and, 223–224
   framework for, 126
   for ill-structured problems, 123–124
   journalling, suggestions, 225
   levels and depth, 139–140
   multi-disciplinary teams and, 138–140
   outcomes, 120
   retrospective, 121, 122, 124, 223–224
   stages (Boud's), 223–224
   strands of reflection *see* Strands of reflection
   strategies to facilitate, 120
   techniques, 141
   terminology and global perspective, 142
   time as important factor, 127, 128
   time-course for introduction, 142
   triggers, 127
   types, 223
   uncomfortable experiences, 129
'Reflection on action,' 223
Reflections, evidence-based, 110–111
Reflective diary, 121, 132, 141
Reflective group supervision, 156
Reflective judgement, 141
   development *vs* education, 142–143
   staged model, 123–124
Reflective learning, 122
Reflective practice, 119
Reflective practitioner model, 148
Reflective practitioners, educating *vs* reflective judgement development, 142–143
Reflective questions, 141
Reflective thinking, 122
Reflectors, 42

Regulation, professional, 286
Regulations, 8–9
   CPD, 265–266
   international differences, 10–14
   parties involved, 10
Rehabilitation, 200
   evaluation tools, 204
   goals, 205
   impairment level change and effect on outcome, 199
   individualization, 202–203
   leisure, 196
   motivation for and occupation, 196–197
Rehabilitation professionals, 5
Relationship, sense of being in, 234
Relaxation, 23
Research
   appraisal, 101–102
   basic and clinical, interactions, 163
   discovery in scholarship of practice, 162
      see also Scholarship of practice
   qualitative, 102, 105
   quantitative, 102
   skills and evidence-based practice, 110
   types of evidence-based questions, 105
Research–practice gap, 93
Responsibilities of healthcare practitioners
   of advanced practitioner, 3, 262, 263, 264
   to advance profession, 272–273
   of consultants, 287, 293
   for CPD, 265, 266
   for lifelong learning, 262–263
Restructuring, organizational, 296
Right-sizing, 296
Risk-taking, consultants, 289–290
Role models, 244
   learning from, 248–249
   in multiple mentoring, 246
   parents and family, 244
   questions about, 242
Roles
   balance in career-planning, 38
   changing, for healthcare practitioners, 6–7
   consultants *see* Consultants
   new, DoH document, 285
   Salience Inventory, 47–48
Role Values, Salience Inventory, 47–48

S

Salience, work (concept), 35–36, 39, 173
Salience Inventory, 47–48
Scholarship, definition, 171
Scholarship of practice, 161–188, 175–176
   application (dissemination/use), 162, 164–165, 171, 175–176
   discovery, 162, 163–164, 171, 172–173
   health science considerations, 170–178
   integration, 162, 164, 171, 173–175
      methods, 168, 169
   integration and application (intellectual debate), 176–177
   interviews with early-career practitioners, 166–170
   teaching, 162–163, 165–166, 171, 177–178
   techniques and exercises for, 178–184

Scholarship of practice (*contd*)
   action research, 180–183
   Fawcett Hill's learning through
     discussion, 178–180
   memoirs, 183–184
   see also Action research
Schön's reflection in action, 137, 138
Scientist practitioner model, 148
Scientists, theorists as, 68
Search strategies
   for evidence, 99–101
   tips for, 100. 101
Self, sense of in practitioners, 234
Self-awareness, consultants, 290, 291–292
Self-concept, 37
Self-congruence, dynamic, 235–236
Self-directed learning, 156, 270–271
   adult learners, 218–219
Self-efficacy, concept, 86
Self-employment, 5
Self-esteem, increase by mentoring, 251
Self-evaluation, as component of reasoning,
   154
Self-knowledge, 41–49, 53–54, 268
   emotional intelligence, 41–42
   increase, 24
   learning style preferences, 42–43
   locus of control, 48–49
   personality style and preferences, 43–45
   Salience Inventory, 47–48
   Values Scale, 45–47
Self-management, 235
   behavioural strategies, 246
   benefits from mentoring, 246–247
Self-monitoring skills, 42
   benefits from mentoring, 246
   self-reflection and, 138
Self-reflection, 123, 138, 182
   see also Reflection in practice
Self-regulation, 286
Self-talk, 246
Sense of purpose, 290
Sensing Types^R, 44
Service, being 'in service' to others, 292
Service-learning model, 165
Service reviews, 113
Skill acquisition, 33
Skills
   broad base prior to professional education,
     174
   inclusion in theory–practice connection
     framework, 82–83, 85
   for utilization of evidence-based practice,
     110
Social care
   career trends, 41
   changes, 284
Social cues, self-monitoring skills, 42
Social sciences, development, 68–69
Social services, globalization, 147, 148
Socio-adaptive theories, 77–78
Socio-political influences, 1–29
Socio-political organization culture, 177
South Africa, regulatory procedures, 12
Spain, healthcare practitioners for UK from,
   15–16

Spatial propositions, 71
Special interest groups (SIGs), networking,
   241
Speech and hearing sciences,
     clinical/professional reasoning, 150
Speech and language therapists (SLTs), 212
   goals, 198
   occupational practice, 201
Spiral career pattern, 50
Spirituality, 176
Sponsors, 250–251
   roles and functions, 250
Standards, professional, 8–9
   international differences, 10–14
State Registered Occupational Therapist
   (SROT), 10
'Steady As You Go' program, 87
Story telling, 228–232
   use and structure, 230–231
   value of, 230
Straker's hierarchy of evidence, 104
Strands of reflection, 128, 139, 141
   connective, 134
   factual strand, 129–130
   practical use, 134
   retrospective, 132, 133
   substratum, 132, 133
A Strategy for the Allied Health Professions,
   Meeting the Challenge (Department of
   Health 2000), 284
Strengths, personal/professional, inclusion in
   theory–practice connection
   framework, 82, 85
Stress (work-related), management, 23–24
Stroke survivors, 195, 196
   consequence of occupational practice,
     204–205
Student exchange programs, 19
Students, choice of education programs, 16
'Success circles,' 51
Succession planning, 285
Super's model of developmental tasks, 36–37
Sweden, occupational therapy, 17
Systems awareness, 298–299

T

Tabled/tabling of items on agenda,
   meanings, 15
Teaching, scholarship of practice *see*
   Scholarship of practice
Team work, networking and, 241
Techniques, new, mastering, 169
Teleconferencing, two-way audio, 83
Temporal nature of reflection, 127, 128
Temporal propositions, 71
Theorists, 42, 68
Theory
   building blocks, 70–72
     concepts and constructs, 70–71
     propositions, 71
   characteristics, 70
   consumers of, 74–76
     active, 74, 75
     concepts and propositions, 76
     passive, 75–76

Theory (*contd*)
  progression skills, 74–75
  definition, 65, 69
  grand, 72
  historical aspects, 67–69
  levels of theoretical information, 78
  meta, 72
  middle-range, 72
  mystique of, 65, 69
    reducing/demystification, 69–74
  practical knowledge dichotomy, 67–68, 69
    reflection in practice and, 142
  practice, 72
  rationale and benefits, 65, 66–67
  reasoning grounded in, 66
  selection, 65–66
  terms related to, 72–74, 77
  types, 72
  utilization, 66
  see also individual theories
Theory-driven patterns of practice, 77
'Theory first–then practice' approach, 77, 79–80
'Theory in training,' 73
Theory–practice interconnection, 64–89, 76–83
  conceptual model role, 73
  differences between health professions, 76–77
  framework for integration, 81–83
  non-linear relationship, 81–83
  practical examples, education and distance learning, 83–86
  practice guidelines, 79–81
    see also Guidelines, practice
  top-down approaches, 77–78
    levels of theoretical information, 78
    three level taxonomy of theory, 77–78
Therapist, concept, 292
Therapists, re-call, 14
Thinkers
  concrete and use of theory, 67
  critical *see* Critical thinkers
  critical thinkers *vs*, 35
Thinking
  deductive, 66
  reflective, 122
    outcomes, 120
    see also Reflection in practice
Thinking and Feeling (T–F) personality types, 44, 45
'Thinking on your feet,' 137, 138
Thoughtful action, 135
Time Continuum Model of Motivation (Wlodkowski), 84–85
Time management, 23–24
  in learning through discussion, 179
  quadrants system (Covey), 23
Titchen's critical companionship, 232–233
Total Quality Management (TQM), 296
Transitory career-path, 50
Transtheoretical Model of Behaviour Change, 73
Treatment models, development, 165
Turning Experience into Learning, 124

U

Understanding, concept/definition, 270
United Kingdom
  continuing professional development, 265, 266
  healthcare practitioners numbers, 14
  regulatory procedures, 12
  shortage of healthcare practitioners, 15–16, 16
  student number expansion at universities, 14
Universities
  access policies, 14
  student number expansion (UK), 14
  see also Academic institutions
USA
  regulatory procedures, 13
  tabled/tabling of items on agenda, 15

V

Validation, reflection and experience, 224
Value endorsement patterns, 47
Values
  definition, 39
  impact on career decision-making, 47
  inclusion in theory–practice connection framework, 82, 85
  personal, consultants, 291, 292
  work, 39, 173
Values Scale, 45–47
Videotaping, development of clinical reasoning, 221–223
Virtuous practice, concept, 175
Vision, need for, 2
Visual deficits, occupations limited by, 207
Visualization, self-management strategy, 246
Volunteer services, 165

W

Websites, 28–29
  career-planning and competency development, 63
  evidence-based practice, 116–117
  see also Internet
White Paper, NHS, 91, 109, 283
Wisdom, 154, 272
Wlodkowski's Time Continuum Model of Motivation, 84–85
Work, as role, 35–36
Workforce, dynamic, 290
Workplace, adult learning and, 220
  ideal place/context for, 233
Work salience, concept, 35–36, 39, 173
Work values, 39, 173
World Health Organization (WHO), 17
  ICF *see International Classification of Functioning, Disability and Health (ICF: WHO 2001)*
Writer's block, 130
Writing
  descriptive *vs* reflective, 131, 132
  free-flow, 130
  memoirs, 183–184
  for portfolio and formal reflection, 132
  professional journals *see* Journals
  reflections in practice, 130–131